Praise for *The Way to Black Belt* . . .

"Without mincing words *The Way to Black Belt* is simply (introduction of martial arts I have read. Amid a glut in the r and 'training' textbooks, authors Kane and Wilder have pulled the switch to illuminate a shining star; one most likely destined to become a classic.

The value in this unique book lies in the ability of the readers to instantly create a roadmap toward their own martial arts success. Because oftentimes the term 'success' is subjective and only relevant to the desires of the individual martial artists Kane and Wilder leave nothing to the imagination and offer numerous 'golden nuggets' of valuable tips and information applicable to every martial arts style and level.

The truth is that I have been searching for *The Way to Black Belt* my entire adult life. After experiencing a myriad of instructional hazards along the way wrought with everything from unethical instructors to martial arts 'cults,' attaining my first black belt (1st *dan*) was the culmination of a long journey begun with disappointment and discouragement. If *The Way to Black Belt* was available at that time I would have eagerly snapped it up.

After nearly ten years of training police officers in control and defensive tactics, and conducting many self-defense seminars for private persons and organizations I am always asked by participants what is the best way 'to get started' in martial arts training. Now I have a definitive answer, *The Way to Black Belt*!" —**Jeffrey-Peter A.M. Hauck, J.D.,** Entrepreneur, Professional Consultant and Trainer, Former U.S. Army 82nd Airborne Infantry Pathfinder, and 15 year retired Municipal Police Sergeant. Co-author of *Ports and Happy Havens*.

"I was impressed with both its content and depth. Kane and Wilder not only succeed in defining a functional path to attaining *yudansha* level they also effectively bring back meaning and lost value to this important journey. The once coveted black belt has seemingly lost its value during this generation of mail order 'accreditation,' internet instruction, and strip mall studios. Reading this work I was reminded of a quote by Indira Gandhi, 'There are two kinds of people, those who do the work and those who take the credit. Try to be in the first group; there is less competition there.' Without question, Kane and Wilder are from Gandhi's first group and I suspect their book will be an instant success. I am certain that this work will be a welcomed addition to the bookshelves of any teacher who places value upon an intelligent and sound delivery system. In fact, *The Way to Black Belt* is so good I wish I had written it myself." —**Patrick McCarthy**, Hanshi 8th *dan* black belt, International Ryukyu Karate-jutsu Research Society (www.koryu-uchinadi.com).

"I could have read this years ago when I first started training. This long overdue book is a must read for anyone who desires to embark on the journey toward martial art mastery, and a book I highly recommend to all serious martial artists.

Drawing from nearly seventy years of combined personal experience, fascinating research into learning, and contributions from world-class martial artists, Kane and Wilder provide a wealth of knowledge to help the reader set goals for training, find the right instructor, determine their learning style, understand important martial art concepts, and maximize their training.

As I read this book and took notes to incorporate Kane and Wilder's advice into my own training and teaching, I couldn't help but think how much faster I would have advanced and how much further along I'd be today if I'd have read this book and applied this knowledge at the beginning of my journey into martial arts years ago. Don't wait! Read and apply the lessons in this book to your training immediately." —**Alain Burrese, J.D.,** former U.S. Army 2nd Infantry Division Scout Sniper School instructor and author of *Hard-Won Wisdom From the School of Hard Knocks.*

"This is one of those books where I find myself nodding at almost every sentence. Above all, Kane and Wilder have succeeded in setting down an all-important approach to training that will stand any martial artist in good stead. Make no mistake, the book is not offering a shortcut to the coveted black belt, but rather a clear guide to the correct path—not the easy way, not the hard way, but simply the right way to achieve success.

The Way to Black Belt is filled with sound advice, valuable insights, and inspiring examples and anecdotes from two lifetimes in the martial arts. Kane and Wilder make excellent mentors and their work will help martial artists of all levels to avoid mistakes, wrong-turns and dead-ends. The authors are not only highly-qualified instructors with real-world experience in security, they are educators of the highest order, offering valuable advice on 'how to learn' for maximum results.

There's first-rate guidance on finding the right instructor and judging the 'personality' of a *dojo*—things to look for, and things to look out for—plus all the little things that make a big difference—how often to train, what to eat, how to cope with injuries. And unlike so many books that limit themselves to techniques and exercises, *The Way to Black Belt* covers important mental and psychological aspects of training too—setting goals, visualized-learning and overcoming self-imposed limits and barriers.

Kane and Wilder draw on sources as diverse as Musashi, Sun Tzu, Bruce Lee, and Von Clausewitz and include contributions from modern-day masters from Okinawa, the U.S., and Europe. There's also an impressive list of Web-based resources where the reader can find a wealth of free information.

If you're serious about your art, I strongly recommend you get your hands on a copy and follow the advice contained in this excellent book. *The Way to Black Belt* is an invaluable guide for any martial artist on the journey to black belt and beyond." —**Goran Powell,** 4th *dan* black belt and author of *Waking Dragons.*

"The authors tell the reader in the book's Introduction they tried to create a book that included everything they would have wanted to know and ask when they were beginning their martial arts journey. They have done just that.

The book is broken down into eight general subject topics: self limitations, finding a good instructor, knowing how you learn, understanding strength versus skill, daily practice, understanding strategy to master tactics, working with injuries, and use of technology.

The organization is interesting. The reader is presented a textual collage of voices starting with an introduction written by a martial arts veteran, plus relevant quotes, discussion, student perspectives and personal histories. Also included are action plans, comments on what to look out for, chapter summaries plus additional educational material, history and insights—a lot to absorb.

It is as if the reader were sitting around talking with a group of senior students who advise him or her, talk about a wide range of subjects and give their different perspectives. This collective experience produces a sort of group mentoring that makes the student's personal journey less lonely—he has heard how others proceeded along the same path ahead of him.

One chapter that I found particularly interesting focused on understanding the strategy of the art studied. In a comprehensive, way it analyzed how reactions in self-defense situations are simplified if the student is, first, well grounded in the strategy of the art, rather than particular tactics. The psychological foundation of this observation is discussed along with a method of decision making. This is then related to the strategies of different arts, such as the striking and grappling arts. The linkage between strategy and training and the relation between *do* and *jitsu* arts are also discussed.

If there is any fault in this work, it is that it is so detailed and inclusive that there is almost too much to digest. But then again, this is the type of work that a student can come back to, read and reread and use as a reference.

This book is thus much more than a simple guide to prospective black belt students. It is also a reference, a work chock full of history, explanations, insights, personal experience, psychological insights, reference material backed by suggesting reading, relevant Web sites and reference material.

While this book targets students who are studying to achieve their black belt, it at the same time illuminates a path far beyond this limited goal. But its discussion of strategy and tactics, the physiological and practical elements of combat and martial history make it a book of interest to martial artists on any level." —**Christopher Caile,** 6th *dan*, Founder & Editor of FightingArts.com.

"Every time I step onto the *dojo* floor I do so with a little hesitation. What business do I, a full-grown adult that never dreamed of putting on a *gi* and has never been notably athletic, have trying to learn something as complicated and physically demanding as karate? Reading this book will help anyone for whom the goal of a black belt seems nearly impossible to consider that maybe you're wrong. That maybe if you just get yourself to class regularly, pay attention, work hard and persevere, that you can reach that goal. Not only do I feel inspired by the stories the book offers of others on the path—people of all ages, shapes, sizes, and abilities—but I now have a ton of great ideas and advice on how to make the most of my training along the way. I'm sure I'll be reading this invaluable book over and over." —**Laura Weller,** guitarist, vocalist, and songwriter for international recording artists, The Green Pajamas.

"*The Way to Black Belt* is a well-written, well-reasoned effort that will no doubt quickly become a standard martial arts reference. The authors have gone beyond the title to define what a black belt is and is not, and the book is as much about why to seek such a thing as how. The book is broad, deep, and covers everything from motivation to diet to physiology and psychology. Serious martial artists will benefit from having this book on their shelves, it is a terrific resource." —**Steve Perry,** 40-year martial artist and bestselling author of the *Matador* and *Net Force* book series.

"An indispensable guide to the how, why, where and who of the first, all-important years of martial arts training. This is the book I wish I'd had when I started out—the authors have forgotten more than most writers will ever know about making your training experience rich and meaningful." —**Arthur Rosenfeld,** martial arts instructor and author of *The Cutting Season* and *The Crocodile and the Crane.*

"I wish I had had this book when I first started training in the martial arts. The direction that *The Way to Black Belt* gives is priceless. The resources and information given are fantastic, the authors having spent years in the arts, and are able to point the way for you and clear away the chaff so you can get more out of your training the moment you open this book." —**Marcus Davila,** 5th *dan* black belt.

"Whether you choose the martial arts for competition or life study, the difference between failure and success is seeing the path, the goal, and the ability to focus. *The Way to Black Belt* points the way, spotlighting key aspects of training like no book before." —Robert Wittauer, Director, Emerald City Judo.

"Easy to read. Simple to understand. Clear and complete information." —**Lt. Stever Reddick,** USN (ret), recipient of Bronze Star Medal for valor.

"Kane and Wilder are quickly becoming one of the most insightful author teams in the world. Already authors of well-known books such as *Surviving Armed Assaults* and *The Way of Kata*, they have added *The Way to Black Belt* to their stable.

This book does what it says on the cover, and more. Not only does it give you techniques and tips on how to ensure you're ready for your black belt grading, it also helps you do self-profiling, seeing whether you're introvert or extrovert, it explores the way that people learn, and even goes so far as to explain how sleep can help you improve. This isn't just a book about martial arts, it's a book about life as well. What you learn in this book you can apply to your life as well. If you understand how you learn, then you can go outside of the dojo and apply that to learning other skills.

Sprinkled with anecdotes, quotes, and with every chapter having introductions from such well-known authors as Iain Abernethy, this book is going to quickly become every black belt wannabe's bible. Not only is it going to be their bible, but I feel that any association that wants true black belt gradings, rather than money-making gradings, should make it mandatory for their prospective black belts to read it.

If you're serious about making it to black belt and being the best martial artist you can be, this book will help." —**Matthew Sylvester,** martial arts instructor and technical consultant for *Fighters, Combat, TKD & Korean Martial Arts*, and *Traditional Karate* magazines.

"As a working executive with frequent travels out of town, and kids soccer games to attend, I was challenged to complete the intense training requirements to earn a black belt. The *dojo* I trained at allowed us additional access on weekends to keep up with the rigorous training schedule. The enthusiastic and consistent support and encouragement of other black belts in the *dojo* allowed us to correct flaws in our techniques and make improvements.

Kane and Wilder's book which addresses the discipline, determination, and planning required to achieve this level accomplishment, is right on target. This book lays out a realistic and frank approach to achieving black belt status. It provides a step-by-step guidelines how to approach your training, mentally and physically. The chapter addressing strategy offers a rich philosophical insight.

Kane and Wilder also provide a wonderful collection of suggested readings to continue your karate education. It's a 'must-read' for anyone serious about studying karate." —**Steven M. Heiser,** IT Director

THE WAY TO **BLACK BELT**

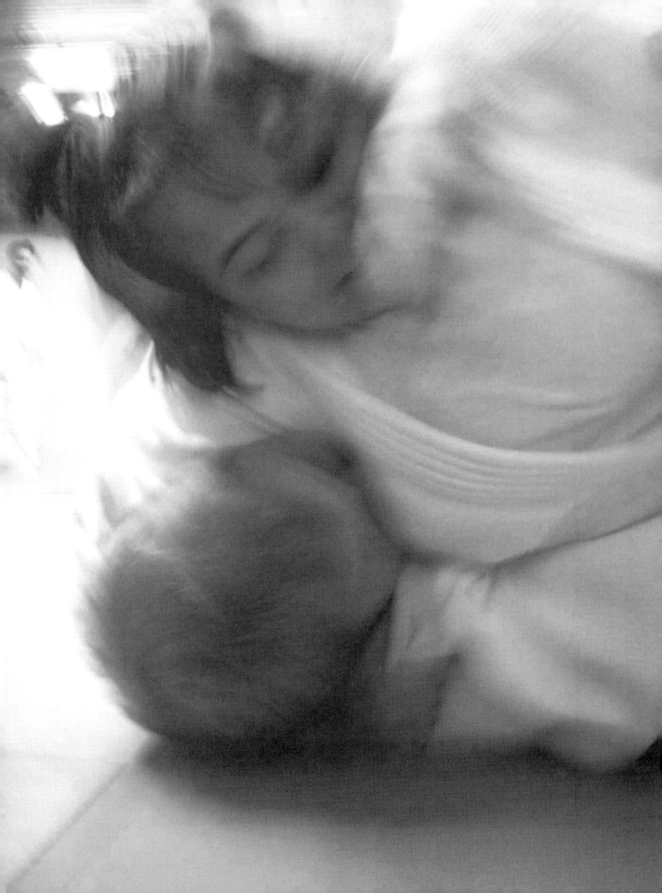

THE WAY TO
BLACK
BELT

LAWRENCE A.
KANE
AND KRIS
WILDER

YMAA Publication Center
Boston, Mass. USA

YMAA Publication Center, Inc.
Main Office
23 North Main Street
Wolfeboro, NH 03894
1-800-669-8892 • www.ymaa.com • ymaa@aol.com

Editor: Susan Bullowa
Cover Design: Richard Rossiter
Photos by Joey Kane, Lawrence Kane, Laura Vanderpool, and Kris Wilder.

ISBN-13: 978-1-59439-085-2
ISBN-10: 1-59439-085-1

10 9 8 7 6 5 4 3 2 1

Publisher's Cataloging in Publication

Kane, Lawrence A.

The way to black belt / Lawrence A. Kane and Kris Wilder. -- 1st ed.
-- Boston, Mass. : YMAA Publication Center, c2007.

p. ; cm.

ISBN: 978-1-59439-085-2
"Foreword by Dan Anderson, 8th degree"--Cover.
Subtitle on cover: A comprehensive guide to rapid, rock-solid
results.
Includes bibliographical references and index.

1. Martial arts--Training. I. Wilder, Kris. I. Title.

GV1102.7.T7 K36 2007   2007938468
796.8/092--dc22   0711

Warning: Readers are encouraged to be aware of all appropriate local and national laws relating to self-defense, reasonable force, and the use of weaponry, and act in accordance with all applicable laws at all times. Neither the authors nor the publisher assume any responsibility for the use or misuse of information contained in this book.

Nothing in this document constitutes a legal opinion nor should any of its contents be treated as such. While the authors believe that everything herein is accurate, any questions regarding specific self-defense situations, legal liability, and/or interpretation of federal, state, or local laws should always be addressed by an attorney at law.

When it comes to martial arts, self defense, and related topics, no text, no matter how well written, can substitute for professional, hands-on instruction. These materials should be used *for academic study only.*

Printed in Canada.

Dedication

To Jackson and Joey, two of the smallest guys that make the biggest difference.

Contents in Brief

Contents in Full

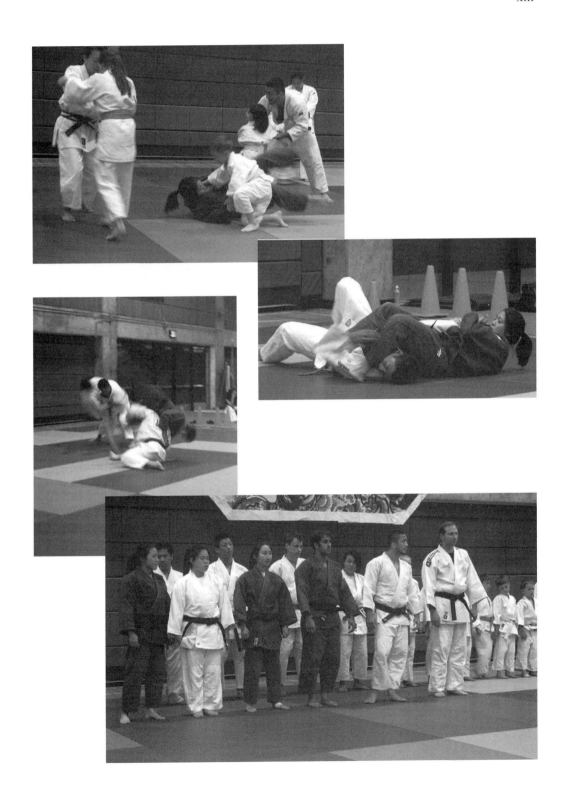

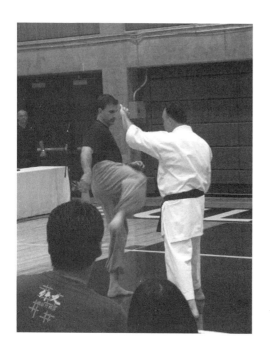

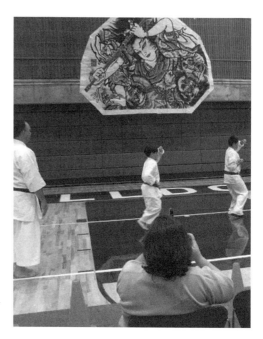

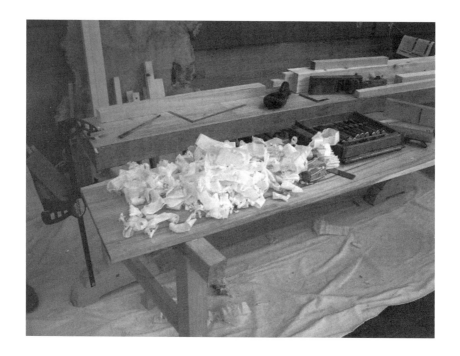

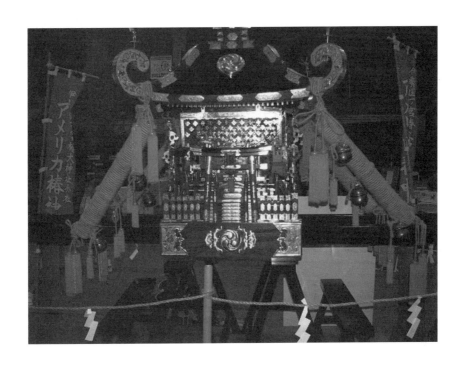

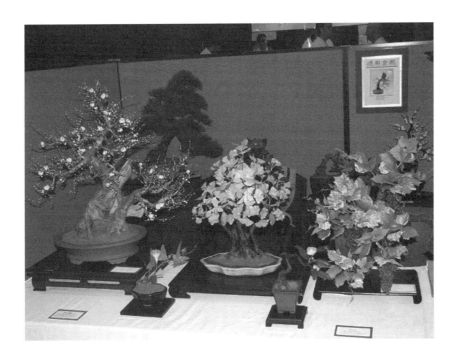

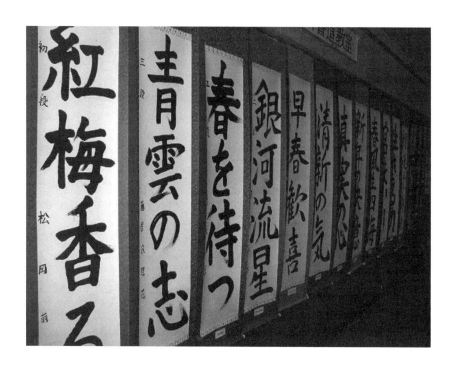

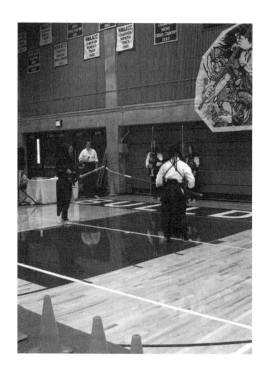
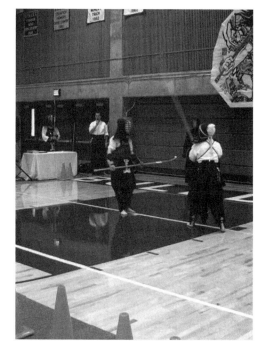

Foreword

by Dan Anderson

Black Belt. What is that, anyway? For many of us who grew up in the 1960s, it was a thing of wonder. Bruce Lee, James Coburn, invincible fighters who could take on an army of foes and defeat them without breaking a sweat. Ahhhh, those were the days. I remember when I was training, my instructor pulling my very gullible leg, telling me how his instructor could do *Heian 4* in one jump into the air. Sounded great to me. I had never seen a black belt. What did I know? Much later on I found that a black belt was a person like you and me who had trained hard to attain a certain degree of skill.

So again, what is black belt? Black belt is like graduating from grade school. Yes, you read right—grade school. I used to think it was high school but 40 years of the martial arts has disabused me of that notion. There is much too much to learn yet. I remember my first-degree black belt test. In the sparring, Wayne Lenore and I nearly knocked each other out. When the grading board left to go over the test in private, Bill Kunkle (the toughest fighter in the school) said, "That's what brown belts should look like." I thought to myself, "If I do not pass the test, at least Wild Bill thinks I'm a good brown belt." That was like a promotion in itself. That night I passed. Although I did not know it at the time, I was now off to middle school.

So what does that memory have to do with this book? Actually, nothing. Why? Because from my first lesson on I was bitten by the bug. There was nothing that I wanted more than to become a black belt. That was me. How about you? One of the things it took me quite some time to recognize was that I was different. I was a nut, so to speak. Karate was my "thing." I was a lifer. I did not need a book like this to get to black belt. I was going to get to black belt no matter how long it took. I found out after I began teaching commercially that most people did karate for vastly different reasons than myself.

THIS IS WHERE THIS BOOK COMES IN! As authors Kane and Wilder state so well in the book, most martial arts teaching was of a "monkey see–monkey do" fashion. They found out, as so many Americans have, that we Westerners do not learn well that way. We need to know the whats and whys of what we are learning. We are a culture of understanding and not one of patience. This is where this book excels. I read page after page and found much that would help any student of any belt level. Whether it is inspiration or physiology or mental preparation, it is all there. The fascinating aspect of this book is that authors Kane and Wilder have summed it down to eight factors. They have applied investigative skills to their research as well as their own experiences teaching the martial arts and they have come up with actually an *instructor's* guide.

Let us take a look at the eight factors they outline from the perspective of when I was a white belt:

Do Not Limit Yourself used to be "Do not be a wimp!"
Find a Good Instructor used to be "You've found one so do not question me!"
Know How You Learn used to be "Watch what I do and do it!"
Understand Strength versus Skill used to be "Get good enough!"
Practice a Little Each Day was limited in its application.
Understand the Strategy to Master the Tactics was nonexistent.
Know How to Work Through Injuries used to be "Tough it out!"
Use Technology was non-existent.

Again, look at the eight factors they outline. Each factor is a *full chapter*! The wealth of knowledge in this book is staggering. I'll let you read on to see what applies to you and what you do already. I have a personal rating scale for any martial arts book I look at. If there is something I can learn from the book then the book has paid for itself. This book will pay for itself many, many times over. From an instructor's viewpoint, what would I add?

Make friends with boredom. You will meet up with it some day in your training.

A black belt is a white belt who never gave up.

Actually set foot in the school. Then train. The hardest thing to do when beginning martial arts is to arrive.

Realize when you have achieved a goal and do not fail to set another.

If you are reading this foreword in a bookstore, pondering a purchase, close the book and head for the checkout counter. This one is a keeper.

Dan Anderson, 8th Degree Black Belt
www.danandersonkarate.com

Professor Dan Anderson is a founding member of the Worldwide Brotherhood of Modern Arnis and the director and chief instructor of the Dan Anderson Karate School. Since beginning his martial arts training in 1966, he has earned a 7th dan black belt in karate, a 6th dan black belt in Filipino Modern Arnis, and an 8th dan black belt in Modern Arnis – 80.* He is a four-time National Karate Champion, having won over 70 Grand Titles! Two of his greatest tournament achievements include winning the 2002 Funakoshi Shotokan Karate Association World Championship and winning two Gold Medals in the 1990 Goodwill Games. Anderson is the founder of American Freestyle Karate, a uniquely American martial art as well as the author of the best selling book, American Freestyle Karate: A Guide To Sparring, which has been in print for 26 years.

---

* The proper name of the art is Modern Arnis – 80. The title "Modern Arnis – 80" has two meanings: 1980 was the year Professor Anderson began his training with Remy Presas, the founder of Modern Arnis. Additionally, if you take the number 8 and place it on its side, you get the symbol for infinity.

His eight other books and four DVDs have proven popular with serious martial artists worldwide. He has been honored by inclusion into the Karate Living Legends, a lifetime achievement honor, as one of the 50 most influential martial artists in the 40-year history of tournament karate. His Web site is www.danandersonkarate.com.

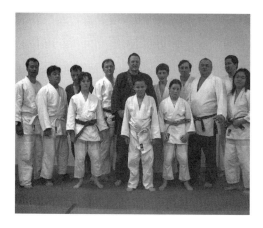

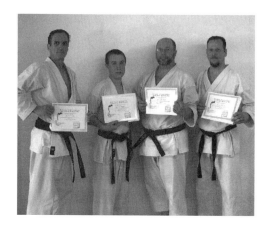

ANYONE CAN BEGIN THE PATH TO BLACK BELT, REGARDLESS OF AGE OR GENDER.

FOUR STUDENTS PROUDLY HOLD THEIR CERTIFICATES AND WEAR THEIR NEW BLACK BELTS AFTER A SUCCESSFUL TEST. THREE EARNED A SHODAN (1ST DEGREE BLACK BELT), WHILE ONE EARNED A NIDAN (2ND DEGREE) RANK AFTER A GRUELING 4½ HOUR TEST.

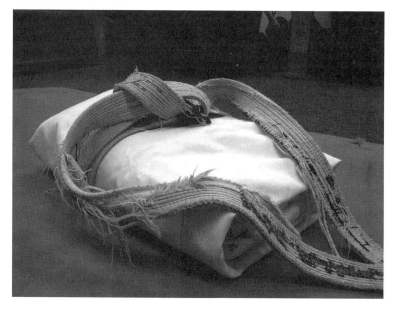

A WELL-WORN BLACK BELT REFLECTS YEARS OF DEDICATED TRAINING.

Preface

*"In Okinawa, karate is not practiced primarily as a sport or even
as an exercise for health. The Okinawans consider karate a life-long pursuit to be
practiced as training for both the body and mind."*
– Morio Higaonna [1]

The old adage goes: "Youth is wasted on the young." This is, perhaps, because many of us gain wisdom and experience only after our strength and vitality have begun to fade. You do not have to be all that old, however, to regret the follies of youth. At every stage in life there are things we wish we had known earlier, lessons that would have kept us from doing something we would later learn to regret as well as lessons that would have enabled us to accomplish something more easily or understand and appreciate it more fully. That is the purpose of this book, not to suggest the meaning of life, of course, but rather to help novice and journeyman martial artists benefit from the wisdom of their older, more experienced colleagues.

Our goal is to help you earn your black belt as swiftly and efficiently as possible while simultaneously enabling you to make the most out of the experience. To be all that you can be, as it were. Among other things, you will learn how to set goals, find a good instructor, monitor your progress, overcome plateaus in your training, take advantage of every learning opportunity, and work through the inevitable injuries that come with rigorous martial arts training. There is no substitute for perseverance and hard work in the training hall (*dojo*, *dojang*, or *kwoon*), yet exertion soon becomes drudgery if you are not developing new skills and making progress toward your goal. We will arm you with the information you need to make the most of your training time and swiftly become a highly skilled, well-qualified black belt candidate.

> *"Learning
> never ends."*
>
> – Japanese proverb

So why should you listen to us? We have been learning and teaching martial arts for a very long time. Wilder began training in *taekwondo* in 1976 at the age of 15, while Kane started judo in 1970 when he was six. When we sat down to write this book, we brainstormed all the things we wished we had known when we first started training so many years ago. We also sought diverse viewpoints, speaking with high-ranking practitioners and senior students from a variety of different martial styles to gain their insight on the topic. This book not only draws upon our experience, but also includes contributions from world-class martial artists such as Iain Abernethy, Dan Anderson, Loren Christensen, Jeff Cooper, Wim Demeere, Aaron Fields, Rory Miller, Martina Sprague, Phillip Starr, Jeff Stevens, and many more.

Acknowledgments

We would like to express our sincere appreciation to Iain Abernethy, Dan Anderson, Loren Christensen, Jeff Cooper, Wim Demeere, Irene Doane, Aaron Fields, Frank Getty, Dan Keith, John McNally, Rory Miller, T. Kent Nelson, Martina Sprague, Phillip Starr, Jeff Stevens, Mark "Blackwood" Swarthout, Michael Thue, Graham Wendes, and Martin Westerman whose contributions have greatly enhanced the content of this book.

The photos herein were taken by Joey Kane, Lawrence Kane, Laura Vanderpool, and Kris Wilder. Laura also reviewed the draft manuscript, gave us discerning feedback, and helped shore-up our grammatical deficiencies. Susan Bullowa did a first rate job of editing and indexing the book.

We would like to recognize the following talented martial artists who posed for the pictures: Andreas Raas and Rex Baggett II from Dragon Center Karate (www.dragoncenterkarate.com); Kevin Chan, Cameron Frenette, Mike Hiatt, Hubert Moebs, Valentin Moebs, Tsutomu Nagoya, Charlie Rackson, Mike Rackson, Rommel Trinidad, and Robert Wittauer from the Emerald City Judo (www.emerald-cityjudo.com); Gordon Abe, Tyler Abe, Joseph Chong, Jan Higaki, Peter Im, Bryan Imanishi, Gary Imanishi, Taryn Imanishi, Alex Lee, Masayuki Mizuuchi, Art Oki, Andrea Pirzio-Biroli, Jonathan Scherer, Robert Shields, Manami Wakuta, Jason Wang, Frank Wessbecher, Roger Yau, Richard Yoon, and Patrick Yoon from Cascade Kendo Kai (www.cascadekendokai.org); Rick Borish, Doug Day, Michael Day, Michael O'Donnell, Jon Oles, and Joe Oles from Magnolia Karate Academy (www.magnoliakarate.com); Aaron Fields, Papken Farrell, Jeremy King, John Litchfield, Erik Miller, Laura Ramirez, and Kiyoshi Shiraishi from Seattle Ju-Jutsu Club Hatake Dojo (www.seattle-jujutsu.org); Restita Dejesus, Marina Kosenko, Ken Smith, and Nancy Wilson from the Ying-Yang Martial Arts Center (www.yyac.com); Ryan Gallagher, Catherine Hildebrand, Bryan Hutchins-Caldwell, Hiroo Ito, Joey Kane, Duncan Lee, John McNally, Andy Orose, Larry Schenck, Laura Vanderpool, and Lindsay Vanderpool from West Seattle Karate Academy (www.westseattlekarate.com); David Engstrom (acupuncturist and body-worker), and Scott Schweizer (Matayoshi Kobudo, Snohomish, WA). Thank you one and all!

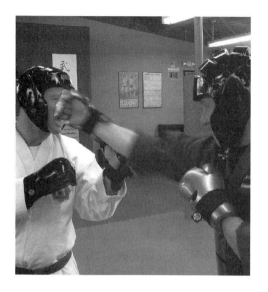

MODERN FOAM PADDING HELPS PREVENT INJURY.

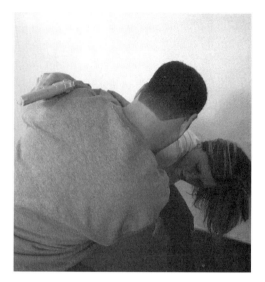

WORKING ACROSS GENDERS AND TYPES OF WEAPONS HELPS
MODERN MARTIAL ARTISTS REALISTICALLY PREPARE TO DEFEND
THEMSELVES ON THE STREET.

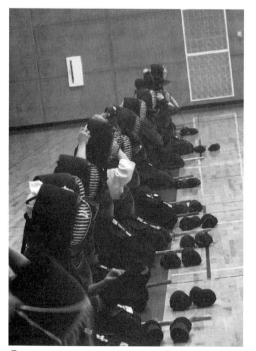

TRADITIONAL PROTECTION CALLED *BOGU* IN JAPANESE.

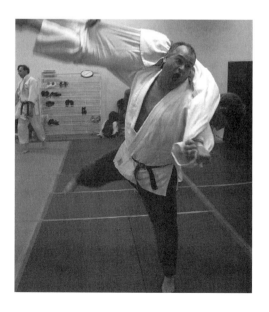

CONTROL, NO MATTER HOW POWERFUL THE TECHNIQUE, IS AN
ESSENTIAL CHARACTERISTIC OF A BLACK BELT.

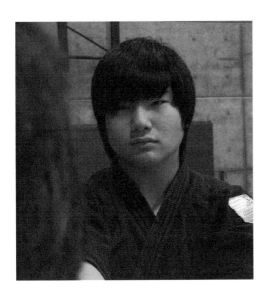

Focus in training, no matter what the art, is essential.

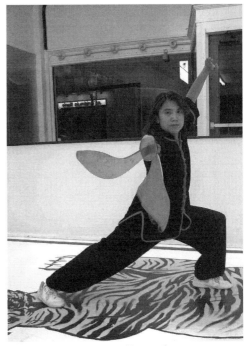

Many arts include weapons. This is a Chinese broadsword form.

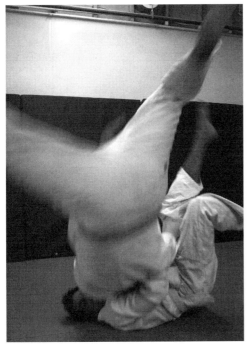

Commitment, speed, and focus, equal success.

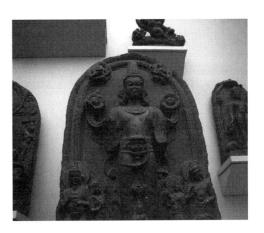

History and tradition are an important aspect of most martial arts. Practitioners often learn a lot about the culture where their art originated.

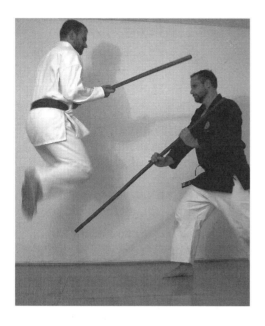

THERE IS LITTLE ROOM FOR ERROR WHEN WORKING WITH WEAPONS.

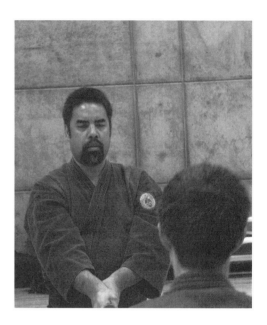

SENIOR PRACTITIONERS ALWAYS HELP JUNIORS.

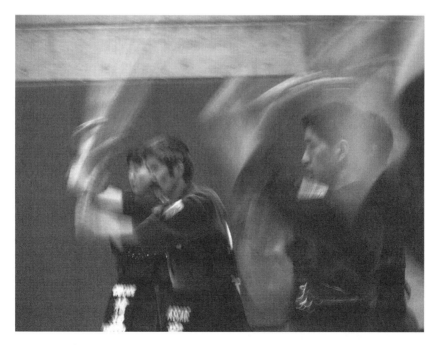

SUPERIOR TECHNIQUE MAKES YOU CONTINUOUSLY STRONGER, REGARDLESS OF AGE.

Introduction

"You become responsible, forever, for what you have tamed."
– Antoine de Saint-Exupéry [2]

Introduction

So you want to earn a black belt. Obviously; that is why you have purchased this book. Before we delve into how you can best achieve that goal, however, let us spend a few moments talking about what a black belt really represents and how it is commonly measured. After all, if all you wanted was the belt you could simply go to your local martial arts supply store or hop online and buy one. But that is not what this is all about, is it? It is really about developing the knowledge, skill, and ability necessary to be considered an expert martial artist.

A Brief History of Belt Systems

First, some history: The founder of judo, Professor Jigoro Kano, codified a system of wearing colored sashes or belts, which was subsequently adopted by most martial arts systems and is widely used today. This *dan/kyu* system distinguishes between advanced practitioners and different levels of beginning and intermediate students. The *dan*, or black belt, indicates advanced proficiency. Those who have earned it are called *yudansha* or *dan* recipients. The *kyu* degrees represent the varying levels of competency below *dan*, and are called *mudansha*, those not yet having received the *dan* rank.

Kano *Sensei** felt it particularly important for all students to fully realize that one's training was in no way complete simply because they had achieved the *dan* degree. On the contrary, he emphasized that the attainment of the *dan* rank merely symbolized the real beginning of one's training. By reaching black-belt level, one had, in fact, completed only the necessary requirements to embark upon a relentless expedition, a journey without distance that would ultimately result in self-mastery.

After establishing the *Kodokan Dojo*, Kano *Sensei* distributed black sashes, which were worn around the standard *dogi* (training uniform) of that era, to all the *yudansha*. Around 1907, this black sash was replaced with the *kuroi-obi* (black belt), which became the standard that is still used today. Of this standard, there was the white belt and the black belt. Later addition of green and brown belts rounded out the traditional ranking system.

By following a structure of merit, such as the belt system, instructors have a way of monitoring the development and skill progression of their students and can teach them according to set standards. While the majority of martial styles use a belt sys-

---

* *Sensei* means teacher, literally "one who has come before." Like all Japanese words, *sensei* is written the same for both singular and plural. There is no "s" at the end to denote more than one.

tem, it is by no means universal—some use badges or patches while others use no formal ranking method at all. A common approach incorporates five *kyu* belts: white, yellow, green, blue, and brown; and three *dan* belts: black, *akashiro* (red/white), and red.

The tips of the belt are decorated on occasion as well. *Dan*-level belts are frequently embroidered with the name of the practitioner at one end and the name of his or her style at the other. This embroidery is typically done in the native language appropriate for the art (e.g., Japanese for karate, Korean for *taekwondo*).

Colored stripes on both ends of a *kyu* belt can delineate gradations between *mudansha* ranks. Some schools use additional colored belts, such as orange or purple, rather than colored stripes to show these gradations. These stripes, when used, take the color of the next level of advancement such that white belts have yellow stripes, yellow belts have green stripes, green belts have blue stripes, blue belts have brown stripes, and brown belts have black stripes. In Okinawa, one or more gold stripes at the ends of a black belt indicate *shogo* (teaching/degree) rank. For children under age 16, stripes are frequently white no matter what color of belt to which they are attached.

Evaluation and Testing

A "belt test" is a critical evaluation of your martial arts knowledge, skills, and abilities, an opportunity to prove that you are ready to move on to the next higher level. You may not pass every test the first time, yet you should know that few instructors will ask you to test for any promotion for which you are not ready or nearly so. So what might the test be like? Wilder, who has earned seven black belts in three different styles, relates some of his experiences:

My old *taekwondo* instructor was some eighty miles away from where I lived and the new teacher that I found was not even teaching at the time I sought him out. I had experience as a teen in *taekwondo* and had also taken some karate in college. I wanted to continue training, so I found out where my soon-to-be new instructor lived and gave him a call.

He lived in the adjacent town and he told me he was flattered by my interest but he was working pretty hard at the time and did not really have much time to run a school. He said that he was not really all that interested. Sensing a "maybe" in his voice, I called back a couple of days later and talked him into agreeing to meet me.

Soon I had an appointment once a week in his basement where he did his personal training. He looked at my basics and awarded me a mid-level rank, a blue belt, if I recall correctly. I spent the time outside of class working on my skills and quickly progressed through the ranks over the next year and a half. Once the black-belt test date was set, I had about two months' notice to polish my skills. I spent hours upon hours working on my kicks, blocks, and forms, drilling the basics on my own.

One Saturday afternoon we began the test. Present at the test were my instructor, a video camera, and me. We started at the first thing I was taught and began to move through the rank requirements, covering every item I was supposed to know. Each form, strike, and block was scrutinized. We then moved on to sparring. He was a good six-feet-two-inches tall, long, lean, and fast. At five-eight with far less skill, I was really put to the test.

After that, the examination moved on to "What else do you know?" I demonstrated anything and everything I had gathered throughout all my training, showing other forms and applications. Some three hours later when it was over, I was awarded my black belt. The certificate followed about a month later. I had made it and was proud!

Over the course of time life changed and I had moved yet again. Living in Seattle (Washington), I had continued my martial training, this time taking up karate. Eventually it came time, once again, for my black-belt test. This time around, three other students would be testing at the same time along with me.

When we arrived at the hotel on the day of the test, we found that a conference room had been reserved for our use. It was centrally located for all the attendees and spectators. The various witnesses included friends, spouses, and other instructors. Some brown belts from the organization were also present to assist when we were short of fresh people.

The number two instructor in the organization had traveled to be present for the test that he was going to supervise. The room was carpeted and well laid out. Our organizational logo with its swirling dragons had been drawn, very well I might add, on the jumbo white board at the head of the room where seats had been placed for the examination board. This was a very formal and intimidating situation.

To add to the stress of the day, I had cracked a few of my left ribs a week earlier while practicing with one of the black belts. Nevertheless, I was as prepared as I could be for the test. It was a new style but the approach was much the same. Once again, we began with the basics and moved through the entire syllabus of the system. About three hours and lots of water and aspirin later, we were done with the physical portion of the test.

There was one further requirement, too. Each time a practitioner tested for a black-belt grade, he or she had to write a research paper and hand it in to the head instructor. The boundaries were wide open: "If you need ten thousand words to get your point across, do it; if you can expresses what you need to in a single dot in the center of the page, do that," we were told. I sweated over that paper just as much as I sweated on the *dojo* floor, going through a good ten drafts before I felt it was ready, and then sheepishly handed it in, feeling in my heart it was not good enough. Nevertheless, it was accepted and I became a new black belt in the organization!

Judo was a different affair altogether. You had to compete and win to receive points. When you reached the magic number, as I recall it was sixteen points, then you became eligible for your *shodan* (first-degree black belt). Consequently, keeping a record of your wins and losses was essential. The tournaments, the dates, who you fought, a win or a loss, how you won or lost, the length of the match, the technique used to win or how you were beat, your rank and your opponent's rank were all meticulously recorded. If you beat another brown belt, it was worth half a point; a *shodan* was one point, a *nidan* (second-degree black belt) two points, and so on. As you might guess, defeating a higher rank was quite a challenge and not very common, as the upper ranks knew you were in the hunt for points and they were not too inclined to lose to a lower rank.

You also had to show proficiency in the *kata* (forms) of the system. The form *Nage No Kata* required two people to perform and involved six throws done by each participant. Precision and body mechanics were of the highest concern when performing the *kata* with your partner. This required much time, both in and out of class.

We chose to demonstrate the *kata* to some other judo *sensei* to pick up tips and perfect our technique. Whenever a visiting instructor came from out of state to visit the *dojo,* we would be sure to show off our form and ask for advice. Once *kata* competency was demonstrated at an acceptable level, it came down to presenting the book of wins and losses.

This record went to a regional board. Membership was checked, the book was reviewed, and a testament of witnessing the *kata* was given both by my *sensei* and by another instructor who had watched us complete the form properly. Once all the paperwork was completed, we waited.

One day, a couple of weeks after the paperwork submission and the regional meeting, my *sensei* called me and another student forward after class with the pronouncement, "We are going to change the colors now." We stepped forward, bowed, took off our brown belts, and put on our new black ones. About a month later, the certificates arrived from Japan and were given to us in a similar, yet even more casual, manner.

These examples come from three different art forms. Kane's experiences have been somewhat similar. He remembers:

My *shodan* (first-degree black belt) was a bit of a surprise. I knew about a year ahead of time that I would be testing for my black belt. During that time, I had written my research paper, studied my *kata* (forms), rehearsed my *bunkai* (applications), practiced my *kihon* (fundamentals such as stances, blocks, and strikes), and worked out very hard. I felt anxious yet reasonably confident. In my heart, I knew that I was ready, but did not know exactly when the test would occur or how it would be handled. Because I had a pretty good idea of what others had gone through, I had been preparing for an arduous, formal test. Then one day my *sensei* called me up in front of the class, asked me to take off my old belt, and handed me a new one. It was as simple as that. He had clearly been watching my preparation, had seen me perform all the requirements adequately, and decided that I was ready.

My *nidan* (second-degree black belt) test, on the other hand, was both arduous and formal. In addition, I was recovering from a serious injury when I attempted it. One hot, humid Saturday morning I tested with three other students. When we arrived at the *dojo,* all the windows were covered with dark paper. An advancement board soberly awaited us, conversing quietly together while we warmed up and prepared ourselves for testing. There were still a few twinges of nervousness even though I knew that I was fully prepared. A bit of meditation and a vigorous warm-up calmed my nerves and I felt ready to go.

We presented our research papers and then went through the entire syllabus, covering *kihon, kata, bunkai, kaisai no genri* (the theory of deciphering fighting applications from *kata*), *kumite* (sparring), *dojo* etiquette, history, and traditions of the art, and a whole lot more. As the day progressed, the room became a sweltering, humid mess. The mirrors quickly fogged over and the floor became slick with sweat. Even though we took a couple of thirty-second water breaks, one candidate nearly succumbed to heat exhaustion before we were finished.

When we got to *shime* (testing of technique and power), the instructors checked our concentration, body alignment, movement, breathing, and the mechanics of our techniques by giving pressure and striking various parts of our bodies while we performed *sanchin kata.** They not only used their hands and feet but also a *shinai* (bamboo sword) as well. It was quite challenging but I managed to maintain my concentration under those stinging blows. I had some interesting bruises to show for it the next few days.

After four and a half grueling hours, the test was finally complete and the testing board retired into a back room to discuss the results. Exhausted and dripping with sweat, we drank water, stretched, and attempted to joke with each other while we anxiously awaited the results.

After several minutes, the board filed back in and called us up to the front of the room one-by-one. Everybody passed! Those who tested for *shodan* were asked to remove their brown belts and tie on black ones in their place. In the same manner as my *kuroi-obi*, their new belts were custom embroidered with the *kanji* (Japanese characters) of their names as well as the name of our style, *Goju Ryu* karate, in red thread. We were all handed certificates and congratulated on our promotions.

Will your tests be like these examples? Yes, they will, and no, they will not. Each test you take will carry with it a certain level of pensiveness, a shallow feeling in the pit of your stomach that you are not ready or will not do your best. There will be surprises, challenges, and even disappointments. Each organization, club, or system, has its own way of going about testing and they will be different in the techniques, and, perhaps, the ritual, but the human experience will be the same.

Know that your instructor is testing you because you appear to be ready. Your time in training and knowledge base are at a level that they see as warranting a test and an acknowledgment of all your hard work. Pass or fail, it is important to remember that rank is always earned, never given. With enough dedication, discipline, and

---

* *Sanchin*, which means "three battles," is a moving meditation designed to unify the mind, body, and spirit. *Sanchin kata* is the foundation of many martial systems to this day. While its techniques appear fairly simple and straightforward, it is actually one of the most difficult *kata* for martial artists to truly master. Techniques are performed in slow motion so that practitioners can emphasize precise muscle control, breath control, internal power, and body alignment.

> **Something to think about:**
>
> A Japanese journalist witnessed a demonstration of *sanchin kata* performed by some of Master Kanryo Higashionna's students. Higashionna *Sensei* founded *Naha-Te* karate. The reporter was deeply impressed by what he saw, particularly the way in which the *karateka* (karate practitioners) moved their hips, contracted their muscles, and controlled their breathing. Inspired by this experience, he wrote the following *haiku:* [3]
>
> *A roll of thunder*
>
> *Seizing the first bolt of lightning*
>
> *With empty hands*
>
> Is your own performance anywhere near as impressive today? By the time you are ready to test for your black belt, perhaps it will be.

diligent training, you will ultimately become worthy of wearing a black belt.

In most systems, there are ten *kyu* levels to pass through before receiving a black belt. So how do you go about earning that rank as swiftly and efficiently as possible while simultaneously making the most out of the experience? Well, that is the subject of the rest of the book.

How to Use this Book

Here is a brief overview of the material to follow:

Chapter 1 – Do Not Limit Yourself

This chapter debunks common excuses that would-be practitioners often have and motivates you to begin your journey into the world of martial arts. It helps you set goals, monitor your progress, and overcome plateaus in your training once you have gotten started. Knowing what you are looking for, clearly articulating your goals, and realizing that they may legitimately evolve or change over time is enormously important to setting yourself up for success.

Chapter 2 – Find a Good Instructor

This chapter helps you choose an art, find an exemplary instructor, and locate a place to begin your training. It also helps you understand how much you might reasonably expect to pay for classes, defines appropriate student/teacher relationships, and steers you away from dangerous martial cults and other adverse situations. Even if you have already found a place to train this information will prove useful.

Chapter 3 – Know How You Learn

This chapter helps you understand your own learning style and personality type in a manner that can expedite the knowledge transfer process. It explains how people internalize new physical skills, teaches you how to ensure a positive learning outcome, imparts powerful visualization techniques, and sets you up to make the most of almost any educational situation in the *dojo* and beyond.

Chapter 4 – Understand Strength versus Skill

This chapter helps you understand the value and recognize the relationship between strength and skill in martial arts training, identifies focus areas appropriate for your age and gender, and demonstrates the fundamental importance of *kihon* (basics) for your success in earning a black belt.

Chapter 5 – Practice a Little Each Day

This chapter demonstrates that advancement is a continuous process and offers strategies to avoid becoming overwhelmed with all you will need to know to earn your black belt. It is packed with creative ways to make the most of your training time and take advantage of every opportunity to learn.

Chapter 6 – Understand the Strategy to Master the Tactics

This chapter demonstrates that a deep understanding of strategy and tactics is a necessary prerequisite to making the most of any martial art. There are simply too many techniques to apply without knowing the context in which they work most effectively. You will learn about Boyd's Law and Hick's Law, understand the linkage between strategy and training, and delve a bit into the relationship between *jutsu* (fighting techniques) and *do* (martial ways).

Chapter 7 – Know How to Work Through Injuries

By their very definition, martial arts are warlike and dangerous. This chapter demonstrates that while injuries are commonplace, getting hurt does not have to interrupt your training substantially. You will understand what happens when you become injured: learn a little basic first aid, develop a good understanding of when you might need to see a medical professional and when you can treat things yourself, discover proactive ways to prevent getting hurt in the first place, and find creative ways to continue practicing while injured.

Chapter 8 – Use Technology

This chapter covers a wide variety of ways to take advantage of modern technology and the vast resources available today to learn more about your martial art, expedite the learning process, and prevent or minimize injuries. Training journals, nutritional recommendations, and exercise routines are covered as well.

Each of the aforementioned chapters begins with an introduction by an experienced black belt and ends with a treatise from a senior student (many of whom are already black belts themselves; learning is a continuous process). In the middle of each chapter, you will find an essay written by a veteran black belt as well. At the end of each chapter, we provide an action plan, suggested reading, and recommended Web sites so that you can put your new knowledge to use right away. Appendices at the end of the book cover common martial arts terminology, review briefly the various martial styles you might wish to study, and, just for fun, give you a list of our favorite martial arts movies that you might enjoy.

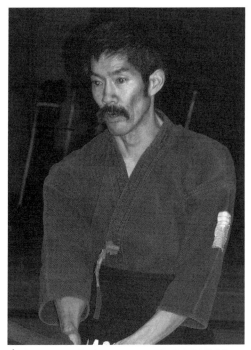

A LIFETIME OF DEDICATION BRINGS A HIGHER QUALITY OF EXISTENCE.

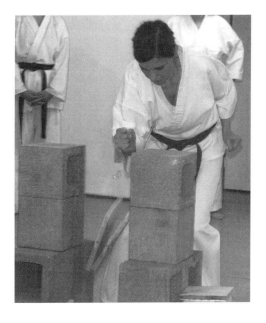

YOU CAN DO MORE THAN YOU THINK YOU CAN. *TAMASHIWARA* (BOARD-BREAKING) IS A GOOD WAY TO TEST FOCUS AND POWER. WITH A LITTLE TRAINING, ANYONE CAN DO IT.

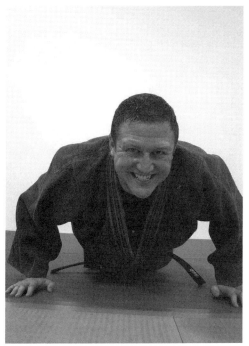

TRAINING SHOULD BE FUN AS WELL AND CHALLENGING. FITNESS IS INTEGRAL TO MARTIAL ARTS TRAINING.

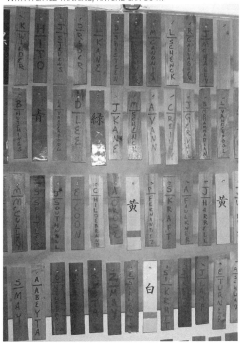

A RANK BOARD SHOWS STUDENT PROGRESSION.

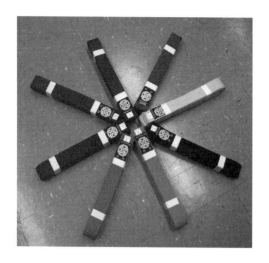

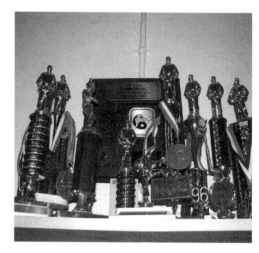

RANK BELTS ARE USED TO BRING ORDER TO THE *DOJO*, ASSIST IN TRAINING, SHOW MERIT FOR HARD WORK, AND KEEP YOUR *GI* CLOSED.

TROPHIES ARE THE RESULT OF GOOD TRAINING AND SPIRITED COMPETITION. THEY SHOULD NOT, HOWEVER, BE THE GOAL OF TRAINING.

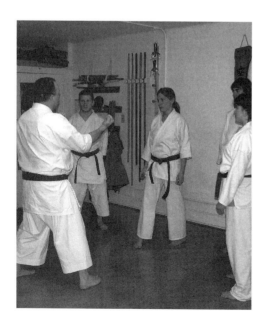

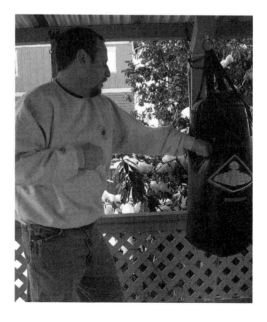

WORKING WITH ADVANCED RANKS IS A SURE WAY OF GETTING BETTER FASTER.

A LITTLE TRAINING OUTSIDE OF FORMAL CLASS GOES A LONG WAY.

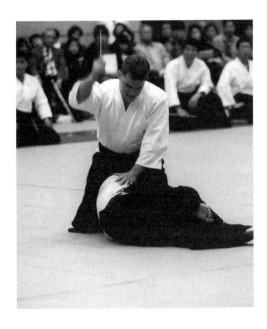

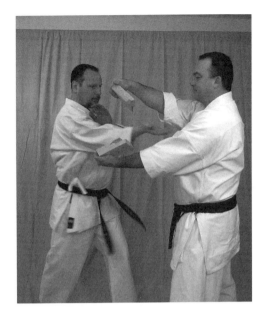

Go to a foreign country and demonstrate their art in front of them. Now that is a no-limit life! (Photo courtesy of David Engstrom)

One board, then two, soon three. Constant improvement is the path to excellence in the martial arts.

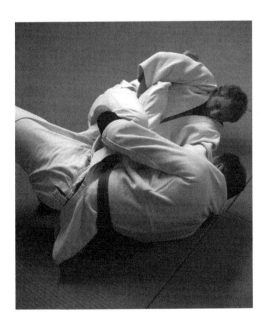

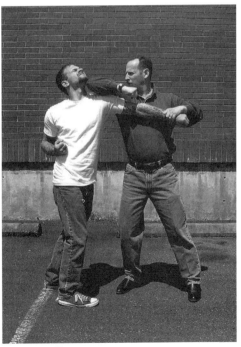

Learning to take advantage of any situation or position is the martial way.

Train hard. You never know when martial skills could save your life. The harder you train in the *dojo*, the easier the application an emergency.

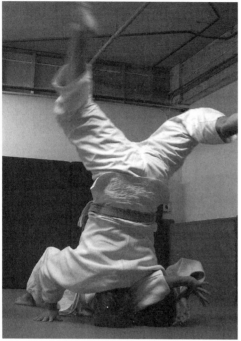

THIS TECHNIQUE DIDN'T JUST HAPPEN, AND IT DIDN'T HAPPEN
ON THE FIRST TRY, EITHER. BE PATIENT WITH YOURSELF.
EVERYTHING COMES WITH TIME.

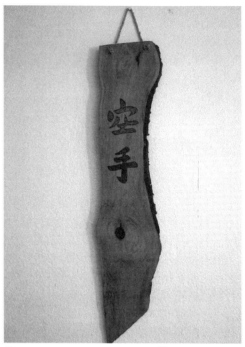

THE *KANJI* FOR KARATE CARVED IN WOOD. YOU SHOULD INTE-
GRATE YOUR ART INTO YOUR BODY SO THAT IT BECOMES PART OF
WHO YOU ARE, LIKE THE CARVING IN THE WOOD.

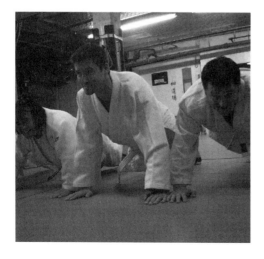

TRAINING AS A GROUP SOMEHOW ALWAYS RESULTS IN GET-
TING ONE MORE REPETITION THAN YOU THINK YOU COULD
DO ALONE. SURROUND YOURSELF WITH PEOPLE WHO CAN
HELP YOU SUCCEED.

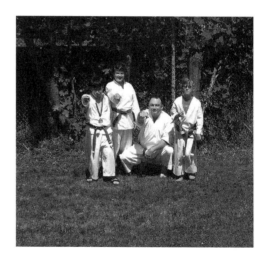

DON'T LIMIT YOURSELF TO JUST ADULT TRAINING, SPENDING
TIME WITH YOUTH BUILDS FOR THE FUTURE.

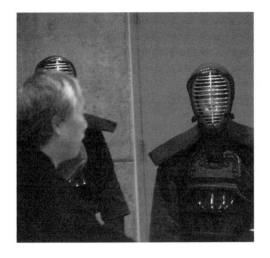

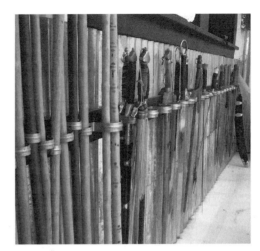

YOUR INSTRUCTORS ARE THERE TO HELP YOU GET BETTER FASTER: LISTEN INTENTLY TO WHAT THEY HAVE TO SAY.

AS YOUR SKILL INCREASES, SO WILL YOUR EXPOSURE TO OTHER ASPECTS OF THE ART.

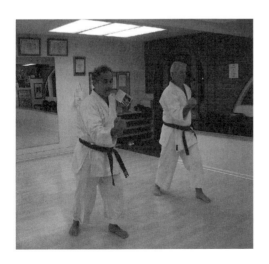

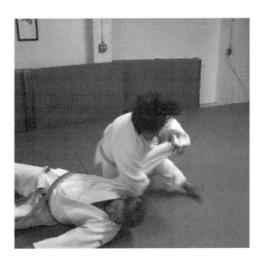

MARTIAL ARTS ADD VITALITY TO LIFE LIKE NO OTHER ENDEAVOR.

GOOD TECHNIQUE HELPS EQUALIZE DIFFERENCES IN SIZE AND STRENGTH.

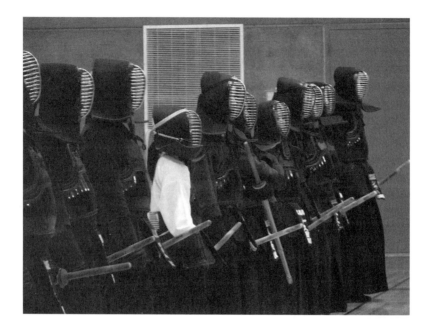

REGARDLESS OF AGE, SIZE, OR SKILL, JUMP IN AND GET STARTED. ATTITUDE AND DILIGENCE ARE GREATLY RESPECTED AND WILL CARRY YOU FAR.

CHAPTER 1

Do Not Limit Yourself

*"The only way to discover the limits of the possible
is to go beyond them into the impossible."*
– Sir Arthur C. Clarke [4]

Introduction (by Iain Abernethy)

Of all the barriers to progress we can face, by far the most potent are the ones we create for ourselves. Negative thoughts and self-imposed limits are poison for your potential! **"I cannot"** *always becomes* **"I never did"** *if left unchecked. To become what we are truly capable of becoming, we must ruthlessly free ourselves from the "brain chains" of mediocre thought and compromised aspirations.*

The martial arts teach us to be bold and courageous. Timid and self-sabotaging thoughts, therefore, have no place in the mind of a martial artist. We need to confidently think **"I will!"** *so that we can then triumphantly yell,* **"I have!"** *Know with all certainty that when you think positively and liberate your potential, you have the potential to achieve anything. If you want to make strong, positive progress in the martial arts, be sure to think strong, positive thoughts.*

The power of your thoughts should never be taken lightly. The human mind is the most complex thing in the known universe: its power is vast. Almost everything you see around you once started as a thought inside someone's head. I know it may sound a tad "mystical" but the fact that our lives are shaped by our thoughts is "profoundly" down to earth. Our lives are shaped by our actions and our actions are the result of our thoughts. What we think about will manifest itself in our lives through the simple process of cause and effect. You are what you think.

If you think that you cannot master that technique, beat that opponent or achieve that grade, those negative thoughts will ensure that you are right! So long as you continue to think negative thoughts, they will create an impassable barrier. The good news is that it also works the other way around! When you truly believe that you can master that technique, beat that opponent, or achieve that grade, you set off a chain of events that will inevitably lead to your success. Your positive thoughts will lead to positive actions. You do the right things and you achieve the right results. Simple!

When we think positively, it is sometimes said that we are being unrealistic, we are daydreaming, or that we are setting ourselves up for a fall or becoming arrogant. However, if we think in a negative way then we may be applauded for having our feet on the ground, for being realistic, practical, and down to earth. All this may lead us to wonder why the majority consider thinking negatively to be realistic whilst thinking positively is considered unrealistic.

The reason negative thinking is deemed more realistic is simply that the majority of people think negatively. These negative thoughts become barriers to progress and therefore the negative thoughts become a reality. Therefore, thinking negatively is realistic… for all those who think negatively! However, for those who think positively, positive thoughts are also realistic. Your positive thoughts free your potential and ensure you will make strong progress.

As warriors, we must never accept an inferior position to anything! We do not accept the limitations of circumstance and we should certainly never limit ourselves. This warrior spirit and refusal to accept any limitations should not only be central to your martial arts, it should be central to all aspects of your life. Be bold, courageous, and positive in everything you do.

– Iain Abernethy [5]

Break the Limits of Possibility

Learning martial arts can be very challenging. It is a lifelong process that encompasses not only internalizing an abundance of fighting techniques, but also learning proper body alignment, breathing, and movement. It is both a physical and mental process. Diligent practice builds the physical strength, endurance, and flexibility necessary to become a black belt. Physical training is arduous yet certainly doable when you dedicate yourself to it. For many practitioners, mental conditioning is an even more challenging endeavor. Tough as mental conditioning may be, however, almost anyone is capable of achieving it if he or she approaches training from the right perspective.

Most people never know the limits of what they can do until or unless they are faced with a seemingly impossible challenge and decide to step up and meet it. Even significant challenges, like earning a black belt, are relatively mild when put in the proper perspective. Which is harder, learning to punch, kick, throw, and grapple effectively or learning to adjust to life as a paraplegic or quadriplegic after a sudden catastrophic accident? Clearly, the latter, yet many individuals in that condition lead long, productive lives. It is all a matter of attitude. Strong, positive thoughts facilitate your ability to overcome most any obstacle while negativity and doubt can impede your progress. Here are a few famous examples:

- Due to a rare birth defect, Kyle Maynard was born a congenital amputee, missing his limbs below the elbows and knees. Despite having neither hands nor feet, he refused to let his condition interfere with his goals in life. He learned how to eat, write, and even type (50 words per minute) all without relying on the hands he did not have. By the age of nineteen he played middle school football as a defensive lineman, became a state high school wrestling champion, and established a new world weightlifting record. Mr. Maynard exemplifies the indomitable spirit of someone who refuses to be limited by his disabilities.

  "It is a paradoxical but profoundly true and important principle of life that the most likely way to reach a goal is to be aiming not at that goal itself but at some more ambitious goal beyond it."

  – Arnold J. Toynbee [6]

- Cycling legend Lance Armstrong discovered he had advanced testicular cancer that had spread to his lungs and brain in 1996. Like many cancer survivors, he refused to let his struggles through surgery, chemotherapy, and rehabilitation place limits on his competitive spirit. Unlike anyone else in the world, however, he not only came back to win the *Tour de France* in 1999, but eventually won that illustrious bicycle race a historic seven times. The field of racers he competed against included world-class athletes who pedaled far enough in training each year to encircle the globe. The daily metabolic rate of a *Tour de France* cyclist exceeds that of most Mount Everest climbers, closely matching the highest rates found in any other animal species, yet he demonstrated the mental discipline and physical prowess necessary to outdistance all competitors and win.

- Passengers and crew on United Airlines Flight 93 found themselves in an unexpected and horrific challenge when terrorists hijacked the airplane, stormed the cockpit, and began killing people. Todd Beamer, Mark Bingham, Sandra Bradshaw, Tom Burnett, Andrew Garcia, Jeremy Glick, Richard Guadagno, Cee Cee Lyles, along with other passengers and crew, armed themselves with a variety of makeshift weapons and stormed the flight deck. While they managed to overcome many of the terrorists, they were tragically unable to regain control of the aircraft before it crashed. Regardless, their heroics thwarted the terrorists' aims, saved countless lives on the ground, and proved that ordinary people are capable of extraordinary valor even in the face of certain death.

- Susan Butcher was one of Alaska's most famous athletes. Competing in a traditionally male-dominated sport, she won the world's longest sled dog race, the Iditarod, a historic four times. Braving grueling conditions such as subzero temperatures, blinding snowstorms, treacherous ice, dangerous wildlife, and sleep deprivation to mush 1,152 miles from Anchorage to Nome, Alaska, she made this trek 17 times during her racing career. In 1985 she was forced to defend herself and her dog team from an attacking bull moose, an approximately 1,200 pound beast, using only her ice ax and parka. The crazed moose stomped two of her dogs to death and injured 13 more before another musher came along and shot it. Butcher, who withdrew after the loss of her dog team, was leading the race at the time. Had that incident not occurred she very well may have won five Iditarod races over her illustrious career, tying an all-time record. While she ultimately lost her struggle with leukemia in 2006, she demonstrated the same bravery and grit in battling her illness as she did when struggling against both nature and the other dog teams during the Iditarod races.

- During a routine hike in 2003, Aaron Ralston suddenly found himself in dire straits when an 800-pound boulder shifted unexpectedly and pinned his wrist to a canyon wall in a remote area of Canyonlands National Park in Utah. After six days of captivity, he realized that desperate measures were needed for survival. Using a cheap, dull pocketknife, he managed to amputate his own arm, rappel one-handed down a hill, and then hike six miles through the wilderness before someone found and rescued him. This extraordinary tale of survival shows what a sufficiently motivated person is capable of doing.

Earning a black belt pales in comparison to these aforementioned challenges. It is by no means an easy task, however. To succeed you need a positive attitude, one in which you can visualize success. You need to clearly articulate why you are embarking on your martial journey, set specific long- and short-term goals for getting there, and follow through to ensure progress. It also helps (a lot) to hang around supportive people who can help energize you along the way.

It is a good idea to begin by making a list of the significant achievements you have already made, athletic or academic endeavors, personal or professional accomplishments, anything that helps you see that you can set and attain goals. It is easier to visualize yourself succeeding in martial arts when you know that you have excelled and/or persevered in other areas of your life as well. Knowing that you have met and overcome other challenges makes martial arts seem a bit less intimidating.

It is also important to realize that while earning a black belt is a truly monumental milestone along the martial path, it is but one of many stopping points. Until you quit, the learning never ends. First things first, however. To begin your journey you must articulate why you want to start and where you want to go. Once you know that, you will already be one step closer to achieving your goal.

> *"Ninety-nine percent of all failures come from people who have the habit of making excuses."*
>
> – George Washington Carver [8]

Begin by Articulating Why

What draws you to the martial arts? People become interested in *budo* (martial ways) for a variety of reasons. Simply stating that you want to earn a black belt is not enough to create a compelling vision to carry you through the challenges along the way. Are you looking for character development, tournament competition, physical conditioning, mental discipline, self-defense skills, weapons forms, any or all of the above, or something completely different? Are you really looking to achieve rank and promotions or just learn some new skills? What are you seeking as you begin your martial journey?

Before you articulate what you want today, it may be useful to know that our interests in *budo* generally evolve and change over time. As children, we may be drawn to the martial arts simply because they are fun. Building strength, balance, and coordination is definitely rewarding, yet the most beneficial aspect for many youths is the enhancement of self-esteem that comes from surmounting challenges and receiving promotions throughout the training. Parents likely appreciate the discipline and conditioning aspects more than their children do. Many of our students' parents have remarked that their child pays better attention in school as a result of his or her karate training.

As young adults, we may be more concerned with the competitive aspects of our art. Social interactions and physical conditioning become more important. The ability to defend ourselves from potential adversaries is often a draw. As we reach our late 30s or early 40s, however, many practitioners begin looking for something deeper,

Advice for New Students

by Martina Sprague [7]

Know your objective. It is difficult knowing the exact reasons for our studies when we first sign up for martial arts lessons. But after a year or two when the information you receive has had time to gel a little, providing you have made a conscious effort at self-discovery, you should have a clear idea of what you wish to achieve and why. Start by heeding the following warning: The martial arts differ from other sports or physical activities in the sense that they come with a split objective. A soccer player wants to join a team, compete, and win. A marathon runner wants to improve her time over last year's run. A gymnast wants to go to the Olympics and take the gold. What does a martial artist want?

The martial artist might want to improve his physical fitness, build self-esteem and confidence, win on the tournament circuit, do stunts for the movies, or learn to defend himself and others against assault. Alternatively, he might want to learn how to fight. In either case, the goal is ill defined. Because the martial arts carry a split objective of sports and fighting, it is difficult or nearly impossible to choose the part that interests you the most and single-handedly focus on this part. You cannot reach your full potential on the street, however, if your main interest is tournament competition. Likewise, you cannot reach your full potential on the tournament circuit if your main interest is self-defense or real fighting. Yes, you can be a jack-of-all-trades, but who finds that attractive?

If you do not know what you wish to achieve, then how can you design a program that takes you there? If you wish to accelerate your learning, then start by identifying your objective. Note that objective is singular. You only have one objective—everything else you learn is support work. If you are unable to identify your objective, then seek to educate yourself until you have the understanding it takes to know what you want. Every time you go to the training hall, keep your objective in mind. When you know your objective, the attitude with which you approach your training will assist your instructor in meeting you halfway and help you accelerate your learning.

such as *ki* (internal energy) training, character development, or even spiritual enlightenment. Knowing what you are looking for, clearly articulating your goals, and realizing that they may legitimately evolve or change over time is enormously important to setting yourself up for success in earning a black belt.

What is your objective in learning martial arts? Take some time to think deeply about your objective and then write down why you want to train. If you are unable to identify your objective, then seek to educate yourself until you have the understanding it takes to know what you want. Once you know why, you will need to take the next step and get started. Believe it or not, this is the first point where many potential black belts fail. They know what they want, yet they keep finding obstacles that keep them from getting started.

There are No Good Excuses

If you really want to become a martial artist and earn your black belt badly enough, there are no good excuses to keep you from obtaining that goal. Black belts come from every ethnic and religious background. They can be tall, short, male, female, old, young, healthy, or disabled. In short, just about anyone can earn the rank through dedication, discipline, and diligent training. That being said, many potential martial artists dwell on all the reasons they cannot begin their training, focusing on the negative rather than looking for the positive. Without that positive mindset, it is nearly impossible to earn your rank. Similarly, many practitioners who begin with a positive mental attitude drop out the first time they encounter a significant barrier along the way.

To earn your black belt you will need to overcome the plethora of excuses that keep you from starting (or finishing) your journey. Here are some common excuses that may be holding you back:

"I really want to get started but I need to get in shape first."
"I am too old to begin such rigorous training."
"I am too small to become a successful martial artist."
"I am disabled; there is simply no way I can perform these techniques because of my condition."
"I have an old injury that prevents me from participating."
"It is just too complicated; I'm simply not smart enough to figure it all out."
"I just do not have enough time to practice."
"I do not have anyone to practice with."
"It is too expensive; I cannot afford the training."

We hear these kinds of things every day, yet for every obstacle, there is a workaround. Here are ways of overcoming the aforementioned excuses, shifting your mindset to a more positive and ultimately successful approach:

Fitness is not a prerequisite. While a high level of physical fitness is absolutely required to earn a black belt, it is by no means a prerequisite to begin training. Most martial arts classes begin with *daruma* (exercises), where students warm up, stretch, and perform basic calisthenics. This helps practitioners not only get in shape over the long run, but avoid training injuries on a daily basis as well. Some instructors include *daruma* with every class session while others expect students to learn the routines and then, once competent, begin performing them on their own to focus limited class time on martial techniques that you cannot learn by yourself. Either way, participation in these activities will dramatically increase your fitness level over time.

You can practice *daruma* in the *dojo* during, as well as in between, formal class sessions. With or without martial arts, daily stretching and moderate exercise are vital components of a healthy lifestyle anyway. If you truly want to get into fighting shape, however, there is more you can do.

Many classes also include *kigu undo*, or supplemental exercises, with traditional training equipment. This works much like modern weightlifting, though it is tailored specifically to strengthening muscles, and moving tendons and ligaments associated with martial arts applications. Traditional Okinawan training equipment, for example, includes *makiwara* (striking post), *ishisashi* (stone padlock), *tan* (wooden log), *tetsuarei* (dumbbells), *chiishi* (weighted sticks), *makiage kigu* (wrist roller), *nigiri game* (gripping jars), *tou* (bundle of sticks), *jari bako* (sand bowl), *tetsu geta* (iron clogs), *kongoken* (heavy rectangular loop), and *sashi ishi* (stone weight). We'll discuss these a bit more in the section called *Incorporate Strength and Conditioning Training* in Chapter 8.

These items are traditional implements used by many karate practitioners for supplemental exercises. There are also modern devices that can be incorporated into your training regimen to strengthen and/or condition your body such as heavy bags, mannequin bags, speed bags, jump ropes, medicine balls, mechanical weight machines, and free weights. Having an instructor present is important. Superior instructors can motivate you to do far more than you ever thought possible, yet they will never let you to do anything that will cause lasting injury. Sore muscles come with the territory, of course, but that happens with any worthwhile fitness program in which you participate.

Most martial arts classes are fairly aerobic as well. We have all seen commercials for *Tae Bo* and other workout routines that utilize movements similar to those performed in traditional martial arts. If you prefer a sword, there is *Forza*, an aerobic workout using *bokken* (wooden sword) movements. Like these adaptations, *kata* (forms), sparring, mat work, and various drills performed throughout a traditional martial arts class will give you an excellent workout.

It is not uncommon to wring sweat out of your *gi* (uniform) after rigorous training. Unless you are already in good shape, it will be a real challenge at first. If you cannot keep up, however, your instructor should accommodate reasonable requests for breaks so long as you are striving hard and continue watching and learning from the class while you take a breather. Do not worry, you will definitely get used to it over time.

While some students cannot do more than one or two push-ups during their first class, they soon find themselves doing ten, twenty, fifty, or a hundred at a time. A lack of fitness is nothing to be embarrassed about when you begin your training. Many students take up martial arts as a fun and interesting way to get into shape. It takes time to get there, however. That is perfectly normal and to be expected.

Just as new practitioners are not expected to be able to do a Chuck Norris-style roundhouse kick after their first lesson, they are not expected to be Olympic-class athletes when they walk in the door, either. Clearly, if you are massively out of shape or have led a sedentary lifestyle, it is prudent to check with a medical professional prior to beginning any training regimen. Having said that, you should never let a lack of physical fitness keep you from beginning your martial arts training.

Age matters not. You are never too old to begin training. One of the most amazing things about traditional martial arts is that the longer you train the stronger you get, regardless of age. Clearly, disease or injury can derail progress, but proper technique requires very little in the way of brute force to be effective. That is why a little old man (or woman) with a black belt can readily defeat younger, stronger, and more agile opponents. We see examples of this in most every martial art, including *aikido*, *arnis*, judo, *jujitsu*, karate, *kobudo*, kung fu, and *taekwondo* just to name a few.*

"Dwell not upon thy weariness, thy strength shall be according to the measure of thy desire."

– Arab proverb

Of course, it takes much work to get there. The adage "use it or lose it" becomes especially pertinent as people age. Sedentary lifestyles eventually lead to a loss of muscle tone, bone density, and mental acuity. Flexibility decreases, accidents, and injuries become more frequent, and a host of other complications arise. Yet, scientific research has shown that prudent exercise programs can slow the effects of aging, helping you live better, more fulfilling, and, oftentimes, longer lives. Recent studies suggest that moderate exercise may even delay the onset of Alzheimer's disease and other forms of dementia, demonstrating mental as well as physical benefits. While physical fitness may not be a prime goal of most martial arts programs, it is a definite side benefit.

Many of the best active martial artists in the world are over the age of 40, many well into their 50s, 60s, or 70s. Names like Dan Anderson, Loren Christensen, Teruo Chinen, Peter Consterdine, Morio Higaonna, Hoch Hochheim, Joe Hyams, Sang Kim, Chuck Norris, Geoff Thompson, and Yang Jwing-Ming come to mind. Some are much older than that. Fourth-degree black belt Paul Owen, who began taking judo at age 40, still teaches today even though he is 91 years old!

Another 90-year-old, Keiko Fukuda, is the highest ranked woman *judoka* (judo practitioner) in the world. A ninth-degree black belt, she has been practicing her art

---

* In this book, we italicize all foreign language words, yet some Japanese terms have become part of the English language. For example, everyone knows what karate is but few have heard of *kobudo*. That is why the latter is italicized and not the former.

for 70 years! No matter what age you are, you are never too old to begin martial arts training. Once you begin, there is really no limit to how long you can participate if you set your mind to it and take good care of yourself.

Size does not matter. Oftentimes, smaller people feel trepidation about training in the martial arts, fearing that a lack of size or strength will set them back. Unlike Western boxing or wrestling, most martial arts have no weight class distinctions. Men and women train together in most traditional *dojo*. The reason for this is that the fighting arts were created specifically to ensure that superior skill could overcome brute force in battle. After all, what good is a martial art that only works on smaller, weaker foes? While this does not always hold true in sporting competitions where safety rules prohibit equalizing techniques like eye-gouges, joint strikes, and vital point techniques, there are numerous examples of smaller competitors defeating larger ones through superior tenacity and skill.

As previously mentioned, judo practitioner Keiko Fukuda is the highest-ranked woman black belt in the world who studies that art. In the 120-year history of the judo, only a handful of people have received a higher rank, tenth-degree black belt, yet Fukuda is not only 90-years-old but she also stands a mere 4-feet-10-inches tall! One of those tenth-degree black belts, Professor Kyuzo Mifune, was only 5 foot 3 inches tall, quite short for a Japanese man, yet he was one of the most feared competitors at the *Kodokan Dojo* in Japan. Both these diminutive masters are proof that superior skill can overcome a lack of size or strength in sporting competitions as well as in self-defense scenarios. Judo, in fact, is an art specifically designed to use an opponent's force against him or her in battle, a great equalizer for smaller practitioners.

Clearly, the previous examples show how superior skill can overcome a lack of size or strength in an art that was specifically designed to use an opponent's strength against him or her, but it may lead you to wonder if this principle holds true for other arts that are less tailored to that approach. Absolutely! It works that way in virtually every martial art. Karate, for example, is primarily a striking art, one where force on force contact is the norm. One of the greatest karate masters of all time was Chotoku Kyan.

Born small of stature, weak of body, and afflicted with both asthma and myopia, Kyan grew up to become one of the most feared masters of *Shuri-Te* karate, specializing in brutal vital point striking techniques. Challenged to a friendly match with a sixth-degree judo black belt, for example, he stuck his thumb into the man's mouth, dug his fingernails into the man's cheek, and yanked him to the ground hard enough to tear part of his face away. Finishing the bout with a hammerfist blow to the face, he chose not to kill his helpless opponent since it was, after all, a "friendly" match. A student of Kyan's, Tatsuo Shimabuku, founded *Isshin-Ryu* karate.

If you truly want to become a black belt and are willing to practice hard enough, it makes absolutely no difference what size you are.

Disabilities can be overcome. Growing up, Kane had a neighbor named Robert who had lost both legs to a landmine during the Korean War. Though confined to a wheelchair, Robert continued to exercise regularly and had terrific upper-body strength with arms like a professional bodybuilder. He also practiced martial arts, earning a black belt after several years of dedicated training.

His *sensei* was able to modify techniques specifically to draw upon the strengths and minimize the weaknesses of Robert's condition. For example, he learned how to remove the armrests from his wheelchair and use them like *tonfa** to execute blocking and striking techniques. He also learned how to fight when lying on the ground without relying on his legs for support or movement, using his enormous upper body strength for striking, grappling, and controlling techniques.

Similarly, he was also able to bring new insight on the application of martial concepts back to his school. For example, he once taught a seminar on how to fight if someone is attacked when sitting on a toilet where one's legs are incapacitated by one's pants.† To ensure proper decorum, they actually practiced these techniques sitting on chairs, fully dressed, with their *obi* (belts) tied around their knees to limit leg movement. This example not only demonstrated effective techniques that might be used when confronted in an unusual situation, but also helped students recognize the obstacles and opportunities presented by various physical challenges.

While the criteria for achieving a black belt remain the same for men, women, disabled practitioners, and everyone else, there are ways of working around most any challenge to perform at that level. There are black belts with most every type of disability you can think of out there, not just folks confined to wheelchairs. For example, martial arts have proven very useful in helping

---

* *Tonfa* are traditional Okinawan weapons similar in form to modern side-handled police batons.
† The *samurai*, always ready to meet an attack, were actually taught to remove one pant leg to avoid becoming entangled when forced to fight in this situation.

> In 1997, I was at a judo tournament in Burnaby British Columbia, Canada, and saw the most profound example of not being limited by your..., well, limitations. A competitor was led onto the mat by a young woman. As he moved, he never lifted his head and he shuffled slightly while he walked. The young lady kind of presented him to the referee, and it hit me… he was blind. Not only was he blind but he was an international competitor in the Special Olympics, and he was competing in an open tournament!
>
> The referee reached out and took his hands and placed them on the other *judoka's gi*. They both gripped each other and as the referee let go, the match began. The match looked a lot like any other match except the referee communicated by touch. When the match was broken and reset, as often happens in a judo match, he would give the score in the hand of the blind man by tapping in his palm for his score and the back of his hand for the opponent's score.
>
> You might ask the same question I was asking, "If he is blind, why didn't the referee just say the score?" A Canadian guy next to me leaned into me and said, "He is deaf, too." "What?" I responded, slightly stunned. "Since birth," he replied. "The woman that took him onto the mat is his wife."
>
> I cannot tell you I recall how the match ended and, frankly, that is not important. What I saw was a great display of not being limited. A blind, deaf person not only learned the sport of judo, quite an accomplishment in and of itself, but also successfully competed in an open tournament.
>
> *— Kris Wilder*

autistic children learn important life skills, improving their ability to function in other settings. You can be hearing, sight, or mobility impaired, or have just about any other type of disability and still become a black belt if you train hard enough and long enough.

Injuries can be worked around. If permanent disabilities cannot keep a man with no hands and feet from becoming a state champion wrestler or a wheelchair-bound person from earning his black belt, injuries should not be able to keep you from participating in martial arts. Clearly, you will not want to do anything that will exacerbate the injury or slow your recovery, but experienced martial arts instructors are experts at finding safe ways to train when injured. See Chapter 7 for more information.

Complex challenges can be tackled in small parts. When new martial artists begin their training, they find they must relearn basic concepts like breathing, standing, and walking. They are taught how to breathe through their diaphragm rather than solely with their lungs, introduced to a variety of uncomfortable stances and foreign postures, and shown how to move in unusual new ways. Balance and coordination take on a new meaning. That is just the beginning.

Soon they are introduced to *kata* (forms), the dance-like movements in which the ancient masters hid the secrets of their unique fighting systems. Almost all Asian martial systems have *kata* of one type or another, from *arnis* to kung fu, karate to judo, and *taekwondo* to *taijiquan*. A *kata* is simply a pattern of movements containing a logical series of offensive and defensive techniques that are performed in a particular order. They are often complex and difficult for beginners to memorize. To truly learn one, you not only need to know the pattern but understand all of the applications as well.

All this new information can easily become overwhelming if it is not broken down into easily digestible component parts. That is the beauty of martial arts, however. Complex elements like *kata* are all built from *kihon* (basics), fundamental building blocks that are relatively easy to learn. You do not have to be a genius to figure it out. Here is an example:

You might learn a basic stance such as *sanchin dachi* (hourglass stance), spending time on all the important elements of body alignment that make it work properly in a static position. From there, you will learn how to move, stepping, shifting, and turning in the stance while maintaining correct posture. Once you have mastered that, you will add a martial technique like a punch, block, or kick into the mix.

From there, you will learn how to breathe properly in concert with the movement to add power to your technique. In a modern *dojo,* this whole effort may only take a couple of hours, and then you will move onto something else to maintain your interest. It is so important to good technique, however, that in the old days in Okinawa or Japan *karateka* could spend as much as a year or two perfecting a single stance. Fear not, however, if you do not get it right the first time there will be plenty of opportunities for more practice. Anything you see once, you will be doing again later on during another class.

Because form precedes speed and both form and speed are necessary for power, you will almost certainly practice all this slowly, taking as long as necessary to master the fundamentals. Soon you will find that you have picked up a rich range of postures, movements, and techniques that you can perform singly or together. Suddenly that complex *kata* is not so challenging. It is merely a series of fundamental building blocks, which you already know, strung together into a set pattern.

As you can see, you are not expected to master the complex form without first learning the building blocks from which it is created. This is the time-honored way to impart vital martial knowledge—one that has worked for hundreds of thousands if not millions of practitioners around the world. This takes time and diligent practice, of course, but it rapidly begins to make sense. You do not have to be a genius to figure it out. All it takes is patience and practice, a lot of practice.

There is always time to practice if you are creative. Training halls are a lot like health clubs; they come in a variety of scopes and scales. Some are open for just a few hours three or four days a week while others run around the clock. If you have an unusual schedule, it may lead you to select one *dojo* over another in terms of lining up your free time with instructor availability. If you travel a lot, your instructor may have associated clubs in other cities so that your training will not be disrupted. Thousands of firefighters, doctors, law enforcement officers, airline pilots, military personnel, and other professionals whose hectic or variable schedules preclude regular daily training have found ways to earn their black belt. If they can do it, you can too. Even if you cannot make a regular class time, most instructors are willing to offer private lessons to fit your schedule.

Another piece of good news is that once you have learned some basic skills, you will not need an instructor in attendance every time you train. There are hundreds of creative ways to practice a little each day and refine the skills you have. See Chapter 5 for more information.

Solo training beats no training. While it is easier to stick with a training regimen when you have a partner to work with, it is certainly not a requirement to earn a black belt. Some types of training, in fact, are easier to perform solo. See Chapter 5 for more information. The road to earning a black belt is long and arduous. You cannot rely on external motivation to navigate it successfully. Intrinsically motivated practitioners find ways to practice on their own.

Creative financing can help you achieve your dream. Martial arts instruction, while not hugely expensive, can be a significant investment for many. Evaluate your priorities and spending. Making your lunch is almost always more cost-effective than eating out. Simply forgoing a daily latte or pack of cigarettes will cover the cost of training at most schools. It is healthier for you, too. If earning your black belt truly is a priority, you can probably find enough disposable income to pay for your lessons.

Scoured your budget and still cannot afford the cost of training? Never fear, there are creative ways to pay for instruction that you may be able to pursue as well, particularly if you run into financial challenges after you have already begun training for a while and the instructor already knows you well. The two most obvious areas to examine are scholarships and trade for services.

Many martial arts schools offer scholarships to promising students who have a financial need. Discreet inquiries to your instructor will let you know if this is an opportunity of which you can take advantage. If you make a living, you undoubtedly have a skill that is worth something. You may be able to trade cooking, cleaning, light construction, Web design, clerical work, massage therapy, bookkeeping, or any of a number of other functions to cover the cost of your classes. Do not be afraid to discuss alternatives with your instructor.

Experienced students often receive opportunities to teach as part of their development. In some schools, it is even a requirement for earning your black belt. If you have advanced sufficiently in your training to merit the position, you may be selected as an assistant instructor. In such capacity, the cost of the lessons you take is often offset by the value of the instruction you give. This is yet another option you may be able to discuss with your *sensei* should you find yourself in financial difficulty late in your training.

The bottom line is that there are no "good" excuses. Could you have come up with excuses we have not countered herein? Of course you could. The important idea is to set the excuses aside, come up with an objective, and visualize success. Keep that objective in front of you as you decide what art to study, where to train, how to get started, and why you will not give up once you have begun.

The next step is paramount: Find a *dojo*, walk in the door, and begin. Repeat as necessary until you have accomplished your goal and tied that black belt around your waist.

"I respect the man who knows distinctly what he wishes. The greater part of all mischief in the world arises from the fact that men do not sufficiently understand their own aims. They have undertaken to build a tower, and spend no more labor on the foundation than would be necessary to erect a hut."

– Johann Wolfgang von Goethe [9]

So we have broken through the excuses and gotten started. Now let us focus a bit on setting you up for success along the way. The best way to accomplish that is to set goals that support your objective and then monitor your progress toward achieving them.

Set Goals and Monitor Your Progress

An important way of setting yourself up for success in your martial arts training is to create a challenging set of stretch goals against which you can monitor your performance and maintain your motivation over time. In his outstanding book *Mental Strength*, Iain Abernethy describes a methodology for setting and achieving goals. He suggests creating SMART goals, those that are Specific, Measurable, Achievable, Realistic, and Time-bound. Okay, it is a goofy acronym but it is easier to remember and it works. Here is how:

Specific. To have any success in achieving your goals, they must be specific. A generic target like becoming rich, successful, or good looking is impossible to achieve simply because you cannot truly tell whether or not you have completed it. Something specific, like earning a black belt, on the other hand, is a reasonable long-term goal. Shorter-term subordinate goals might be things like perfecting a stance, learning a new *kata*, achieving an interim rank promotion, or any number of other steps in the long-term process. Having both short- and long-term goals helps ensure progress.

Measurable. In addition to being specific, goals must be measurable if they truly are going to have meaning. It is important to know empirically whether you have successfully met your target. A specific yet unmeasurable goal, for example, is developing the ability to hit hard. A quantifiable method of measuring your ability to punch effectively, on the other hand, is being able to break a wooden board or a brick with your fist.* Measurable goals are more motivational because you can definitively know when you have achieved success.

Achievable. Goals should inspire you to achieve success. Consequently, they must be achievable or they will quickly defeat the whole process of creating them in the first place. Goals should be stretch targets, things that make you strive your hardest because they are not easy to reach. Even so, earning a black belt in one year goes beyond a stretch and is simply not achievable (at least not a black belt that is worth having, anyway). Even superior athletes with a natural affinity for the martial arts are bound by "time in rank" and other promotion standards. Earning an interim rank such as a green belt after a year of training, on the other hand, is reasonably achievable by many practitioners. Setting specific, measurable, and achievable stretch goals to carry you through your training is an excellent way of setting yourself up for success.

Realistic. Goals must not only be achievable, they must also be realistic. For example, while practicing ten hours a day is an achievable goal, it is probably not realistic, particularly if you have job, family, or other commitments. A goal of practicing for an hour or two a day, on the other hand, may very well be reasonable to strive for. To be truly motivational, you must realistically be able to achieve your goals.

Time-bound. Open-ended goals are rarely achieved. There is an old saying in the business world, "what gets measured gets done." Set realistic milestones along your martial path, specific events that you can measure along the way. This is especially important as you progress throughout your training. Instructors will generally have routine testing and promotional steps that can serve to measure your progress, yet the higher your rank the longer the gap between tests becomes. Creating and monitoring your own development along the way, therefore, is very important. It helps you become intrinsically responsible for your own motivation.

Extrinsic motivation (inspiration from others) is nice to have, yet intrinsic (self) motivation is essential for long-term development, particularly as you reach inevitable plateaus in your training where you struggle for long periods of time

---

* *Tamashiwara*, or breaking techniques, are something that you should never attempt without appropriate supervision by a competent instructor. It can be a good way to measure the strength of your technique, but it is also an easy way to seriously injure yourself if you do it incorrectly.

without perceptible progress. Any black belt worth wearing must be earned. You simply cannot rely on anyone other than yourself to keep you focused and inspired along the way.

Know How to Overcome Plateaus in Training

Martial arts can be pretty complex. Watching an experienced practitioner perform a *kata* or compete in a sparring match is almost magical as that person flows from one technique to another with effortless grace. Getting to that point requires mastery of all the fundamental building blocks that make that performance possible, then integrating them into a cohesive whole.

"It's good to have dreams, but disaster to live off them. Make goals; goals are nothing more than dreams with dates on them."

– Graham Wendes [10]

Even fundamental aspects like punching, for example, are far more complex than you might imagine. To execute a powerful punch, you must begin with a proper fist, assume a correct stance, align your body precisely, move smoothly, and breathe properly. You must decide what type of punch your want to throw (e.g., fore fist, standing fist, knife hand, finger thrust, hammerfist, knuckle strike, swing strike, or uppercut), know where to aim, determine the proper arm rotation (if any), accurately gauge the distance to your target, and coordinate your timing. Throughout the entire process you need to know and precisely control when your muscles must be relaxed and when they should tense, something that varies on a muscle-by-muscle basis.

Because of this complexity, even practitioners who approach their training with a positive mental attitude and have set specific, measurable, achievable, and realistic goals will eventually reach plateaus in their training. During these plateaus, you may be working for long periods of time without the perception of improvement. If you feel stymied while you struggle to make obvious progress, you are more likely to abandon your dream.

It is important to understand that this feeling is perfectly natural. It happens to everyone. The challenge is that only those individuals who can successfully work their way through these plateaus will eventually become black belts. This may be part of the reason why so many practitioners drop out in the middle ranks where dramatic improvements in knowledge, skill, and ability begin to take longer to develop.

It helps to know that progress in the martial arts rarely follows a continuous upward curve. It frequently takes the form of a step function. Here is why: There are two aspects to training, mental and physical. Both the mental and physical components need to move in synch in order to make significant progress. When one moves without the other, you rarely notice your own progress, though you should be aware of the fact that any experienced instructors who watch you will undoubtedly notice that you truly are incrementally improving.

> *"Do not turn back when you are just at the goal."*
>
> – Publilius Syrus [11]

So how do these aspects get out of synch? Practitioners frequently understand what to do long before they are physically able to perform, so mental usually comes first. That is easy to understand, yet even the mental aspects of martial training can become so complex that they take time to internalize. From an instructor's perspective, while teaching children can be a lot like filling empty vessels with facts and ideas, teaching experienced adults is much more complex. Concepts can no longer be poured in; they must be fitted into what is already there. Consequently, it can take a while to integrate new ideas with what you already know, particularly when it comes to esoteric concepts like deciphering *kata bunkai* (fighting applications from *kata*) or utilizing *ki* (internal energy, also known as *chi* or *qi*).

The body needs time to burn the techniques into muscle memory just as the brain needs time to integrate the new knowledge. In other words, while there may be exponential improvement in the early stages of training during which you learn fundamental building blocks, the mental and physical aspects need time to coalesce around the more complex techniques.

Working with others is an excellent way to keep yourself motivated while you are struggling to overcome a plateau. Not only do supportive, positive people reinforce your self-esteem, but two heads are also often better than one when it comes to solving complex problems. Focus on more than just the physical aspects of the training (e.g., punching techniques, *kata* patterns, tandem drills) but discuss mental aspects as well. Talk about the strategies and theories behind the techniques you practice. Discuss what works for you and why. You can frequently reach an epiphany that facilitates monumental improvements in your technique simply by experimenting with a training partner and discussing what you found afterward.

Variety is also important. Students and teachers alike can benefit from exposure to a variety of teaching styles. Take advantage of seminars, workshops, and one-on-one sessions with senior students and instructors as they become available. Exposure to multiple styles is good, but do not jump around so much that you confuse yourself. While many instructors recommend achieving *shodan* (first-degree black belt) prior to picking up another style, there is nothing wrong with practicing two or more complementary arts at the same time, as long as you can make it fit into your schedule and do not lose focus. Keep your goals firmly in mind and do whatever is necessary to move forward in your training.

Believe it or not, a critical plateau in training is earning your black belt. A first-degree black belt is really a marvelous milestone in your martial journey, the point at which you have mastered enough of the basics to begin your training truly in earnest. It opens doorways to advanced techniques you never thought were possible and certainly had no hope of understanding, let alone mastering, beforehand. You may need, however, to revise your goals at this point or begin to struggle for new meaning in your journey. Some practitioners begin to teach, others select a secondary art to practice, while still others simply see it as an important milestone along the way. Whatever you decide, you will need to reevaluate where you are going with your training or you will likely drop out.

In most martial systems, the skill differential that separates first- and second-degree black belts is humungous, comparable to the gap between a rank beginner and a *shodan*. Once you truly understand the magnitude of that gap, you may become discouraged, deciding that it takes too much effort to bridge it. During these times, it is especially important to look inward for motivation, reinforcing your introspections with feedback from your instructor along with other external sources of inspiration.

It is often hard to see how far you have come all by yourself. We recommend keeping a training log that captures your notes and charts your progress along the way. This can help you truly understand and appreciate the magnitude of the improvement you have already made and help you stay on track for more learning to come.

Student Perspective (by Graham Wendes)

I was always a procrastinator. I knew I had to deal with it, so I always planned to… the next day. The best thing I ever did was to sit down and look back over my life. It is no good at all to dwell on the past, but to ignore it is just plain foolishness. I did not beat myself up; I just worked out all the "if onlys." If only I would have done such and such, I would be in that position by now (educationally, financially, work-wise, etc.), if only I would have taken control of this, or that, where could I be now?

It is a sobering exercise, and I would not recommend it to the fainthearted.

It made me realize how long one year, or even three years, is when viewed in the future, but how fleeting they are in retrospect. Albert Einstein said something along the lines of "All time is relative. A moment in pain or misery is like a lifetime, but a week in the arms of a lover passes in the wink of an eye."

So, I finally got stuck into something I had always wanted to make my career—and was surprised to find it did not suit me at all. The realization came as a shock, but that was not the issue. The main issue was that I would not commit myself to either my career, or karate training, because I suffered with the "when I've" affliction. When I've got this, done that, achieved the other, then it will all be okay.

Had I reached out for what I thought I wanted to do earlier, instead of hoping it would just "happen" to me one day, I would have realized sooner it was not for me, and left more time to get on with my life.

Now, I'm committed to my original career path, but I look at it through different eyes. I do not see it as a necessary evil that depresses me anymore. In fact, I do not "feel" about it at all; I got rid of the emotional attachment and I'm better all around for it. It is just what I do, but I am working hard to make it better for me and my family. Helen Keller, the gifted poet and author said, "You may not be able to change your circumstances, but you can always change your attitude towards them." Did she practice what she preached? I think so; she was deaf and blind.

The qualification I could have earned less expensively five years ago, the professional membership it would have afforded me with associated benefits, and the employment choices are now nearly mine because I got my priorities sorted out and went back to college at my own expense. Do I expect to work in construction all my life? Not on your Nellie, but I'll be the best I can while I'm in it, it is just a job, but if I practice doing the minimum I can get away with in this job, what skill have I perfected? Exactly; so I'm practicing being a winner, even at something that does not really enthuse me. I call it my shugyo *(hardship) training, if I can suffer this and make it a success, I can achieve anything. I know it is "traditional" to do your* shugyo *by practicing* kata *under an ice-cold waterfall, but it does not pay that well.*

The point is that it is good to have dreams, but disaster to live off them. Make goals; goals are nothing more than dreams with dates on them. Hit the date targets, and if you were mistaken about whether the achieved goal was right for you when you got there, who cares? Think what you have learned about yourself, life, the universe, and everything along the way. The sooner you find out the better.

Notice earlier that I said "mistaken." You are not "wrong" if you make a mistaken decision. You were RIGHT to make a decision at all and act on it, if it turns out that particular decision was a mistake, you do not need to punish yourself for it.

Attach emotions only to the people in your life, never to things or situations. Things wear out, break or just get used up or lost. Situations are always controllable to some degree. Mushin, live in the moment, everything is as it is, it can be no other way. People can make you happy or sad, furious to delirious, but you can choose whether to associate with them.

My wife and I both come from negative family environments. Some years ago, we sat down (always think sitting down, you never know how long you will be thinking, and a cup of tea helps lubricate the brain cogs) and decided there was no benefit to either of us, or our son, in pursuing such an elusive grail as "family harmony" outside of our happy threesome, so we pulled away. Peace at last!

I'm not saying you should do that; it was right for us, and no one else's business, but WE had a choice, and WE made it.

The point is to do what needs to be done as soon as you realize or decide what it is. Do not wait or procrastinate. Someone once told me that we all have invisible "use by" dates stamped on our arses that only fate can see. Live each day like it is your last, even if you work in a boring office block. It is one of those strange coincidences that as I write this, today is 9/11. Four years ago, we watched the Twin Towers drop thinking our son was on top having breakfast with his mates before flying back from Camp America. As it turned out, after four hours of his phone not responding, they had all changed their plans, and are all making the most of their lives today.

Einstein was right, they were the longest four hours of our lives, and we have endured some crap.

Our son has a large print of New York on his bedroom wall with the Towers intact. Underneath is a plaque with his creed, "Carpe Diem (seize the day), because you just do not know."

Since I looked over my shoulder and got my act together, I have increased my income without really trying, helped my wife find her way and increase her income, finally got my 1st dan (black belt) after taking my 9th kyu (brown belt) on February 22, 1976 and messing around for 28 years, and written two-thirds of the book that "everyone has in them."

Life is not easier, but I get more out of it. I can actually see the light at the end of the tunnel, which I can now believe is not just another train coming to knock me back again.

I could list many more benefits to my family life of moving forward rather than just looking forward, but I would rather you took strength from this… and went out and saw the benefits in your own life.

In closing this epic, I would offer you these words of caution: When you get moving on your life, you will find, "When you make moves, providence moves with you," and things will snowball. If you feel out of control of your progress, that is because you are making some. Unfortunately, as you rise to the challenges and opportunities, and race forward, you may find other people in your life may not be able to keep up, or may just get jealous. Only you can decide whether to help them along with you, or leave them behind and hope they catch up.

Success brings its own responsibilities.

– Graham Wendes [12]

Something to think about:

It is really as simple as this: Find a *dojo*, walk in the door, and begin. Repeat as necessary until you have accomplished your goal and tied that black belt around your waist.

Summary

You never know what you can accomplish until you try. Earning a black belt is a significant challenge, yet a surmountable one. You will never achieve it, however, if you limit yourself or your imagination with negative thinking. Put aside your excuses, find a *dojo*, walk in the door, and begin. Repeat as necessary until you have accomplished your goal and tied that black belt around your waist.

To optimize your chances for success, it is paramount to identify your training objective in writing, documenting the exact reasons why you want to sign up for lessons. Keeping that objective in mind, visualize success and eliminate any obstacles to beginning and continuing your training. Maintain your motivation by creating a set of stretch goals against which you can monitor your performance over time. These goals need to be SMART; that is, specific, measurable, achievable, realistic, and time-bound.

Action Plan

Make a list of the significant achievements you have already made such as athletic or academic endeavors, personal or professional accomplishments, or anything else that helps you see that you have set and achieved goals in the past. If you could do it before, you most certainly can do so again.

Write down your objective for training in martial arts, identifying the reason you want to earn a black belt. Think about it a while and articulate as clearly as possible.

Keeping your objective in mind, create a specific list of short- and long-term goals for meeting that objective. Be sure that each of these goals is specific, measurable, achievable, realistic, and time-bound.

My top three specific, measurable, achievable, realistic, and time-bound short-term goals are:

_____

_____

_____

My top three specific, measurable, achievable, realistic, and time-bound long-term goals are:

_____

_____

_____

Answering the following questions can help you articulate your goals:
What are the three most important elements of your role as a student?

_____

_____

_____

What are the three most important things your instructor can do to help you succeed?

_____

_____

_____

What are the three specific challenges you know that you will face?

_____

_____

_____

What are three ways to overcome these challenges?

_____

_____

_____

What three indicators will serve as mile markers to demonstrate progress on your journey toward earning a black belt?

_____

_____

_____

Armed with this information, find a *dojo* and begin your training (see Chapter 2 for more information about how to go about doing this).

Suggested Reading

Abernethy, Iain. *Mental Strength: Condition your Mind, Achieve your Goals.* Cockermouth, U.K.: NETH Publishing, 2005.

While most of us know that mental strength can be developed in the same manner as physical strength, very few of us really know how to go about doing it save for serendipitous discovery. Based on his considerable success as a martial artist and author, Iain Abernethy lays out a step-by-step methodology for overcoming doubt, building self-confidence, and achieving your dreams. Nothing in this book is rocket science, yet his codification of a straightforward, understandable, and implementable process is nothing short of brilliant. Abernethy's clear, encouraging guidance will show you how to develop a strong, powerful mind, grow your talents, become the person you want to be, and live the life you want to live, too. This information is extremely well laid out, masterfully written, and, most importantly, it works.

Armstrong, Lance. *It's Not About the Bike: My Journey Back to Life.* New York, NY: Penguin Putnam, Inc., 2000.

Much more than just a biography of the world's best (and most famous) cyclist, Lance Armstrong provides a heartfelt look at his amazing life. He writes about his cycling feats (of course); growing up without a father; his illness, treatment, and recovery from cancer; his struggles to have a child (wife's in vitro fertilization); and more. He outlines his triumphs and challenges, setbacks and victories in a compelling and interesting manner. Even martial artists with no interest in the sport of cycling cannot but be inspired by this fascinating book.

Maynard, Kyle. *No Excuses: The True Story of a Congenital Amputee Who Became a Champion in Wrestling and in Life.* Washington, DC: Regnery Publishing, 2005.

Born a congenital amputee, the author nevertheless managed to succeed in everything he has put his mind to, accomplishing amazing feats such as becoming a state champion wrestler and typing a 250-page book, all without the use of his hands or feet. This inspirational autobiography that shows how a positive attitude can give someone most would see as disadvantaged every advantage in life. It is a useful resource for those who need inspiration to meet their own seemingly impossible goals.

Powell, Goran. ***Waking Dragons: A Martial Artist Faces His Ultimate Test.*** Chichester, U.K.: Summersdale Publishers, 2006.

This outstanding book retells the author's pinnacle karate achievement, completing a 30-man *kumite* (sparring competition) during which he successfully fought against 30 progressively skillful opponents in consecutive full-contact bouts. Despite the fact that this feat is rarely undertaken, let alone pulled off, by even master martial artists, the accomplishment is far less important for the reader than the way in which he got there. Powell aptly demonstrates how he learned and grew through various trials and tribulations in a way that is entertaining, easy to read, and, thankfully, never self-aggrandizing. The sum of these experiences helped him develop the quintessential martial virtue, an indomitable spirit necessary to take on and overcome nearly any challenge, even the brutal 30-man *kumite*. He compares this spirit to a pilot light. No matter how battered and beaten you may become, with the right mental attitude your pilot light can still burn brightly. No opponent can ever reach in and blow it out.

Siddle, Bruce. ***Sharpening the Warrior's Edge: The Psychology and Science of Training.*** Millstadt, IL: PPCT Research Publications, 1995.

This was a groundbreaking book ten years ago and it is still relevant and highly recommended today. Siddle's work examines survival and combat performance from a scientific perspective. It explains why performance and reaction time deteriorates under survival stress conditions and, more importantly, explains how to tailor your training to minimize these adverse effects in a real-life confrontation. Further, it helps you develop a mindset that can give you an edge in most any dangerous situation.

Recommended Web Sites
The American Success Institute (www.success.org)
The American Success Institute (ASI) is an educational publishing and philanthropic organization founded by Bill Fitzpatrick, a 5th *dan* black belt, small business expert, and motivational speaker. He created a self-improvement program called

"An understanding heart is everything in a teacher, and cannot be esteemed highly enough. One looks back with appreciation to the brilliant teachers, but with gratitude to those who touched our human feeling. The curriculum is so much necessary raw material, but warmth is the vital element for the growing plant and for the soul of the child."

– Carl Jung [15]

Action Principles®, which has proven popular with corporations, professional groups, and college audiences throughout the world. A non-profit group, ASI donates thousands of motivational books to schools, social agencies, and correctional facilities each year. Their Web site has an abundance of free articles, motivational quotes, and classes, including a Master Self-Defense course that was featured in *Black Belt* and *Martial Arts Professional* magazines. You can also buy some of their products through the site.

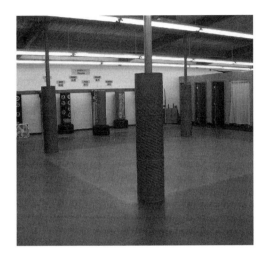

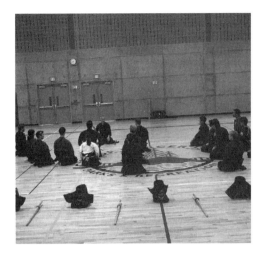

A WELL-MAINTAINED, CLEAN, AND ORDERLY ENVIRONMENT MAKES A GREAT PLACE TO SPEND YOUR TRAINING TIME.

GENERAL COMMENTS FOR THE ENTIRE CLASS SET THE DIRECTION OF THE CLUB DURING TRAINING.

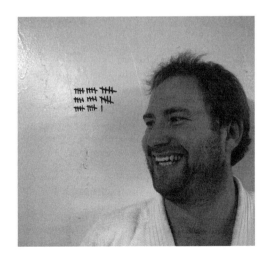

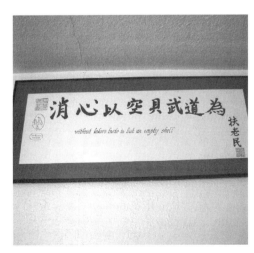

DIFFERENT TRAINING FOR DIFFERENT FOLKS. THESE HASH MARKS ON THE *DOJO* WALL REPRESENT THE NUMBER OF STUDENTS THAT HAVE THROWN-UP DURING INTENSIVE TRAINING.

WITHOUT "HEART," THE MARTIAL ARTS HAVE NO DEPTH. IT IS IMPORTANT TO MAKE EVERY EFFORT AGREE WITH HEART AND TECHNIQUE.

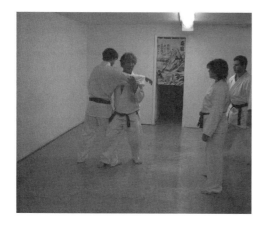

EXAMPLE IS THE KEY FORM OF INSTRUCTION. IN INSTRUCTOR-
SPEAK THIS IS CALLED, "MODELING."

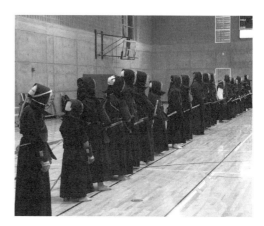

ALL EYES ARE ON THE INSTRUCTOR. ALL EARS ARE LISTENING.
THAT IS HOW YOU LEARN.

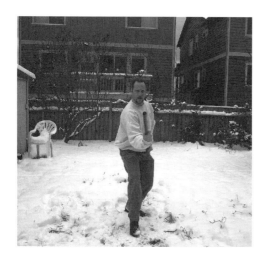

A GOOD INSTRUCTOR WILL INSPIRE SOLO TRAINING AT HOME.
INDIVIDUAL EXPLORATION OF TECHNIQUE CAN EXPEDITE YOUR
PROGRESS IN THE MARTIAL ARTS.

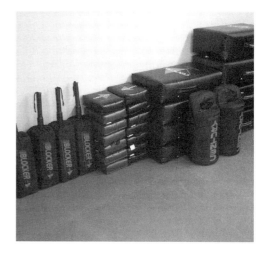

WHEN LOOKING AT POTENTIAL SCHOOLS, LOOK FOR ORDER AND
CLEANLINESS. ESPECIALLY LOOK AT ANY ITEMS THAT ARE NOT IN
USE DURING A TRAINING SESSION. ARE THEY WELL-MAINTAINED
AND TIDY? THIS WILL TELL YOU A LOT ABOUT THE SCHOOL.

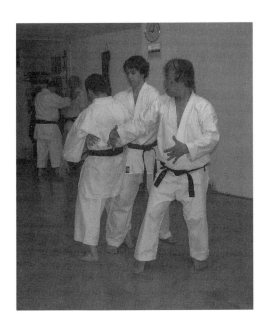

WALKING THROUGH TECHNIQUES SLOWLY IS ONE WAY TO BUILD A SOLID FOUNDATION NECESSARY FOR QUICKNESS AND POWER LATER ON.

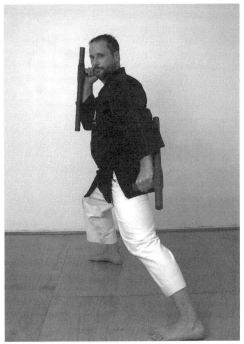

WEAPONS, WHETHER EDGED OR BLUNT, ARE DANGEROUS. A GOOD INSTRUCTOR WILL TREAT BOTH THE WEAPONS AND THE STUDENTS WITH RESPECT.

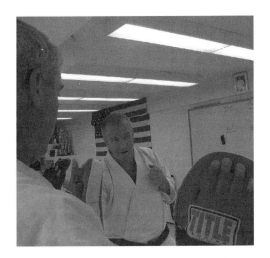

CLEAR EXPLANATION IS IMPORTANT TO LEARNING WELL. A GOOD TEACHER CAN MAKE WHAT THEY WANT CLEAR AND UNDERSTANDABLE, UTILIZING A VARIETY OF EFFECTIVE METHODS TO COMMUNICATE WITH EVERYONE.

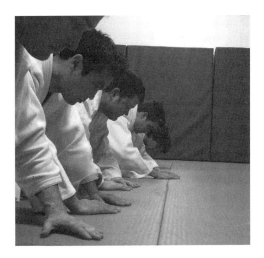

MARTIAL ARTS ARE BY NATURE WARLIKE AND DANGEROUS. CONSEQUENTLY, ETIQUETTE BECOMES VERY IMPORTANT. MANY CLASSES BEGIN WITH SOME FORMAL ACKNOWLEDGEMENT OF RESPECT SUCH AS BOWING TO TEACHERS AND OTHER STUDENTS.

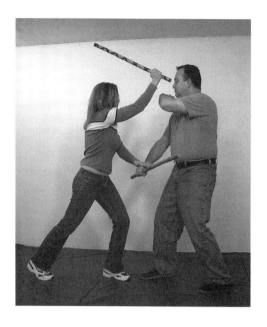

SOMETIMES AN INSTRUCTOR HAS TO TRUST THE STUDENT TO NOT MAKE AN ERROR. THIS IS A JUDGMENT CALL, WHICH CAN BUILD THE STUDENT'S SELF-ESTEEM AND BELIEF IN THEIR SKILLS.

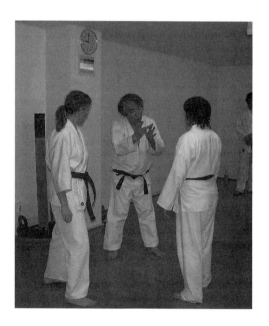

HAVING A PASSION FOR THE ART IS AN ESSENTIAL CHARACTERISTIC FOR AN INSTRUCTOR TO HAVE.

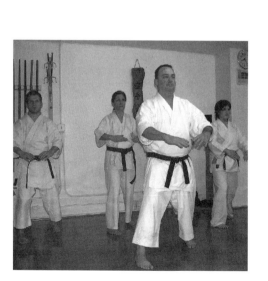

LEADING A SMALL GROUP OF STUDENTS, MOVING FROM GROUP TO GROUP IS ANOTHER METHOD TEACHERS WILL USE. WHILE YOU CANNOT ALWAYS GET INDIVIDUALIZED ATTENTION FROM THE HEAD INSTRUCTOR, YOU CAN LEARN FROM EVERYONE IN THE GROUP.

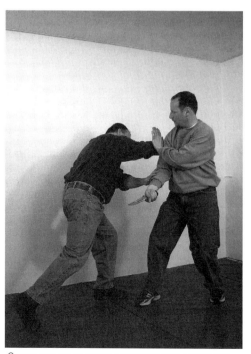

ONE-ON-ONE IS A GREAT WAY TO LEARN CRITICAL TECHNIQUES FROM YOUR INSTRUCTOR. BE PREPARED, HOWEVER, TO MAKE SPECIAL TIMES AND PAY ACCORDINGLY.

CHAPTER 2
Find a Good Instructor

*"Teaching should be such that what is offered is perceived as a valuable gift
and not as a hard duty."*
– Albert Einstein [13]

Introduction (by Martin Westerman)

Two stories come to mind when I think about teaching. The first: When someone asks my father, the artist, how long it took him to paint a picture, he replies, "About 50 years." The second: An old Japanese ceramicist, long ago, created a bowl that people hailed as a masterpiece. His assessment: "From this, I learn to do better work."

I like knowing that we grow and improve over time. It fills me with optimism, which is the real foundation for teaching and learning. If we never thought we could improve, there would be no reason to learn or teach anything. So, that is the first thing I seek in a teacher – optimism. The next two things I want to see in a teacher are: (1) a love of the subject that inspires and engages me and (2) the ability to structure in small steps, from simple to complex, which enables me to get from where I am to where I want to go

I always feel nervous about whether I can meet the challenges a teacher sets, but I know the rewards can be big. We can create things bigger and more wonderful than either of us expected; bigger than either of us could have done alone. That is the final thing I seek, a partner in learning. Teaching and learning are Yin and Yang, driven by endless curiosity, throwing off sparks of recognition and insight, arriving at clarity and economy of movement.

The best teachers become your partners in making your best future come true. It takes time, and it is always worth it.

– Martin Westerman [14]

The Teacher is More Important than the Art He Teaches

The Japanese word for teacher, *sensei*, literally means "one who has come before." The instructor you select is a person who has advanced further along the martial path than you have. He or she will be your guide as you strive to learn new concepts, understand the subtle nuances, and master new skills necessary to earn your black belt. Choosing the right person to lead you down this path is paramount.

A common question asked of long-term martial artists is, "Why did you choose to train where you did?" More often than not, the reply is shockingly simple, something along the lines of, "It was the only class available." Sometimes the closest instructor really is best, but it is important to have a good way of making that determination. After all, if earning a black belt takes a minimum of four to six years, you are going to be working with that person for a very long time indeed.

"A bad wound may heal, but a bad name will kill."

– Scottish Proverb

In his sophomore year of college, Wilder was leaving the university for the summer yet wanted to continue his training so he asked his instructor where the closest affiliated *dojo* to where he was moving might be. His *sensei* replied that he did not know, adding that it did not make any difference. He said, "You should find a good instructor, regardless of style." This is very good advice.

We believe that new students should choose the art they wish to pursue in large part by choosing the person who will be teaching it. Because there are only a limited number of vital areas on the body that can be manipulated, struck, or otherwise damaged by a martial practitioner, and there are only a limited number of ways that each joint in the body can move, every martial art shares certain common components. Emphasis and strategies will differ, of course, but techniques (e.g., punching, kicking, grappling, throwing) always overlap.

*Tai chi,** for example, metaphorically boils an egg from the inside out with its focus on internal energy. Karate, on the other hand, boils that egg from the outside in as it begins with an emphasis on external power. Advanced practitioners of both arts are able to harness both internal and external energy, so either way you ultimately get the same (metaphorically) boiled egg.

The fundamentals of fitness are universal as well. No one should feel forced to learn from an instructor who does not fulfill his or her needs just because they are the only local source of whatever style you have set your heart on. Finding the right teacher is far more important to effective learning than discovering the perfect martial art to study. In today's world, it is easy to find a variety of teachers who can lead

*Also known as *tai chi chuan* or *taijiquan*, a Chinese martial art.

you down the martial path. Making the right choice, the best choice, is what this chapter is all about.

Getting Started

Finding a teacher is not always easy. In some cultures, particularly those that believe that spending time with an adequate instructor is, in essence, a waste of time, it can take one or two years to find a teacher. Historically, this was certainly the case in China, Okinawa, and Japan. The goal was to find a truly excellent practitioner, someone with a distinguished name and a superior reputation. Instruction was more about what the teacher knew than anything else, particularly the student's interests or needs. Because these masters were so admired, students would adjust their ways to accommodate the teacher's requirements.

Dojo in feudal Japan, for example, were very selective. Gaining admission was an onerous process. Aspirants had to approach the *dojo* with letters of introduction and recommendation from someone well known and respected by the head of the school. Far-reaching background checks were conducted on each candidate. When someone's application was accepted, the applicant proceeded to swear a blood oath or *keppan,* to guard the school's secrets and uphold the honor of the *ryu* (system). This loyalty oath was placed in writing, then signed and sealed with the applicant's blood. Small scars on the inside of their arms (or sometimes their fingers) reminded them of the great honor it was to have been granted this opportunity.

Once the aspirant had sworn his oath and been accepted as a member of the *ryu*, the application was still not complete. A period of *hodoki* (unleashing or untying of the hands) followed where the applicant proved that he was worthy of training. During this probationary stage, he was given all manner of menial chores to perform (e.g., sweeping the floor, chopping wood, washing uniforms, preparing meals) as instructors tested how much the aspirant could tolerate to determine how badly he wanted to learn. If the beginner performed the assigned tasks with patience and perseverance, he could be inducted into the ranks of the *ryu*.

Once accepted, the student became a *monjin* (person at the gate), one who was eligible to actually begin their training. After this, it still took years of faithful service and vigorous effort before the student could learn, or even know about, the *okuden* (hidden teaching) or secret techniques of a school or martial style. In the old days, training was clearly more than simply attending lessons and picking up new skills. *Budoka* (martial artists) were part of a privileged group who followed a lifelong path toward becoming better people as well as highly skilled practitioners.

Today, anyone can pay an initiation fee, buy a uniform, and join almost any *dojo* in the country. Although there is no longer any *keppan* or formal *hodoki*, turnover rates among students being what they are, few instructors devote their full attention to new *budoka* until they have proven that they are worthy of such training. The rare student who demonstrates, discipline, perseverance, and a positive attitude will gradually be given access to more and more of the instructor's time, attention, and specialized guidance.

To find an instructor, first you generally need to find a school. Finding a school can be a surprisingly easy affair. Begin by asking your family, friends, co-workers, and acquaintances. You may be amazed at how many people have some sort of experience in the martial arts, or can refer you to somebody they know who has had some training. The best source is obviously a referral by someone who knows you well, understands how you learn, and also knows someone appropriate who teaches martial arts. If you do not have friends or relatives who can refer you to an excellent instructor, however, you can start your search simply by looking in the Yellow Pages (Web or hardcopy) for your local area.

There's Much in a Name

Dr. Hayward Nishioka, a world-class judo instructor, once wrote "The word *dojo* in Japanese means 'the place to learn the way,' and Orientals consider it a valuable place of many lessons where a practitioner may learn to master himself as well as his opponent." Similarly, this training hall is called *dojang* in Korean and *kwoon* in Chinese. For the sake of brevity, we will simply call the school a *dojo* from this point forward.

The name of a *dojo* can tell you an awful lot about the school. More often than not it was selected by the head instructor so that can tell you a bit about him or her too. It is useful to categorize *dojo* as marquee schools, new name schools, Asian schools, mythic schools, regional name schools, chain schools, affiliations, or combination schools. This categorization along with a little research to validate your assumptions can give you important insight that will help you align your goals with the type of instruction you are likely to receive:

"Marquee" School. These schools have the head instructor's name in their title. Someone who is willing to put his or her name on the school is not necessarily a self-aggrandizing megalomaniac. He or she is likely a recognizable figure in the martial arts world (e.g., famous movie actor, tournament competitor, or author) and uses that name recognition to draw new students into the art. While it is likely a commercial endeavor, you should reasonably expect to receive a certain amount of instruction directly from the marquee instructor. If you choose a school because of a marquee name, be sure to ask about how much time you will actually receive directly from the owner. His or her senior students will often lead daily sessions, particularly if the marquee individual has a busy road schedule or numerous *dojo* locations, so you cannot expect to see the marquee individual every day. If he just pops his head in now and again though, you might want to take that into consideration when deciding if such a school is the right place for you to train.

"New Name" School. You may be new to the world of martial arts but should be familiar with the names of many if not all of the most common martial arts forms (refer to Appendix B for a good starting point). An unfamiliar name should raise some questions and lead to some research on your part. Just because it is a new name to you does not necessarily mean it is a new name in general, though it certainly might be. Even judo was a new name at one time, of course, but a new name or a combination of a new and old name should lead you to take a hard look at what is being taught. The Japanese took a very hard look many times at the upstart sport of judo prior to incorporating it into their school system. Today, it has become an Olympic sport practiced throughout the world.

Because there are plenty of reputable "known" arts out there, choosing an unknown one may carry an unwarranted level of risk. While some instructors who invent their own art form are truly visionaries, others have washed out from traditional styles and created their own to inflate their rank or prowess artificially. Others commingle techniques from a variety of styles, creating a hybrid they feel is superior to its predecessors. Again, sometimes these forms have merit whereas oftentimes they lack a core strategic foundation that binds the individual components together into a synergistic, practicable whole. *Caveat emptor* (let the buyer beware); if you have never heard of a martial style and have trouble finding its origins/history, beware before you buy.

"Asian" School. Many martial arts originated in the Orient. Consequently, Okinawan, Japanese, Chinese, Thai, and Filipino names are frequently attached to a school. If you are looking for traditional instruction, this type of name may lead you toward your goal. Be cautious, however. Some are steeped in tradition while others are nothing more than made-up nonsense. Asian names are often confusing for Westerners, so it is important to ask questions such as, "What does it mean?" *Goju Ryu Karate-do*, for example, means "hard/gentle way of the infinite fist." It is not strictly a hard form but rather incorporates both hard (e.g., punching, kicking) and soft (e.g., throwing, pressure-point manipulation) aspects as the name implies.

Some instructors create Asian-sounding names to trick unwary prospective students into thinking that they have found some secret, ultimate martial art while they ultimately find dubious instruction. Others, on the other hand, make amusing wordplays for perfectly practical arts. For example, Marc MacYoung and Dianna Gordon founded an art called *Dango Jiro*, which means "Mulligan Stew" in Japanese, an apt description since it borrows highly effective techniques from a variety of different arts. Understanding what the foreign language means can give you insight into the kind of instruction you might expect from the art.

"Mythic" Schools. Some schools use mythic symbols like mascots, reflecting the nature of the training you can expect to receive. Dragons, tigers, snakes, and similar beasts are relatively common. A teacher will choose this type of name, for good or bad, because it represents the attitude they want to convey about their school. Consequently, the name gives you important clues about the type of training you might receive.

"Regional" School. Regional names like "West Seattle Karate Academy" demonstrate a local flavor. With a regional name, you are often dealing with a smaller school that is most likely involved in local community, supports local events, and has instructors that live and work in the immediate area. This type of school is more likely to be independent than to be affiliated with a national or worldwide organization. Like any other type of school, this can be good or bad (see "Affiliated Schools" below for more information).

> *"Teachers open the door. You enter by yourself."*
>
> – Chinese proverb

"Chain" School. If you search the Yellow Pages and find a listing for numerous locations under the same umbrella name, you have almost certainly found a chain school. Their ads often sound a bit like those for a tire store and the comparison is not a bad one. When you walk into a national chain tire store, you know exactly what you are going to get: tires that are properly installed and carry a national warranty and, perhaps, a cup of bad coffee or free popcorn while you wait. Those tires are going to be good for the prescribed mileage and will be worth what you paid for them. You will very likely find similarly consistent standards at a chain martial arts studio, but also a revenue-oriented organization that comes along with them.

"Affiliated" School. A good question to ask a potential *sensei* is, "What is your school's affiliation?" Affiliations are both coveted and reviled in the martial arts world. Some schools pride themselves on being affiliated with a larger group. These organizations provide consistency, uniformity, and standards, but can also become stagnant, didactic, and rigid. It is the classic line, "An unguarded strength can be a weakness." Joining an affiliated organization means that you are getting a package deal, whether you realize it or not, with everything positive and negative that implies.

Combinations of the above. You can have various combinations of these names too. Because the first part of the name is generally the most important, it can help you determine what to expect. For example, marquee schools frequently have several branch *dojo* linked together to create an affiliated organization.

Drive-by First Impressions

In their excellent book *Starting and Running Your Own Martial Arts School*, Karen Levitz Vactor and Susan Lynn Peterson tell the prospective *dojo* owners to find their potential school's location and drive a radius out seven minutes away from it to see the neighborhoods. The goal of this exercise is to determine who is most likely to attend the school. Most people, according to the authors, will not drive more than seven minutes to attend a martial arts class. As you look for a potential school at which to train, consider this same process. It is much harder to attend classes regularly if the drive is long. The longer the drive you have to make to get there, the lower your likelihood of regular attendance at the *dojo*. That's just human nature. Because most Yellow Pages Web sites let you rank results by distance, begin with *dojo* that are within that magic five- to seven-mile radius from your home (or however far you can travel in seven minutes). If necessary, you can go further out, of course, but starting closest to home makes sense.

The bottom line is if it is the best school in the world, you are not going to attend if it is halfway across the world…, well, you might. Wilder has a relative who quit his job, sold his house, and moved to China to study. Because most of us have a job and responsibilities that help define out lives, however, access does become an issue. The farther you are from the school, the less likely you are to attend regularly. Without regular attendance, you will almost certainly be unable to earn a black belt, so look for convenient locations first. Make a list of *dojo* nearby and visit them. A good initial approach is to ascertain the emphasis of each *dojo*.

Just as you can learn a lot by the name of the school, much of this can be understood simply by walking through the door. Schools whose front windows are crowded with trophies most likely have an emphasis on tournament fighting and sports competition. The presence of pads and headgear may reinforce this initial impression. Depending upon your age and interests, this may or may not be attractive.

Stacks of *tatami* or other practice mats indicate a propensity for grappling techniques. Racks of weapons offer an obvious clue to the availability of such training. The presence of *kigu undo* equipment, traditional tools used for conditioning exercises such as *nigiri game* (gripping jars) and *makiwara* (striking posts), suggests a traditional approach—one that bodes well if your goal is character development.

Hours of Operation

Hours of operation are important, but not necessarily in the way the school will try to sell them to you. The pitch is often something like, "Sure, the monthly fee is $X, but you have unlimited access to the school during business hours. You can train six days a week or once a week for the same price." That may sound wonderful at first blush, yet we all have busy lives so it is not necessarily a good thing. Although the idea of drop-in training may be attractive, few students actually exercise that option over the long run. Most find that maintaining a routine schedule, training at regular hours on select days, is far easier to stick with than dropping in whenever you have a free moment.

Think about what fits best into your schedule. Will you have training time in the morning before work or school? Afternoons? Evenings? Weekends? Decide what your hours of training are going to be and be sure that your potential school will be open when you need to train. While some schools teach everyone at once, many schools segregate new students from experienced ones, assuring that fundamental skills are known before metaphorically throwing you into the deep end. Separating adult and children's classes is common, too. If your prospective *dojo* has different schedules for beginning, intermediate, and advanced classes, be sure to check on all the various timeslots, not just the one you will be attending right away. Over time, you will progress from one class to the next.

Once you have set a schedule, it is very important to adhere to it. Consistency in the time(s) of day you practice can help you make a habit of your training. It is far easier to continue over a long period of time when training becomes part of your regular routine. Keeping your training time and honoring the promise you made to yourself is core to reaching your goal of becoming a black belt as quickly as possible.

Watch a Class in Progress

Once you have found a potential school in your area, it is important to observe a class in progress. You can learn much about how a school is run by looking across the *dojo* floor while training is in session. Ask the instructor if you can observe a class. If he or she will not allow you to observe, you have almost certainly not found a place where you would want to train. Be courteous and unobtrusive while you observe. If the teacher comes over to talk with you from time to time, you can quietly ask questions about what you are seeing. It is inappropriate, however, to disrupt a class in progress.

"The mediocre teacher tells. The good teacher explains. The superior teacher demonstrates. The great teacher inspires."

– William Arthur Ward [16]

Here are some things to look for:

- Are students standing around looking confused or does everyone appear to be actively engaged in the learning process?
- Are students talking or working?
- Do students and teachers interact in a respectful manner?
- Are students corrected in a positive way when they make a mistake?
- Is there an appropriate level of supervision, a student to teacher ratio that facilitates personalized attention for everyone who needs it?
- Does there appear to be an appropriate emphasis on safety?

- Is this a fun, energetic environment in which to train?
- If the *dojo* rules and/or *dojo kun* (precepts or virtues) are posted on the wall, do what they say make sense to you?
- Are students training in traditional uniforms or modern street clothes?
- Assuming shoes are not worn during class, are they lined up neatly in front of the floor?
- Is the place neat, orderly, and in good repair?
- Is there adequate room to train?
- Is attendance strong?

Interviewing the Instructor

Be prepared to interview the instructor to understand his or her teaching methods. If properly approached, teachers should be happy to discuss their styles, testing methodologies, and teaching philosophies with prospective students. If the *dojo* has a Web site, you should be able to use the instructor's biography or *curriculum vitae* to establish his or her credentials and get a good understanding of his or her approach to teaching. Be respectful of his or her time, however, by preparing questions ahead of time and making an appointment when necessary. Just as you are forming an initial impression of a potential instructor, your future *sensei* is forming his or her impression of you.

Exemplary instructors are firm yet polite when disciplining students, informative when explaining new skills, and persuasive when teaching the more esoteric aspects of their art. They should be approachable for answering questions and polite no matter how silly the inquiries might appear. Above all else, exemplary educators are always prepared and ready to teach each class in a professional manner.

It is perfectly acceptable to ask a potential instructor about his or her teaching style or experience but it is generally considered tactless to ask a martial artist about his or her rank. Some *sensei* will offer that information themselves, but not all. One way to approximate an instructor's experience is to look at his or her belt. A smooth, glossy black belt is obviously fairly new, perhaps indicating a recent promotion to *yudansha* rank, while a tattered, discolored belt may be an indicator of long years of training.* Taking the age of the practitioner in conjunction with the way he/she handles the class, you can get a fair idea of a person's experience level. Rank is far less important than the quality of instruction you will receive.

Characteristics of an Exemplary Instructor. After interviewing an instructor, it may be possible to talk with students and/or parents of students to gather more information. Exemplary instructors have nothing to hide and should not mind

---

* A new belt may also be a gift, particularly if it is embroidered with the practitioner's name, or a replacement for one that has been stolen, lost, or worn out. Conversely, unscrupulous practitioners sometimes artificially "age" their belts to make them look battered and worn, a rare albeit extraordinarily tacky practice.

such additional scrutiny so long as it is not disruptive to their students. Be tactful and polite. Things to look for include following:

Communication. William Ward's the famous saying goes, "The mediocre teacher tells. The good teacher explains. The superior teacher demonstrates. The great teacher inspires." Good communication in the *dojo* begins with a passion for teaching. It is the ability to relate complex materials in a clear and understandable manner. A good understanding of personality differences among students, and a demonstrated willingness to accommodate them as necessary to ensure good communication, are very important. Superior teachers have an intuitive ability to select the most effective teaching style for any situation or student and a willingness to change course midstream if things are not working as anticipated. Finally, an ability to communicate a sense of direction and purpose for his or her school and art form is essential.

Respect. Students' attitudes can tell you much about their instructor. Real respect is always earned, never demanded. Demanding respect never works for any significant amount of time. It is the equivalent of building a house on sand. Respect cannot be manufactured. If the students are respectful of the teacher and, this is important, respectful of other students in turn, then it is real. Oftentimes the respect flows one way to the instructor and the students are treated poorly. This is an indicator of a less-than-positive learning environment, one that you will ultimately regret being involved with.

Ability. Superior instructors must have deep, well-rounded knowledge of *budo*, preferably beyond a single art form. Whatever they ask of their students they must be able to do themselves. If an instructor is unable to do a technique due to injury or age that is certainly understandable. Yet being unable to perform because they simply cannot do what they are attempting to explain should raise some serious concerns and make you question the skills of the instructor. If you cannot do it, you almost certainly cannot teach it. Unfortunately, rank alone is no guarantee of skill, so you will need to observe the person demonstrating a variety of aspects of their art in order to draw any meaningful conclusions.

Enjoyment. Enthusiasm is important. Does the instructor enjoy what he or she is doing? Is he or she genuinely happy being an instructor? Some folks love their art, but only teach out of a sense of duty or to earn a living. It is important that a *sensei* enjoys teaching, so that should be a consideration when looking for an exemplary instructor. One way to test this is to ask yourself, "Would this teacher be a student in his or her class?" If the answer is yes, then you are looking at someone who enjoys both the art and the learning process. If the answer is no, then you may want to look further before settling on this school or club. Like any profession, you excel at what you enjoy.

Integrity. Strong moral character is an essential attribute of any martial arts instructor. A high degree of integrity, personal honor, and common sense are paramount. Never forget that regardless of whether or not you ever use them on the street, you are learning warrior skills in the *dojo*. All such training comes with some risk of injury or even death. Consequently, you will want to train with someone who handles this dangerous activity in a prudent and responsible manner. (See "Student/Teacher Relationshipss" below for more information.)

Professionalism and appearance. Martial arts instructors are professionals. You are giving them money for a service, a unique service, of course, but a service nevertheless. Like any other profession from which you purchase a service, you should expect a certain level of standards. Does the instructor act in a professional manner? Is his or her uniform neat and clean, at least at the beginning of class?* Is the instructor well groomed and presentable?

A good test for this question might be, "Could this person be successful at another job looking and acting the way they do here?" If the answer is yes, continue on; if the answer is no, you may want to take some time to ask another question or two. There may be legitimate reasons why someone looks unkempt, but personal hygiene is a significant indicator of how a person sees themselves, a foreshadowing of what you might expect when learning from him or her. If a person does not care about himself or herself, how can they possibly care about you?

Try Before You Buy

Once you have made a preliminary decision, many *dojo* offer one or more free classes to help you decide whether or not training there will be right for you. It really takes a minimum of two to three months to know for sure (especially if you have not done this sort of activity before), but much can be intuited with a single class.

Most instructors are perfectly happy to give you a brief trial run. We would not personally join any school that did not give a minimum of one free trial class. Do expect to be required to sign a liability waiver for insurance purposes, though. That is a standard procedure.

Student/Teacher Relationships

Student/teacher interactions are complex, especially in the field of martial arts where instructors hold a higher degree of power over their students than in other disciplines. While a math or science teacher can flunk you, manipulate you, threaten you, or otherwise mess up your life, he or she works for an institution with strict bylaws, governance, and oversight. If a student's professor does something inappropriate, there is generally a review board and dispute resolution process to follow.

A martial arts instructor, on the other hand, can kill you. Furthermore, he or she often runs his or her own school with limited, if any, oversight by an associa-

---

* If it's not at least a little rumpled and sweaty by the end of class, that's a whole other issue.

Advice for New Students

by Jeff Stevens [17]

Many years ago, I thought a good martial arts instructor was someone with attitude and aggression. As time went on, I found that this was not required. In fact, it can actually be detrimental to the learning process. When looking for a *dojo* or instructor, listen to your inner feelings about the personality of the *dojo* and that of the instructors. Spend some time watching a class you are thinking of joining. Watch the attitude of the instructors. Ask yourself if you feel comfortable in this environment.

Personally, I was very lucky to have stumbled upon a good instructor and *dojo*, the very first time I went looking. But, in my travels I have seen and heard of a few that could hardly have been called fair. I also thought years ago that a large-sized *dojo* was representative of good instruction. A large school should only tell you that their marketing, or location, has been successful. A good instructor can be found in both large and small *dojo*. I saw a *dojo* once that had around fifty students with just one black belt! Now I'm not against large chain *dojo*, per se, but I'm not sure I would join one now, knowing that a more intimate class affords a more personalized type of instruction. There is nothing wrong with someone making a living teaching martial arts, just be sure that you are getting good value for your dollar with a reasonably sized class.

Some other warning signs would be too much formality, or attention to rituals that are outside the norm for a martial arts class. I heard of a *dojo* once in a shopping mall that spent more time with *sensei* honoring rituals than with actual instruction. Now do not get me wrong; as you might already know, there are a few rituals that go hand-in-hand with learning the martial arts. Just watch for it in excess. It may be a diversion from a poor instructor. Your ideal environment should be respectful, but slightly informal. Lastly, I would keep an eye out for an instructor that unduly brags about accomplishments and trophies (although there is nothing wrong with a *dojo* trophy cabinet).

The information on the instructors should be available in pamphlets or on their Web site (in some schools it may be impolite to ask the instructor directly what rank they are). You do need to know this information as you want someone qualified to teach you, but if in person the instructor appears to be a bragging sort, this could be a warning sign of an overly strong ego. And that means you are there for the instructor's benefit, not yours. Think humble.

tion of that style. Consequently, such relationships need to be founded on a deep sense of trust, integrity, and honesty, untainted by even the appearance of impropriety. Most teachers feel that it is imperative to separate personal and professional relationships. It is important that students understand and respect that division. Tribulations in one's personal life simply do not belong on the *dojo* floor. It is unwise and potentially dangerous.

Expect a Mentor, Not a Friend

Most instructors find that a certain degree of professionalism and detachment is prudent when interacting with students. We live in a highly litigious society where even an unfounded accusation of harassment or sexual misconduct can ruin one's reputation and livelihood. Expect your teacher to be professional and polite, but not necessarily friendly. That does not mean that he or she does not like you. It is just a practical response to real potential pitfalls.

Try to respect your instructor's boundaries. Given turnover rates among new students, teachers will usually distance themselves, at least a little, from all but the most senior, dedicated practitioners. Most *budo* instructors will not go out of their way to provide "secrets" or special assistance to those who have not proven themselves worthy over a significant period of time. That is just human nature.

Your instructor should be your mentor in all things martial arts. He or she is uniquely qualified to excel in that arena. However, *sensei* are neither omniscient nor omnipotent, no matter how frequently students treat them as such. Do not place him or her in the position of becoming your priest, counselor, or psychologist. That is the purview of other professionals.

Beware of Cults

No discussion of martial arts schools would be complete without addressing the phenomenon of cults. Like any group activity, there are good things and bad things that can happen with martial arts instruction. Bumps, bruises, and minor physical injuries come with the territory, but brainwashing should not. Beware of martial arts cults; they are somewhat rare yet incredibly hazardous should you find yourself caught up in one.

Many books have been written on cults with much greater depth than we need to touch upon here. We will focus on the high points while you search for a school and an instructor.

The Merriam-Webster online dictionary lists five different meanings of the word *cult*:

1. Formal religious veneration
2. A system of religious beliefs and ritual; also: its body of adherents
3. A religion regarded as unorthodox or spurious; also: its body of adherents
4. A system for the cure of disease based on dogma set forth by its promulgator
5. Great devotion to a person, idea, object, movement, or work
   (as a film or book)

Now, clearly, we are talking about martial arts so let us change the dictionary definitions around a little bit. Here are a few identifying characteristics to watch out for:

Instructor Knows All (i.e., the "guru" effect)

Your *sensei* is a martial artist. He or she is not your parent, priest, counselor, or psychologist. Nobody knows everything, but sometimes we forget that. Just because an instructor can hit hard does not mean that he or she knows the meaning of life. Watch for instructors that intentionally seek this guru effect: the appearance of having all wisdom. Either these people have let their egos get in the way of their common sense, or they are out and out charlatans. Either way, they are attempting to make themselves into something they are not. Do not get caught up in this game, very little good can come out of it.

The Poser

Beware of instructors who seek to gratify their own ego rather than professionally conducting the business of training martial arts students. We often call these folks "posers." Benito Mussolini (1883 – 1945) was the malevolent dictator of Italy from 1922 until his overthrow in 1943. He was known for striking impressive and inspiring postures while giving colorful speeches, as well as posing for self-aggrandizing pictures and portraits. He was also kicked out of church for throwing rocks and pinching people. He stabbed a fellow student in boarding school. He looked like a good guy but clearly was not. Observe your potential instructor. We are not implying that he or she is a mass murderer, of course, but he/she could certainly be a petty dictator, at least in the *dojo*. Is this instructor a poser or martial arts professional? Do his or her words and actions match?

Respect vs. Blind Obedience

The difference between respect and blind obedience might appear to be thin but it is not. Respect flows both ways—the instructor respects the students and the student respect the instructor. If an instructor does not respect his or her students, you will observe the following kinds of behaviors:

Yelling at students. Constructive feedback is fine, but shouting and public embarrassment are out-of-bounds. Instructors should generally hand out praise in public while dealing with discipline in private. Publicly berating a student is almost never appropriate, save for extreme incidents such as unsafe weapons use in the *dojo* or bullying behavior amongst students.

Striking students in an abusive manner. Physical contact is part of most martial arts training, yet it needs to be commensurate with each individual's ability to receive impact. An instructor who "tees off" on his or her students or who regularly "dishes out" abusive beatings is not taking the student's best interests to heart.

Talking down. Speaking to students in a demeaning or belittling manner is unprofessional at best. Courtesy, etiquette, and respect are important aspects of martial training. There is no call for such behavior in the *dojo*.

"Martial arts and self-defense organizations often tend to be extremely cliquish. That is to say that they are often built around a particular way of thinking or more often, one person's persona. In fact, these are indeed cults of personality. These programs often fall into three basic categories. One, because the 'founder' of the system, or current grand pooh-bah, is thought by the disciples to walk on water and be the messiah of the martial arts. Two, the person presents himself as some kind of killer kung fu comman-do street fighter who has used his devastating fighting system to defeat hordes of attackers in countless combat situations. The third mess is a combination of the first two. Putting it bluntly when you encounter this you have not found an effective self-defense system, you have found a church."

— Marc MacYoung [18]

Gossip. Talking about people behind their backs is downright rude. Subversive instructors use gossip to debase, control, and manipulate their students.

Demands. *Dojo* relationships belong in the training hall. Beware of instructors who make demands beyond what is required for you to learn your martial art. This can include demands for work without recompense, sexual favors, or any other inappropriate activities.

Arbitrary rules. Important "rules" such as advancement criteria, safety conventions, fee structures, and other regulations or guidelines should be consistently applied amongst the population of students. Instructors who arbitrarily and capriciously change the rules are best avoided.

Acute military behavior. You can expect to wear a uniform during class and spend a certain amount of time practicing on your own between training sessions, but your instructor does not run your life. Your free time is your own. *Dojo* practice is not boot camp.

Others carry out the dirty work. Any school that has a group of enforcers, an "elite" squad, or a clique who have the job of carrying out the punishments meted out by the head instructor are a clear indicator of cult-like behavior. Do not confuse this with helping with administrative actions. Do be aware of punitive measures assigned and carried out by "The Squad." It is perfectly normal to have elements of training that are provided solely to senior practitioners who have the knowledge, skills, and ability to handle advanced training. Other than that, all students should be treated alike.

God, Family, Work, and School. Martial arts come after these items in your life. If you are asked to place martial arts ahead of these items, then you are in the wrong place. It is that simple.

It is hard to tell if you are in a cult, particularly once you have already become inculcated into the group. It is important to ask yourself, therefore, how susceptible you are to this malevolent influence. If you are looking for fulfillment in martial arts—that is to say you believe it will address the holes you think you have in your life you are ripe for a cult.

Notorious serial killer and cult leader Charles Manson filled the holes in his followers' lives.* He led them not toward something, but away from their personal pain. Manson provided an insulated environment with all the answers, he used drugs to weaken his followers' resolve, caused confusion, and employed emotional blackmail. Charles Manson, Adolf Hitler, and Benito Mussolini are extreme examples of cult figures.

> *"I knew of a group of martial artists that actually went out as a group and got the club patch tattooed on themselves. I would have to say that comes frightfully close to cult behavior, but then I have friends that have their fraternity letters tattooed on them as well. Is that cult behavior or is it just a tribal act?"*
>
> – Kris Wilder

Look at yourself honestly. If you are seeking to have a hole in your life filled, or seeking to hide from something using the martial arts, you are setting yourself up for an unscrupulous instructor to take advantage of you. While the path to black belt (and beyond) can have a profound impact on your life, it should not become the only focus of your life. If you are looking for fun, self-exploration, new skills and maybe a new friend or two, you have the right attitude. Combine that attitude with an excellent instructor and you are on your way.

At What Price Training?

While exemplary *sensei* have special knowledge, skills, and abilities that are well worth paying for, you should strive to avoid getting ripped off. After all, you are signing up to learn skills that literally take a lifetime to master so this can be a long-term deal if you find the right art form and stick with it. Unfortunately, even with a good teacher it can easily take a year or more to learn enough about a style to ascertain whether it really is a good fit. On top of that, some instructors whose only source of income is teaching martial arts may use unscrupulous or manipulative tactics to bring revenue through the door.

To a certain degree, you get what you are paying for but a higher price does not always indicate higher quality of instruction. Some of the best *dojo* we have trained at cost half the price of their nearest competitor. This is because the owner was not running the school to make a living; he already had a day job. The goal was simply to have enough students to cover the cost of maintaining a convenient place to train. These ladies and gentlemen were passionate about their arts and sincerely wished to find others to share their skills with.

---

* A career petty criminal (e.g., car theft, forgery, credit card fraud), he became the leader of a group known as "The Family" in the early 1960s. In that capacity he masterminded a series of brutal murders. His cult's most famous victims included movie actress Sharon Tate (who was eight and a half months pregnant at the time), Leno LaBianca, and Rosemary LaBianca. According to many former members of the group, Manson implied to his followers that he was Jesus, saying he had died before, some 2,000 years ago.

Nevertheless, you are buying a service when you select a teacher and begin to train so you will need to be prepared to pay a reasonable price for your education. Month-to-month arrangements are best. In the United States, prices tend to run between $45 and $130 per month depending upon where you live, what art you choose, and how many days per week you wish to practice. Anything in that price range is reasonable for quality instruction.

Regardless of the reasonableness of any monthly training fee, we strongly suggest that you be wary of long-term contracts. In fact, if someone offers you a "special" one-time only deal (typically for more than a thousand dollars) that covers all of your training through black belt, it is best to politely turn down the offer and walk away. You have almost certainly found a "McDojo," an instructor's moneymaking machine, rather than a legitimate and reliable place of instruction. Short-term contracts may be acceptable if that is your only alternative, but read carefully, think deeply, and have your attorney give it a thorough review before signing one.

Training costs more than just your dues unfortunately. Initiation fees, uniforms, patches, and testing fees are quite commonplace as well. Requirements to pay a moderate initiation fee of roughly one month's dues and purchase a uniform (~ $20 to $80) are perfectly reasonable. Even if you already have a *gi*, if it is not the same type as that used by the rest of the class you can expect to be required to purchase a new one. While there are a variety of online sources for purchasing a uniform, most schools can provide them for you at a reasonable cost. They can also help with sizing or tailoring when needed.

Uniforms are generally sized numerically in a fashion that does not correlate with any other method of calculating clothing dimensions (e.g., small, medium, large, or numerical size). For example, a size 6 *gi* is typically designed for someone who is about 6'1" tall and weighs roughly 200 pounds, while a size 5 *gi* is appropriate for someone who is about 5'8" tall and weighs about 175 pounds. To add to the confusion, online conversion tables do not always account for shrinkage accurately. Some schools will also require that you purchase a club patch to sew (or iron) onto your *gi* for a nominal fee too (~$5).

If all that was not enough, be sure to look into testing and/or advancement fees as well. Most schools charge a small amount, perhaps $10 to $20, to cover the cost of your new belt and/or certificate for each *kyu* (colored belt) rank you achieve. In nearly every system, it takes nine *kyu* promotions to become eligible for a black belt. There is a larger fee, typically somewhere in the $200 to $400 range, for black belt tests. This fee often covers an embroidered belt and a nice certificate in addition to reimbursing the instructor and/or testing board for their time. Anything significantly larger is suspect. Further, most legitimate schools only charge a testing fee once per grade, regardless of whether or not you pass a promotion test on the first try.

Student Perspective (by Mason Campbell)

Finding a good martial arts instructor was a challenge. To be frank, there are many nuts out there teaching martial arts. Moreover, there are many really good ones too. I started with what was local to me, something that I guess is not uncommon. It was karate and I loved it. I really liked the instructor and the others in the class. We were treated firmly and fairly. He made us all feel as if we where part of a special group, and we were. I had to move a couple of times, so I ended up trying several different arts and instructors. Here are a few of the types I found:

Psycho-Macho – this guy watched too many films or something. He was good at posing in front of the class; I did not stick around to see the rest.

Day Care – And I mean for Adults! These students had a great sense of themselves and not one ounce of technique amongst them.

Crazy Secret Sensei – "We break our bones so they heal harder and we can hit harder." Honest!

You-Can't-Watch – "You join our club before you can see what we do." Well, guess what, I never did either one.

In addition, the list goes on, I am sure.

I did finally find a teacher and he taught an art that was not really at the top of my list, but he was pleasant, professional, and found something inside me that I was not sure existed. I am quite happy and enjoy my training, I hope you, too, are as fortunate as I was.

– Mason Campbell [19]

Summary

When you think about it, people will shop for a health club, but in doing so often choose the one closest to home, and secondarily, choose by price. Looking at colleges and universities distance is often far down the list of criteria on which a choice is made for higher learning. People will choose proximity for the health of their body and go to nearly any geographical extent for the health of their mind. Martial arts in the best environments combine both the mind and the body.

A relative of Wilder's sold his house and moved to China in pursuit of *tai chi*. He chose to go where he was able to find the best instruction that suited him, but he had to give up a lot to get it; in this case selling his house to finance the new life he chose. Those that choose a club at the local community center because it is close may not get the best instruction. Then again, neither path is a guarantee now is it?

Ultimately choosing your instructor is a personal choice and the information in this chapter can only aid you in sharpening your pencil as you begin to check off the reasons for and the reasons why not to choose the school and instructor you just visited.

Action Plan

• Make a list of the schools in your area, regardless of what you think you want to learn.

_____

_____

_____

• Call ahead, make an appointment, and keep the appointment. It demonstrates commitment on your part and it will put the school/instructor in their best presentation mode.

_____

_____

_____

• Once you have completed your visits, look at your information, and make a decision about where you want to train.

_____

_____

_____

• Do not wait until next month or next quarter to sign up. Do it at the first available moment.

_____

_____

_____

Suggested Reading

Heckler, Richard Strozzi. ***Aikido and the New Warrior.*** Berkeley, CA: North Atlantic Books,1985

Heckler has compiled a fascinating collection of essays from *aikido-ka* about what they have learned and/or are learning from their training. The contributors effectively communicate their thoughts and emotions in an interesting and compelling manner. These writings not only illuminate *aikido* concepts, but also provide insight into a variety of important subjects such as martial arts training, competitive sports, harmony with nature, dealing with anger, aging, death, and so on. Essays include such titles as *Aikido and the New Warrior, Blending with Death, Getting a Black Belt at Age Fifty-Two, Aikido and Healing: Does this Stuff Really Work, A Turn to Balance*, and *A Kind Word Turneth Away Wrath.*

Lowry, Dave. ***In the Dojo: A Guide to the Rituals and Etiquette of the Japanese Martial Arts.*** Boston, MA: Shambhala Publications, 2006

A great resource for martial artists and Japan aficionados alike, this book covers all aspects of etiquette and tradition in the classical Japanese martial arts. If you plan to study *aikido, iaido*, judo, karate, *kendo*, or *kyudo*, this is a must read. Subjects include layout of the traditional *dojo*, accommodating visitors, wearing traditional uniforms, handling weapons, the *Shinto* shrine, contemplative meditation, ritual bowing, martial language, interacting with teachers and other students, and training fees. This book is a very easy read filled with colorful vignettes to entertain as well as educate.

Twigger, Robert. *Angry White Pyjamas: A Scrawny Oxford Poet Takes Lessons From the Tokyo Riot Police.* New York, NY: HarperCollins, 1997

Entertaining and clever; if you enjoy the title, you will like the book. An Oxford-educated intellectual moves to Japan and, with no martial arts experience, steps onto the floor of one of the toughest martial arts schools in the country, the *aikido* school for the Tokyo riot police. Readers will be entertained and enlightened by award-winning poet Robert Twigger's journey from corporate UK to a traditional Japanese *dojo*, his foibles, follies, failures and eventual successes in learning about Japanese culture and the martial art of *aikido*.

Vactor, Karen Levitz and Peterson, Susan Lynn, Ph.D. *Starting and Running Your Martial Arts School.* Boston, MA: Tuttle Publishing, 2002

See what it takes to run martial arts schools and gain a new appreciation of your instructor, who in many instances is the owner and teacher at the same time. You will also learn the earmarks of a quality-run school along with one that is not so well run, helping you in making your decision about where to train.

Wiley, Carol A. *Martial Arts Teachers on Teaching.* Berkeley, CA: Frog, Ltd., 1995

There are some real gems in here. The author interviews a good cross-section of martial arts instructors from a variety of different styles and portrays their collective wisdom in an entertaining and informative way. You get great insight into how instructors think, why they teach, how they teach, and what they have learned from doing it. Though suitable for students and teachers alike, it is more valuable to students in more ways than it is for teachers.

Suggested Web Sites

Minnesota State University – Mankato: What Makes a Good Teacher article (http://www.mnsu.edu/cetl/teachingresources/articles/goodteacher.html)

Another insightful essay on what it takes to be a good teacher by Richard M. Reis, Ph.D. The author asserts that exemplary instructors want to be good teachers, take risks, have a positive attitude, never have enough time, treat teaching like parenting, give students confidence, try to keep off-balance, try to motivate students, do not trust student evaluations, and listen to their students. Find out more by visiting this Web site.

System for Adult Basic Education Support: What Makes a Good Teacher article (http://www.sabes.org/resources/adventures/vol12/12hassett.htm)

The introduction to this excellent essay by Marie F. Hassett, Ph.D. includes the following quote, "Good teaching is not about technique. I have asked students around the country to describe their good teachers to me. Some of them describe people who lecture all the time, some of them describe people who do little other than facilitate group process, and others describe everything in between. But all of them describe people who have some sort of connective capacity, who connect themselves to their students, their students to each other, and everyone to the subject being studied." According to the author, good teachers have a sense of purpose, have expectations of success for all students, tolerate ambiguity, demonstrate a willingness to adapt and change to meet student needs, are comfortable with not knowing, reflect on their work, learn from a variety of models, and enjoy their work and their students. Find out more by visiting this Web site.

UNICEF Teachers Talking (http://www.unicef.org/teachers/teacher/teacher.htm)

This interactive Web site contains the contributed opinions of over 500 students from more than fifty countries, attempting to answer the question, "What makes a good teacher?" You can review these responses as well as submit your ideas on the topic.

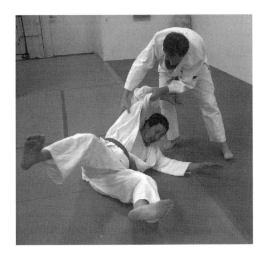

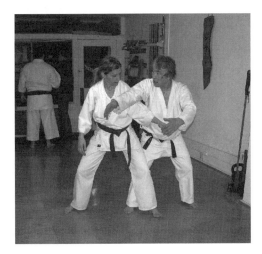

BEING ON THE OPPOSITE END OF A TECHNIQUE CAN HELP YOU "FEEL" WHAT THE MOTION IS SUPPOSED TO BE LIKE.

SOMETIMES THE EXPERIENCE CAN BRIDGE THE LANGUAGE BARRIER.

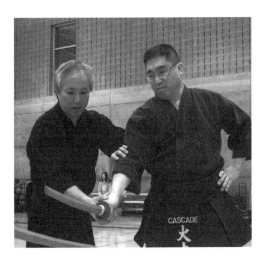

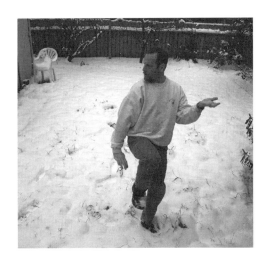

SOME PEOPLE LEARN KINESTHETICALLY BY FEELING THE MOTION. HERE, THE INSTRUCTOR GUIDES THE STUDENT THROUGH THE MOTION.

QUIET TIME WITH ONESELF REPEATING A TECHNIQUE IS ONE WAY TO INTEGRATE A MOVEMENT. TRAINING IN THE SNOW HELPS VALIDATE WHETHER OR NOT YOU'VE INTERNALIZED IMPORTANT FUNDAMENTALS OF STANCE, BALANCE, AND MOVEMENT.

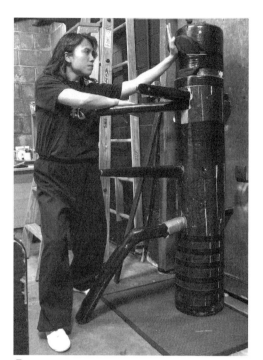

TRAINING TOOLS CAN AID IN SOLO PRACTICE.

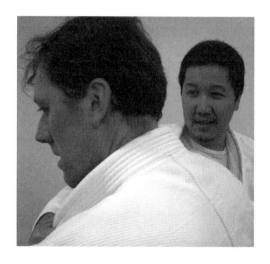

WORKING WITH PEOPLE AT THE SAME LEVEL OF TRAINING CAN BE BENEFICIAL IN THAT YOU ARE NOT OVERWHELMED BY THOSE OF ADVANCED SKILL AND FRUSTRATED BY THOSE OF LESSER SKILL.

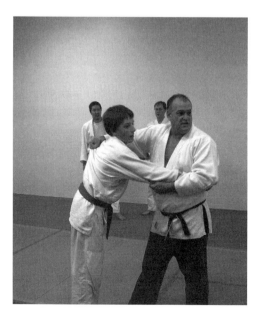

ASKING QUESTIONS CAN HELP IN UNDERSTANDING WHAT MUST BE DONE AND HOW IT SHOULD BE ACCOMPLISHED. WHILE IT IS THE TEACHER'S DUTY TO COMMUNICATE, IT IS YOUR DUTY TO LISTEN AND ASK THOUGHTFUL QUESTIONS.

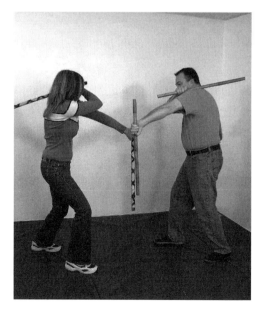

GOING OVER AND OVER A SERIES WILL IMPRINT THE TECHNIQUE INTO YOUR MIND.

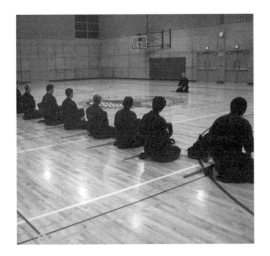

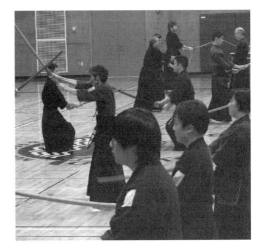

A FORMAL, STRUCTURED FORMAT IS BEST FOR SOME PEOPLE.

ALWAYS BE READY FOR THE NEXT REPETITION, STAYING FOCUSED. IF YOU ARE NOT WORKING, YOU SHOULD BE WATCHING AND LISTENING.

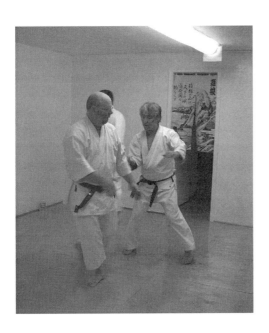

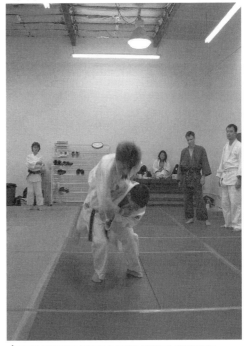

MIMICKING YOUR INSTRUCTOR'S MOVEMENTS CAN BE HELPFUL. IF YOU DON'T KNOW WHAT TO DO, COPY SOMEONE WHO DOES. YOU WILL FIGURE IT OUT SOON ENOUGH.

ALMOST ANYTHING CAN BE A GOOD LEARNING EXPERIENCE. WATCHING OTHERS DO IT RIGHT, OR EVEN WRONG, CAN BE A GREAT AID TO UNDERSTANDING.

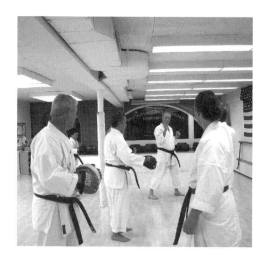

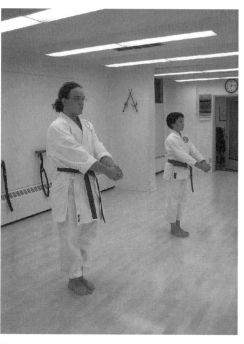

SMALL CLASSES CAN BE A REAL BOON. SOME NIGHTS, FOLKS JUST DON'T SHOW UP. TAKE ADVANTAGE OF THESE OPPORTUNITIES TO SPEND FOCUSED TIME AND RECEIVE PERSONALIZED ATTENTION FROM YOUR INSTRUCTOR.

VISUALIZE APPLICATIONS AS YOU PRACTICE YOUR FORMS. IT DOES NOT CHANGE THE PHYSICAL MOVEMENTS, YET FOCUSED INTENT MAKES ALL THE DIFFERENCE IN YOUR TECHNIQUE.

CHAPTER 3

Know How You Learn

"For the things we have to learn before we can do them, we learn by doing them."
– Aristotle [20]

Introduction (by Aaron Fields)

The biggest problem in the teaching of combatives or combative sport is instructor ignorance with regard to the "how-to's" of teaching. As the educational world has contin-ued to develop and quantify learning methods, strategies, and brain mechanics, the budo *world has continued to blindly mimic. Too often, instructors fail to realize that the acqui-sition of any given physical skill is more similar than different to the acquisition of any other given physical skill.*

From a learning perspective, karate and volleyball are not worlds apart. In addition, for some reason, many in the world of martial arts feel that budo *skills are outside the realm of sport. The truth is that the human body is finite and advancements in sport sci-ence have opened new and refined means and methods of skill acquisition. The context of skill sets may vary (combative sports, combative application, ball sports, swimming, track and field, etc.), but the methods used to achieve high levels of performance should remain constant.*

Alas, most budo *instructors woefully lack the requisite skills to uphold their end of the teaching bargain. The first step to being a good teacher is being a good learner. The second is the ability to say, "I do not know" in response to a student's question. The third is to be honest and secure with one's own skills and abilities and therefore not in compe-tition with one's students. A teacher must always be taking apart the pieces of their sub-ject to further their own understanding and subsequently be able to pass along their own findings. They must be striving to find the core concepts of their practice. In time, stu-dent-teacher relationships will turn into a relationship of training partners, as skill levels get closer between the two. In no arena is a teacher always a teacher. At some point, the student, more or less, reaches the teacher's level and the relationship must change.*

One of the major challenges faced by each student, therefore, is educating themselves on what their learning style is, in other words, how they best learn. Very often, people think of learning as a passive activity. A teacher presents you with information and makes sure you understand it. They present the information in various forms with various methodologies to ensure student comprehension. This approach is a fallacy. The act of learning itself is an acquired and practiced skill. A passive approach will reap mediocre results at best.

Students must walk a fine line in order to understand what they are doing, why, and where they should end up. At the same time, they must put in the sweat equity it takes to actually reach the application level of the skill outside of the context in which it was originally learned; that is, reaching the point that the skill is intuitively applied rather than following rote-memorized patterns. The great truth in budo *and all things is application. "Doubt me, and try me" is a superb way to maintain honesty and practicality in practice.*

I am not suggesting we throw the "traditional" methodology out entirely. Rather, I am suggesting that blind mimicry ends in low-level performance. We have a saying in the fire service, "We must respect the past, while embracing the future." I am sorry to say that many martial artists, for a wide variety of reasons, do not fully understand their particular discipline. They fail to realize that the key to success is a methodology of movement, rather than a collection of techniques. It is likely that this is how they themselves were taught.

Within the context of budo, *a student must learn the skill in question, while fitting it to their specific body type and physical ability. No two people should look identical. The form is not the "look" of the technique; rather, it is the biomechanical principle being applied. That is what instructors should actually be evaluating. Students should strive to not only intellectually understand a technique, but also to know the place where that specific technique falls within the greater context of the sport*

Stress is an important feature of performance-based skills, or more to the point, the ability to function while under stress. We can quantify the effects of stress upon a person concerning the performance of skills. Unfortunately, too often stress is not a teaching tool used to empower the student to higher function levels, but instead is a tool used to overwhelm and confuse the student. At all levels of training, stress must be introduced as a component. The balance for the teacher is ensuring that the student possesses the requisite skills and an avenue to succeed. All levels of training must have goals, be it a simple skill, a combination, or success in randori *(free-style sparring) and* shiai *(competition; literally "to try each other").*

Finally, the human mind strives for analogy. Hard work, discipline, and dedication will, in time, lead to the practice of what we call "do" (the way). Many people practice budo *for the emotional and spiritual components present in some disciplines. In truth, it makes no difference if we kick, throw, choke, punch, or drive nails into two-by-fours; if a person commits to their practice, whatever it is, they will eventually begin to develop the* do *nature. Nevertheless, the most basic nature of combat and combative sports is martial. It is the exertion of one's own will and ability against that of an unwilling opponent. In short, at some level, it is about combat and success, or it is not martial. Therefore, true tradition is one of success, not historical recreation. If your* budo *is sound in biomechanics and applied kinesiology, it will stand the test of time. Meanwhile, let everything else fall where it may—talk less and practice more.*

– *Aaron Fields* [21]

Know What Works for You

Let us assume for the moment that you have found an outstanding martial artist with whom to begin your training. Is that enough to guarantee your success in earning that coveted black belt? Absolutely not! Sadly, some of the best practitioners out there are also some of the worst instructors. They are not all bad, of course, but skill in martial endeavors is no guarantee of prowess in the educational realm. Because you are probably not going to devote your life to martial arts, traveling wherever you would need to go to find the best teacher in the world, you are probably going to make do with the best instructor you can find at a convenient location near you.

So, if you find out a few months down the road that your teacher is less than optimal, what can you do about it? Obviously one choice is to leave and find another one, but that is a rather extreme choice and will likely push back your goal of obtaining a black belt as you start over under a new program. Most of the time the best answer is to look to yourself, understand how you learn, and use that knowledge to make the most of the learning process.

First Lady Abigail Smith Adams (1744 – 1818) once said, "Learning is not attained by chance, it must be sought for with ardor and attended to with diligence." She was absolutely right. Different people learn in different ways and process information differently. Even when you place the most enthusiastic students in the capable hands of the very best instructors, learning does not happen all by itself. You cannot delegate everything to the instructor. Rather, you must own the process yourself. Some folks internalize new information faster than others do, not because they are smarter or harder working, but simply because they are more attuned with how they process information and use that knowledge to make the most out of each training session. Further, they take proactive steps to find an instructor who can fulfill their needs.

To add another layer of complexity, while teaching children can often be a lot like filling empty vessels with facts and ideas, teaching experienced adults is much more complex. Concepts can no longer simply be poured in; they must fit into what is already there. Learning must be meaningful and directly applicable to a student's goals. Rote memorization is not enough. Curricula must present opportunities to apply new skills in meaningful ways with appropriate feedback from fellow learners and instructors.

The first steps, as we have discussed previously, include knowing what you want to learn and finding an instructor who can fulfill your needs. That is just the beginning. You also need to know how you learn and use that new knowledge wisely. Practitioners who understand their own predilections and can take best advantage of new information they receive will make progress in the *dojo* much faster than those who do not. Predilections are tendencies to think favorably of something in particular, in this case a predisposition for a particular way of learning.

There are an abundance of learning style theories out there, many of which we will not cover here. We will focus instead on certain factors that, once understood, can be used directly to improve how you learn. Our goal is not to cover the vast range of academic theory and research, but rather to give you some important pointers that, once understood, you can use to develop a solid appreciation for how you process information in a manner that lets you take action to implement that new knowledge immediately.

To begin, it is important to know that we are all capable of learning in multiple ways. We also have hardwired preferences, however, that help us become most efficient when doing so in a particular way. Consequently, we all learn better in certain ways than we do in others. Learning theory can become a bit academic, certainly not the most exciting reading in the world, so we will try to be brief by focusing solely on the important elements.

"We now accept the fact that learning is a lifelong process of keeping abreast of change. And the most pressing task is to teach people how to learn."

– Peter Drucker [22]

Two learning style factors that are especially pertinent to mastering martial arts are modality predilections and personality type. Modalities are any of the various types of sensation such as taste or touch. Modality predilections, therefore, refer to the way in which you prefer to receive sensory information, such as auditory (sound), visual (sight), or kinesthetic (touch). Personality type refers to the way in which you process information most effectively in a learning environment. This is a very broad field, one that we will only touch upon here. The personality factors most relevant to learning style include two dichotomous scales, extraversion/introversion and sensing/intuition.

Let us begin by delving a little deeper into modality predilections so that you can develop a better understanding of how that works and how to use it in the *dojo*:

Understand Your Modality Predilections

Physiologically, the five human senses—sight, smell, touch, sound, and taste—are all pathways to the brain. Studies show that people retain more information as more modes (pathways to the brain) are accessed during a learning experience. Furthermore, the more times that material is reviewed and reinforced the more readily it is retained.

Active involvement in the learning process accesses more senses and facilitates better recall. In general, people remember:

- ~ 10% of what they read
- ~ 20% of what they hear
- ~ 30% of what they see
- ~ 40% of what they both see and hear
- ~ 70% of what they say
- ~ 90% of what they both say and do

That is a powerful argument for active participation in the learning process. So how does that work in the context of martial arts? Auditory, visual, and kinesthetic modes are commonly utilized in the *dojo*, as instructors discuss (auditory), demonstrate (visual), and encourage students to practice (kinesthetic) various techniques. Knowledge is most effectively communicated when all three of these learning modes are combined during instruction, yet individual students will be more receptive to certain modes than they are to others.

Two other learning modes really do not apply. While the olfactory sense (smell) can trigger a powerful emotional linkage to memory, it is challenging to incorporate the sense intentionally into most instructional situations beyond the culinary arts. Likewise, the sense of taste simply cannot be used all that much in the *dojo*. It may not help you learn martial arts, but you will undoubtedly discover the smell of sweat and the taste of blood at some point during your training though...

To be a bit more practical, many people have strong predilections along a single mode for learning, though most tend to have both a primary and a secondary pathway preference for processing new information. Any combination of auditory (sound), kinesthetic (touch), and visual (sight) processing preference is possible and will vary by individual. Visual/kinesthetic and auditory/kinesthetic are the most common combinations.

The more you know about how you learn the better you can use that information to facilitate knowledge retention. It is useful, therefore, to understand your modality preferences so we will discuss the primary ones in a bit more detail. Once you understand your preferred learning mode, you can formulate an action plan to augment your *dojo* training in ways that take the best advantage of it.

Auditory Learners

The temporal lobes of the brain process aural information. Auditory learners internalize information by hearing or repeating it. They tend to forget faces yet remember names and often prefer using the telephone for conversations. They spell phonetically, sounding out words they cannot remember how to spell. They prefer verbal instructions to written descriptions or demonstrations.

When learning complicated pattern drills, *kata* (forms), and other combination techniques, it is useful for them to hear a brief description of each movement just before doing it. Details like left/right, front/back, high/low, up/down, and so on are very important, since seeing a technique is insufficient in and of itself for these individuals. Japanese (or other foreign language) terminology tends to resonate well with these folks.

If you are an auditory learner, you will undoubtedly find yourself asking many questions, often repeating your instructor's answers aloud or silently to yourself to help lock them in. Unfortunately, you may have a propensity to want to talk with other students about new techniques rather than physically practicing them. A proper balance must be maintained to assure that you receive (and discuss when appropriate) reasonably detailed verbal information to facilitate learning while not disrupting classroom flow with idle chatter. It is often prudent to inform your instructor if you exhibit these tendencies to help him or her understand the behaviors that facilitate your learning. Take responsibility to monitor your actions to ensure that you are not overdoing it too.

Kinesthetic Learners

Proprioception* is the sense of the position of parts of your body relative to other neighboring parts of your body. Unlike the six exteroception† human senses of sight, taste, smell, touch, hearing, and balance that give us feedback about the outside world, proprioception is a sense that tells us about the status of our own body internally. It indicates whether the body is moving with required effort and helps us understand where the various parts of the body are located in relation to each other. Equilibrium and balance are good examples of this sense.

Kinesthesia,‡ on the other hand, is a key component in muscle memory and hand-eye coordination. While proprioception is innate, kinesthesia can be improved through training and feedback. The cerebellum and motor cortex (at the posterior of the frontal lobe of the brain) handle much of our physical environment. Kinesthetic learners often have the easiest time with martial arts, as they learn and improve physical skills primarily by doing.

---

* *Proprioception* is the unconscious perception of movement and spatial orientation arising from stimuli within the body itself.
† *Exteroception* is sensitivity to stimuli originating outside of the body.
‡ *Kinesthesia* is muscle sense, the ability to feel movements of the limbs and body.

They tend to remember physical experiences and like engaging in conversations while doing other activities rather than talking alone. They tend to write words they cannot remember how to spell down on paper to see if the result feels right. Until these folks have practiced a new technique several times they tend to find little value in understanding the concept behind it or the subtleties inherent therein. They usually find great benefit from partner exercises such as flow drills, sparring, and pre-arranged sequences such as *kiso kumite* (pre-sequenced sparring).

It is particularly important for kinesthetic learners to get the "feel" of doing movements properly, internalizing solid body mechanics. Misalignment by a mere fraction of an inch may mean the difference between brutally effective and hopelessly ineffectual technique. Such minor nuances can often be felt even when they cannot readily be seen, a truism that folks with other modality predilections may not appreciate as much as kinesthetic learners.

If you are a kinesthetic learner, you will often have trouble staying still, a trait that could be interpreted as not paying attention even when you are completely focused on the instructor. You may also have a propensity to copy your *sensei's* demonstrations in an attempt to internalize new lessons, another habit that could be misinterpreted as a lack of respect. Fidgeting amongst these individuals is normal, yet you need to pay attention to what you are doing so that it does not become disruptive to other students. It is often prudent to inform your instructor if you exhibit these tendencies to help him or her understand the behaviors that facilitate your learning. Take responsibility to monitor your actions to ensure that you are not overdoing it too.

Visual Learners

The occipital lobes at the back of the brain manage visual sensation while both the occipital and parietal lobes manage spatial orientation. Visual learners tend to forget names yet remember faces. They prefer conversing with others face-to-face and generally dislike using the telephone, though they are often comfortable with e-mail and instant message communication. They tend to visualize words they cannot remember in their minds to figure out the proper spelling. For many, reading an interesting book is very similar to watching a movie. They see moving images rather than individual words.

In order to understand new information, visual learners must clearly see demonstrations. They tend to derive much extra benefit from supplemental reading materials, Web sites, videotaped training sessions, and/or DVDs. Many instructors intersperse senior and junior students during moving drills or *kata* such that students can see and emulate technique from whichever direction they are facing. Furthermore, many *dojo* have mirrored walls because they facilitate improvement for all students, especially visual learners.

If you are a visual learner, you will probably find yourself moving around a lot to be sure that you can see what is going on, particularly during demonstrations. When learning complicated pattern drills, *kata*, and other combination techniques, you may find yourself sketching the patterns you have just seen in your mind rather than focusing on what is going on at the time. Creating a training journal and taking many notes will help lock things into your mind as well as create a resource for future reference, but etiquette generally demands that you do so after class. It is often prudent to inform your instructor if you exhibit these tendencies to help him or her understand the behaviors that facilitate your learning.

A Practical Example—Modality Predilections and Kata Instruction

A *kata* or "form" is a logical sequence of movements containing practical offensive and defensive techniques that are performed in a particular order. The ancient masters embedded their unique fighting systems within their *kata*. These forms became fault-tolerant methods* for ensuring such techniques could be taught and understood consistently over the generations. While the basic movements of *kata* are widely known, advanced practical applications and sophisticated techniques frequently remain hidden from the casual observer. To the uninitiated, those who do not understand its practical applications, *kata* looks a whole lot like dancing.

The uniform *gi* that *karateka*, *judoka*, and many other types of martial artists wear is patterned after underclothes worn during the feudal period in Japan. When a *samurai* left his home, he wore outer layers that covered these garments. A *hakama* (divided skirt) was worn over the pants (and still is in some arts such as *iaido* or *aikido*). A *haori* (coat) or *kimono* (jacket) was worn over the shirt.

Kata does look like dancing and your *gi* was derived from underclothes. If you think these things through to their logical conclusion, you can make the following declaration: "If you do not understand the applications, *kata* is nothing more than dancing around in your underwear." That would be somewhat embarrassing, wouldn't it?

So how do you learn a *kata* and discover how to use it effectively? By learning a *kata* we mean that the practitioner knows the pattern, understands the movements, and can perform the applications with a reasonable degree of proficiency. This can be a very challenging process, particularly for newer practitioners who have little martial arts experience upon which to draw.

Many instructors utilize a five-step approach to help ensure that their students have the best shot at picking things up systematically yet expeditiously:

Step 1 (Visual): Sensei begins by performing the *kata* in front of the class, repeating it a second time slowly so that everyone can closely observe the pattern and pick up some of the movements.

---

* Fault-tolerant systems are designed to operate successfully regardless of whether or not an error or defect occurs, as opposed to those that can be broken by a single point of failure or even systems that rarely have problems at all. They are highly robust.

Step 2 (Visual/Kinesthetic): Sensei leads the group through the form until everyone has the basic pattern down or at least has walked through it a couple of times.

Step 3 (Auditory/Visual): Sensei talks a bit about the *kata bunkai* (applications), demonstrating something for each major movement in the first section (a section is a logical chunk, say four or five moves or wherever there is a clear change in the pattern, direction, or application set).

Step 4 (Kinesthetic): Students perform at least one of the applications with a training partner, getting a feel for how the *kata* might be utilized in a real fight.

Step 5 (Visual/Kinesthetic): Sensei leads the class through a portion of the *kata* again, changing nothing but asking students to keep the application(s) firmly in mind as they perform the movements.

This five-step process is repeated over and over again, not just in any given class session but over weeks, months, or even years of practice. Over time, the class will work through every section of the form until they have seen the *kata* in its entirety, performed it themselves, tried out some tandem applications with a partner, and completed the *kata* solo once again. This approach touches on all three modalities and almost always provides solid results.

By the time you are finished, you not only know the movements but also have a reasonably good idea about what they might mean in practical application and be able to apply them in a real-life fight. Pretty cool, yes?

> *"Only the curious will learn and only the resolute overcome the obstacles to learning. The quest quotient has always excited me more than the intelligence quotient."*
>
> – Eugene S. Wilson [23]

Know Your Personality Type

Understanding your personality type, at least to the extent that you appreciate how you learn best, is very useful in expediting the learning process. Standardized tests such as the Myers-Briggs Type Indicator (MBTI)® or the Insights Personality Profile® can provide terrific insight into all aspects of your character, though you really do not necessarily need that level of depth to excel in the *dojo*. Two character aspects are particularly helpful in understanding learning-style preferences in an actionable way:

Extraversion or Introversion. The extraversion–introversion dichotomy indicates whether a person prefers to direct his or her attention toward the external world of people and things or toward the inner world of concepts and ideas. Some learning models call these personalities Social (extraverts) or Solitary (introverts).

Sensing or Intuitive. The sensing-intuitive dichotomy indicates whether a person prefers perceiving the world through directly observing the surrounding tangible reality or through impressions and imagined possibilities.

Knowing your predilections in these two areas can not only help you find a suitable instructor, but it can also enable you to better articulate your learning needs with your *sensei*. We will discuss them in more detail:

Extraverts

The frontal and temporal lobes of the brain handle much of our social and solitary activities, though the limbic system plays a large role, too, particularly when it comes to emotions, moods, and aggression. If you are extraverted, you tend to draw energy from outside yourself, thriving on interactions with people, activities, and things. You feel eager to spend time with others and may become bored when isolated or alone. As a student, you are likely to be action oriented, learning well in a "do–think–do" environment. You actively participate, ask questions, and enjoy becoming involved in the learning process. You probably enjoy speaking much more than writing.

An inherent strength of this personality type is that instructors immediately know when you need additional understanding or are confused about a lesson or instruction. The downside is that you can have a tendency to monopolize a teacher's attention by asking a disproportional number of questions or engaging in prolonged discussions. If you find yourself in this situation it is critical that you are respectful of everyone else's needs as well as your own, especially those less gregarious than yourself.

Introverts

If you are an introvert, you tend to draw energy from the internal world of ideas, emotions, and impressions. You are eager to spend time alone and may become anxious when meeting with others, typically needing time to yourself to unwind and decompress afterward. As a student, you are likely to be reflection oriented, learning best in a "think–do–think" environment. Even when you are thoroughly engaged in the learning process, those who do not know you well may believe that you are distant, distracted, or a step behind the other students. You probably enjoy writing much more than public speaking.

Introverts prefer to learn complex subjects in an integrated and connected format, learning the big picture through logical chunks of interconnected facts. These individuals generally prefer to think and reflect on coursework, typically excelling at written assignments while being challenged by interactive discussions. They tend to excel at independent study.

Introverts are often uncomfortable asking for help and must sometimes be actively drawn into conversations. Exemplary instructors are good at maintaining enthusiasm and participation from extraverts while actively engaging reticent introverts whose needs might easily be overlooked when they do not speak up. If your instructor does not actively engage your input it is imperative that you push yourself to ask about those things that you need to understand, even if it means stepping outside your comfort zone.

Sensing

Sensing involves observing and gathering data through the senses. If you are a sensing personality type, you are likely to have good motor skill development but may be challenged by logical abstraction and language skills. Learning patterns naturally gravitate toward the practical and the immediate. Your learning styles are is characterized by a preference for direct, concrete experiences, moderate to high degrees of structure, linear or sequential learning, and a need to know why before doing something. Your learning goals tend to revolve around immediate needs. You may be less independent in thought and judgment and may require frequent coaching or direct instruction to achieve them.

Sensing students thrive in an "application–theory–application" approach to learning. They typically appreciate an early understanding of instructional objectives so that they can prepare for what they must know in advance. They prefer to work with "givens" in the real world rather than with abstract theories or possibilities.

If you fall into this category, you will benefit from a syllabus. Many instructors provide a list of advancement criteria, a student handbook, a course outline, or other useful data that will help you map your learning requirements and take the best advantage of your training. If this type of information is not provided in the first couple of months, it may be useful to ask your instructor about his or her expectations to help you set learning objectives.

Intuitive

Intuitive personalities are generally "big picture" types who prefer to focus on imaginative possibilities rather than on concrete realities. Intuition involves indirect perception by way of the subconscious through memories and speculations. If you are an intuitive personality type, you are likely to have solid language and logical abstraction skills but may be challenged by tasks requiring complex motor skills.

This personality type likes to move from theory to practice, typically disliking the highly structured learning environments that work well for sensing individuals. If this is you, you can readily accommodate ambiguity, usually demonstrating a high degree of autonomy in your learning, and valuing knowledge for its own sake. Your learning goals tend to be long term and far-focused. You are more likely to be independent and require less frequent coaching or direct instruction to achieve them.

Intuitive students like generalized concept maps and learn well using a "theory–application–theory" approach. These individuals are comfortable working with hunches and other unexplainable ways of knowing, looking for patterns, meanings, and future possibilities. While they excel at creative coursework, they are often bored by, and resistant to, routine assignments. Curricular variety is essential to maintaining their interest.

If you are intuitive, you may derive great benefit from studying the strategy, history, and traditions of your art so that you can readily place the tactics and techniques within a greater context. Your instructor should be able to provide a list of resources that can help.

While it is impossible to accommodate both the sensing and intuition simultaneously, exemplary instructors are good at striking a balance between the two. For example, intuitive practitioners can be afforded "open *dojo*" time to work on their advancement requirements while individuals with a sensing preference can simultaneously perform structured drills (e.g., *kata*) that cover what they need to know. If your instructor does not do a good job of accommodating your preferences on his or her own, it may be appropriate to suggest ways for him or her to do so tactfully.

A Quick n' Dirty Learning Style Analysis

There are several academically proven ways of determining your learning style and understanding how to use and apply that knowledge. The following table (page 69) can help you identify your predilections more quickly, easily, and inexpensively than taking a standardized test. Read the various descriptions and see where the majority of your answers lie. The answers with the best fit should denote your style preferences. You should be able to determine your modality predilection (auditory, kinesthetic, or visual) as well as your personality type (extravert or introvert, sensing or intuitive).

> *"There are no secrets to success. It is the result of preparation, hard work, and learning from failure."*
>
> – Colin Powell [24]

Learning Outcomes (Domains)

Let us switch gears a bit now. Learning style and personality predilections aside, how do you know that you have actually learned anything from your instructor? How can you facilitate your ability to absorb new skills and information?

To answer these important questions, educational psychologists have analyzed learning behaviors for more than fifty years. They discovered that there are three interrelated outcomes, or learning domains, that help students and teachers understand how effectively knowledge has been absorbed and retained. You can use this

FIGURE 3.1: LEARNING STYLES TABLE

Learning Style Preferences	When talking with another person or presenting to a group at work you:	Meeting someone you like, but don't know well, after a long absence, you:	When asked to build something, put something together, or do a project you:
Auditory	Describe thoughts and sounds. Enjoy listening yet are often impatient to talk. Often prefer using the phone where appropriate.	Tend to forget faces but remember names and what you talked about. You often recognize people by the sound of their voice.	Ask someone to explain what or how to do it or describe expected results. Prefer verbal instructions to written documentation.
Kinesthetic	Gesture frequently and expressively. Fidget a lot. Prefer talking while walking or doing something active when possible.	Tend to remember what you did the last time you were together more than what you talked about or where you went.	Prefer to jump right in and get started, ignoring written instructions to figure it out as you go along whenever possible.
Visual	Use vivid, pictorial descriptions when talking. Dislike listening for too long. Prefer face-to-face interaction when possible; comfortable with e-mail and instant messages too.	Tend to forget names but remember faces and places where you met or locations you visited together. Note physical characteristics and attire.	Like to see others demonstrate if possible. Read available instructions carefully, seeking charts, diagrams, or pictures. Visualize how things go together before assembly.
Extravert	Look forward to conversations, frequently leaving energetic. Prefer group settings. Tend to dominate conversations when able to do so.	Look forward to renewing the acquaintance. Easily able to pick up where you left off before. Tend to maintain a hectic social calendar.	Like to work with a group whenever possible. Prefer to "do" first, often thinking out loud or brainstorming with others rather than formally planning.
Introvert	Have to psych your self up before conversations, frequently feeling drained afterward. Prefer one-on-one to large groups. Tend to listen more than talk.	Unlikely to initiate a conversation. Tend to have few close friends but are able to form very deep, lasting bonds after long association.	Like working independently to finish projects. Prefer to think about everything that is necessary and make comprehensive plans before getting started.
Sensing	Discuss facts, logic, and experiences. Prefer an agenda and structure in work settings. Like to know exactly what is expected ahead of time.	Interested in knowing where the person has traveled, what he/she has done since the last time you met, and sharing interesting experiences.	Determine the sequence and then follow a logical, step-by-step process to completion. Prefer to know "how" before "why" becomes meaningful.
Intuitive	Discuss theories, possibilities and creative concepts. High tolerance for ambiguity and informality in work settings. Work autonomously.	Interested in knowing what the person will be doing; relationships, future plans, and ideas. Sensitive to body language during conversations.	Imagine possibilities and results before delving into and accomplishing the project. Prefer to know "why" before "how" becomes meaningful.

information not only to track progress, but also to ensure that prerequisite experience is obtained so that missing fundamentals will not inhibit your development.

The three learning domains are cognitive (knowledge/thinking), affective (attitude/feeling), and psychomotor (skills/doing). There is a Chinese proverb that states, "Tell me and I'll forget; show me and I may remember; involve me and I'll understand." As this axiom signifies, learning within any one domain is often interdependent with another domain or even with all three. For example, complex psychomotor skills utilized by martial artists require cognitive knowledge of the underlying techniques, overarching strategic concepts, and application processes to be most effective.

Within each domain is a hierarchy that categorizes the degree to which you have learned. As you progress from one level to the next you acquire a deeper and fuller understanding of the information, mastering increasingly complex aspects. We will briefly cover the cognitive and affective domains and then delve a little more deeply into the psychomotor domain as it is frequently the most influential for learning in the *dojo*.

Cognitive Learning (from Benjamin Bloom's[25] Taxonomy*)

The cognitive domain focuses on intellectual skills and abilities, didactic information such as knowledge and facts. Cognitive learning behaviors are characterized by both observable and unobservable skills such as comprehending information, organizing ideas, and evaluating information and actions. The cognitive domain is hierarchical with six levels of mastery, each becoming increasingly more sophisticated. Ranked from low to high, these levels are:

Knowledge. This level is characterized by memorization and recall of new materials. It is the ability to remember or recognize information, ideas, facts, or principles in the approximate form in which they were initially learned.

Comprehension. This level is characterized by interpretation and understanding of the meaning behind the information as well as by the ability to make simple predictions based on the materials where applicable. It is the ability to translate, comprehend, or interpret information based on prior learning.

Application. This level is characterized by the ability to use the materials in new situations, particularly in real-life outside of the classroom. It is the ability to select, transfer, and use data or principles to solve a problem or complete a task independently or with a minimum of guidance

Analysis. This level is characterized by the ability to break the material into its component parts, analyze their individual meaning, and understand their importance within the larger structure of the overall materials.

Synthesis. This level is characterized by the ability to combine the pieces of information into a new or different whole, grouping materials to yield new structures or patterns.

Evaluation. This level is characterized by the ability to judge the value of the material or its suitability for any given purpose as well as to make thoughtful decisions about the information originally presented, adapting it as necessary.

---

* A taxonomy is simply a system of classification, a logical grouping of categories.

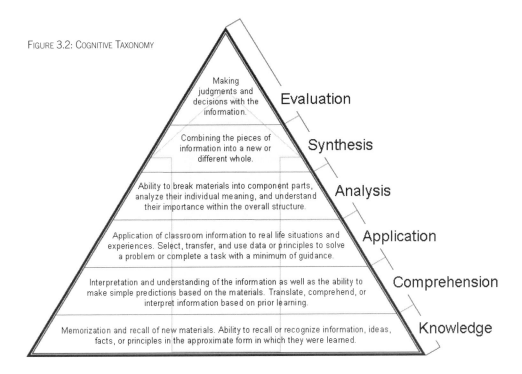

FIGURE 3.2: COGNITIVE TAXONOMY

Making judgments and decisions with the information. **Evaluation**

Combining the pieces of information into a new or different whole. **Synthesis**

Ability to break materials into component parts, analyze their individual meaning, and understand their importance within the overall structure. **Analysis**

Application of classroom information to real life situations and experiences. Select, transfer, and use data or principles to solve a problem or complete a task with a minimum of guidance. **Application**

Interpretation and understanding of the information as well as the ability to make simple predictions based on the materials. Translate, comprehend, or interpret information based on prior learning. **Comprehension**

Memorization and recall of new materials. Ability to recall or recognize information, ideas, facts, or principles in the approximate form in which they were learned. **Knowledge**

Affective Learning (from Bloom's Taxonomy)

The affective learning domain addresses your beliefs, behaviors, and emotions toward a learning experience. A person's interest, attention, awareness, and values are all demonstrated by affective behaviors, though they can be hard to measure objectively. Consequently, this domain is not necessarily as strictly hierarchical as the cognitive domain. Nevertheless, there are five levels of mastery within the affective domain, each becoming increasingly more sophisticated. Ranked from low to high, these levels are:

Receiving. This level is characterized by a willingness to pay attention to instruction and/or an understanding of the importance of the information one is about to receive. This includes being aware of or attending to something in the environment.

Responding. This level is characterized by a willingness to participate actively in the learning process and to derive satisfaction from doing so. This includes exhibiting new behaviors as a result of the learning experience.

Valuing. This level is characterized by placing value on a learning activity or perceiving that the newly learned behavior has worth. This includes showing definitive involvement or commitment.

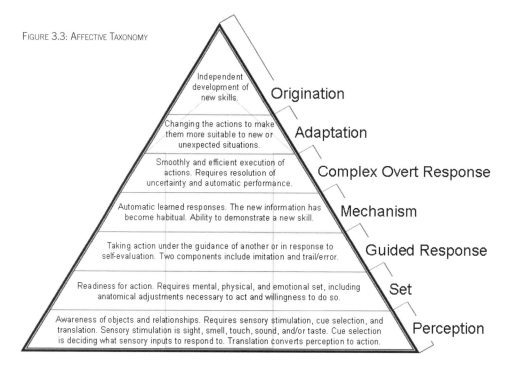

FIGURE 3.3: AFFECTIVE TAXONOMY

Independent development of new skills. — Origination

Changing the actions to make them more suitable to new or unexpected situations. — Adaptation

Smoothly and efficient execution of actions. Requires resolution of uncertainty and automatic performance. — Complex Overt Response

Automatic learned responses. The new information has become habitual. Ability to demonstrate a new skill. — Mechanism

Taking action under the guidance of another or in response to self-evaluation. Two components include imitation and trail/error. — Guided Response

Readiness for action. Requires mental, physical, and emotional set, including anatomical adjustments necessary to act and willingness to do so. — Set

Awareness of objects and relationships. Requires sensory stimulation, cue selection, and translation. Sensory stimulation is sight, smell, touch, sound, and/or taste. Cue selection is deciding what sensory inputs to respond to. Translation converts perception to action. — Perception

Organization. This level is characterized by bringing together different values and resolving conflicts between them. It is the integration of different beliefs, building consistent values, and reconciling differences.

Characterization. This level is characterized by the development of your own value system in a way that it governs your behavior. It is also the maintenance of this system of values over a long period of time in a manner that is consistent, pervasive, and predictable.

Psychomotor Learning (from Elizabeth Simpson's[26] Taxonomy)

The most important domain for martial arts instruction is, of course, the psychomotor taxonomy. This domain is used whenever we learn physical skills, though the cognitive and affective domains still play an indispensable role in all types of learning. Gross motor skills involve large muscles (e.g., walking, running, jumping, swimming) while fine motor skills involve hand-eye coordination (e.g., writing, carving, playing videogames, or hitting a baseball). There are seven levels of mastery in the psychomotor domain, each becoming increasingly more sophisticated. Ranked from low to high, these levels are:

Perception. This level is characterized by an awareness of objects and relationships. It begins with sensory stimulation, sight, smell, touch, sound, and/or taste.

The next step is cue selection, deciding to what sensory inputs you must respond to in order to satisfy a particular requirement or objective. Finally, it ends with translation, relating perception to action by performing a motor act. A good example of this might be a timing drill where you learn how to sense a partner's punch or kick before it is too late to react.

Set. This level is characterized by preparatory adjustment and readiness for action. This state of readiness has three aspects: mental, physical, and emotional. You must be mentally ready to act, physically able to proceed, and emotionally inclined to do so, particularly when a fear of pain or other repercussions may inhibit your willingness to act. A good example of this might be a line sparring drill where you are prepared to block or otherwise respond to a pre-defined technique such as a right-hand punch to your head.

Guided Response. This level is characterized by execution of an overt action under the guidance of another person such as your instructor or in response to self-evaluation when following another's guidelines. There are two components of a guided response: imitation and trial and error. Imitation is the execution of actions mimicking another's performance while trial and error is the testing of a set of various responses to ascertain which are the most effective for any given situation. A good example of this might be a flow drill, form, or *kata* where you imitate a sequence of techniques modeled by your instructor.

Mechanism. This level is characterized by the development of automatic learned responses. The new information has become habitual. A good example of this might be the ability to utilize a wide variety of *kata* techniques in a tandem exercise such as *kiso kumite* (prearranged sparring).

Complex Overt Response. This level is characterized by execution of a complex set of actions smoothly and efficiently. There are two components of complex overt response, resolution of uncertainty and automatic performance. Resolution of uncertainty means that the act can be performed without hesitation. In other words, you can do it without thinking about it. Automatic performance means that the act can be performed with finely coordinated muscle skill and a great deal of control. A good example of this might be executing a variety of effective applications or combinations of techniques during *randori* (free sparring) or a tournament match.

Adaptation. This level is characterized by changing the execution of actions to make them more suitable to new or unexpected situations. A good example might be the ability to use *kata* techniques to survive a real-life street fight. Because there are no rules or safety measures and you are operating under the influence of adrenaline, the dynamics of street fighting are orders of magnitude beyond sparring or tournament competition.

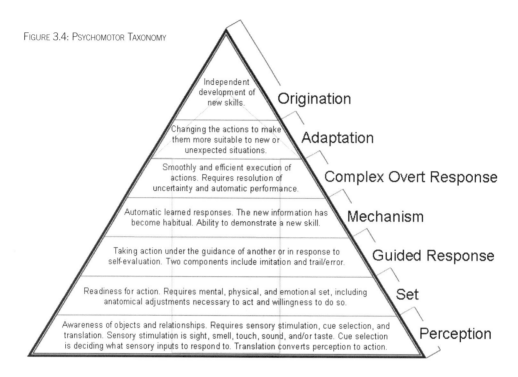

FIGURE 3.4: PSYCHOMOTOR TAXONOMY

Independent development of new skills. **Origination**

Changing the actions to make them more suitable to new or unexpected situations. **Adaptation**

Smoothly and efficient execution of actions. Requires resolution of uncertainty and automatic performance. **Complex Overt Response**

Automatic learned responses. The new information has become habitual. Ability to demonstrate a new skill. **Mechanism**

Taking action under the guidance of another or in response to self-evaluation. Two components include imitation and trail/error. **Guided Response**

Readiness for action. Requires mental, physical, and emotional set, including anatomical adjustments necessary to act and willingness to do so. **Set**

Awareness of objects and relationships. Requires sensory stimulation, cue selection, and translation. Sensory stimulation is sight, smell, touch, sound, and/or taste. Cue selection is deciding what sensory inputs to respond to. Translation converts perception to action. **Perception**

Origination. This level is characterized by independent development of new skills. This includes creating new ways of manipulating the materials you have learned, implementing your knowledge, skill, and ability in original and creative ways. A good example might be creating your own *kata* based upon things you have learned in actual combat.

Visualization

Mental rehearsal, especially involving imagery, appears to facilitate performance in sports and other physical activities. This is most likely because it bolsters memory processing related to physical tasks while reinforcing your motivation for participating in an activity. Mental rehearsal can also be called mental imagery or, more commonly, visualization.

Visualization is defined as an occurrence that resembles a perceptual experience, but which happens in the absence of the appropriate stimuli for the relevant perception. In everyday English, we are pretending to do something, imagining what it would be like, and visualizing our success. This mental imagery is not exclusively defined to the visual learning mode, though it is most prevalent in that domain as it is harder to reproduce kinesthetic, tactile, olfactory, or auditory experiences in your mind.

Football, baseball, basketball, and soccer coaches emphasize to athletes that success is 90% mental, particularly at professional levels where fundamental skills can be performed without conscious thought and minor mental errors can change the momentum or outcome of a game. The same idea applies to participation in martial sports such as judo, *jujitsu*, or *taekwondo* tournaments as well as to street encounters and self-defense situations.

Done properly, visualization can improve athletic performance, enhance motivation, reduce anxiety, instill confidence, and potentially even ameliorate mental trauma associated with injury, speeding recovery. It can help you prepare for a performance, think through potential problems, and formulate associated plans and mitigation strategies. Visualization can be performed on or off the *dojo* floor before, during, or after a competition or practice session, and can last from a few seconds to as long as fifteen or twenty minutes.

Imagining yourself performing any physical skill perfectly can create or reinforce neural patterns in your brain in the same manner as if you had actually performed the physical action. Consequently, martial artists can help train their minds in ways that teach their muscles to perform techniques more effectively. There are several theories as to why this works. One popular model is the Visuo-Motor Behavior Rehearsal (VMBR) approach. This method has been used successfully in a number of sports including racquetball, tennis, cross country running, track and field, gymnastics, diving, basketball, and karate.

An empirical study involving karate demonstrated that practitioners using VMBR over a 16-week period showed significant performance improvements among participants in all aspects of their karate over those who did not take advantage of the technique.* Furthermore, they had lower anxiety levels even though they initially performed poorly in sparring and *kata* drills. VMBR involves three phases:

- Relaxing, establishing a mental state conducive to mental imagery.
- Visualizing, using mental rehearsal to imagine yourself performing flawlessly.
- Performing, applying the physical skill under realistic conditions.

Research concludes that the combination of relaxation and visualization together are more effective for martial artists than either by itself. *Karateka* who routinely practice VMBR ten minutes a day do better than those who only practice it immediately before a competition. There is no difference between instructor-guided imagery and self-guided visualization, though internal imagery works better than

* Weinberg, R. S., Seabourne, T. G., & Jackson, A. Effects of Visuo-Motor Behavior Rehearsal, Relaxation, and Imagery on Karate Performance. *Journal of Sport Psychology*, 228-238, 1981.

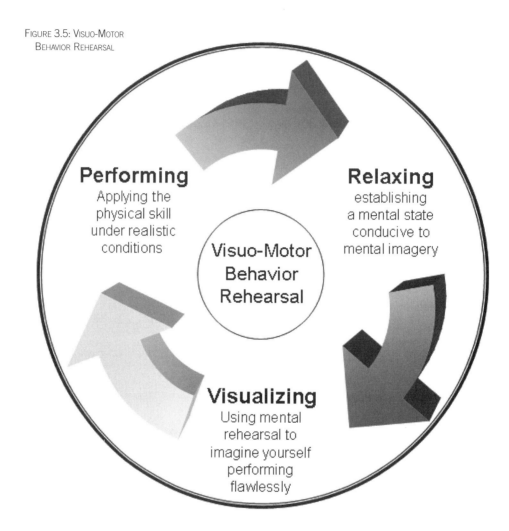

Performing
Applying the
physical skill
under realistic
conditions

Relaxing
establishing
a mental state
conducive to
mental imagery

Visuo-Motor
Behavior
Rehearsal

Visualizing
Using mental
rehearsal to
imagine yourself
performing
flawlessly

external. Internal imagery is visualization from the perspective of the practitioner whereas external imagery is from the perspective of another person watching the practitioner perform. In other words, picture yourself accomplishing the feat from your mind's eye, rather than viewing yourself from the perspective of someone in the audience watching you perform.

You can facilitate relaxation through focused diaphragmatic breathing. Inhale through your nose and exhale through your mouth using expansion and contraction of your stomach to move air deeply into your lungs. Consciously relax your muscles and think about nothing beyond your breathing. Once a state of relaxation has been obtained (which can take place as quickly as a few full breaths once you become good at it), you are ready to begin visualization techniques. After your mental rehearsal, you are physically ready to perform.

By repeating this process cyclically, visualization reinforces physical performance that in turn, enhances your ability to visualize more effectively. It is a benevolent cycle. Real-time feedback between the imagery component and the actual performance helps assure that both skills increase in parallel, allowing you to fine-tune both processes simultaneously. On the downside, visualization can actually hurt your performance if your understanding of the fundamental strategies and tactics of your art is deficient or incomplete. It is best, therefore, to focus on the things you know reasonably well.

Only visualize perfection, focusing on form first, then speed and power. If necessary, elongate the component movements as you think about them, breaking things down into small enough pieces to imagine doing each one flawlessly, even if it takes significantly longer than a real-life performance. It is okay to imagine doing things in slow motion until you feel comfortable that you have captured all the important nuances properly. Once you are confident that you have covered everything important, increase the speed at which you see yourself performing in your mind.

Improving Your Visualization Skills

Visual learners tend to be really good at forming mental images. Auditory and kinesthetic learners, on the other hand, often need help with this skill. However, with sufficient practice, they can sometimes generate more holistic mental imagery than visual learners. Here are some tips for those of you who have difficulty with visualization:

- Visualization is most effective when it is as realistic and holistic as possible. Imagine what all your senses would perceive, not just your eyes. Think about all the emotions that you might feel when you actually achieve in real life whatever success you have imagined.

- Watch a live performance or DVD reenactment by someone who is good at what you want to learn before visualizing yourself performing the task. If you cannot find the exact same techniques, anything similar will help. Worst case, watch a Bruce Lee, Jet Li, Chuck Norris, or Jackie Chan film (see Appendix C for reviews of some martial arts movies we like). It is easier to imagine visual images if you have recently seen something similar that you can adapt.

- Think in pictures rather than words, imagining how you might do what you have seen in another's performance. The more movie-like the mental images the better. Once the images are formed, try to flesh them out with sound, smell, touch, and other sensations.

Advice for New Students

by Martina Sprague [27]

One of the best things you can do in addition to physical training is educating yourself on combat scenarios and the elements that lead to fighting. The beauty with visualization exercises is that you can stop an attack at any point and take whatever time you need to consider a course of action. Visualization exercises help you discover possibilities that you may ordinarily not think of. Is the attacker reaching out to grab you? Is he reaching out to strike you? Does he have a weapon? What is his other hand doing? What are his height and build? What is his physical condition? What does he smell like?

Do not be afraid to visualize yourself losing the fight. It is often argued that you should always visualize yourself the winner to avoid negative learning. I disagree. You gain insight also by visualizing the fight the way it could go rather than the way it should go. Visualizing the possibility of failure allows you to ponder dangerous situations and be wary of them. Visualizing defeat, or at least exploring it, prepares you to deal with an encounter that goes sour.

Vivid visualization creates a feeling of familiarity and prepares you for doing the exercises in real life. You will also create some muscle memory, since your muscles respond to visual imagery. I recommend the use of visualization exercises prior to and after training rather than during training; too much thinking tends to interfere with physical performance. Note that not everybody has equal ability with respect to visualization. Some people are better auditory or kinesthetic learners than visual learners.

- Picture yourself accomplishing the feat from your mind's eye, rather than viewing yourself from the perspective of someone watching you perform from an audience. This will help you align your mental imagery more closely with real life.

Until you are good at visualization, find a quiet, relaxed environment to avoid distractions while you concentrate. Breathe diaphragmatically. Keep focused yet relaxed attention while visualizing.

The Value of Sleep for Learning

Dojo training is normally a holistic experience. You receive visual input from watching instructors and classmates perform techniques, auditory data from listening to explanations, and kinesthetic feedback from practicing the movements yourself. In general, the more often you practice under the guidance of a competent instructor, the better you are able to perform on your own, particularly when you add visualization to the equation. The process of internalizing new information is, however, a bit more complicated than that.

As we have seen from Bloom's and Simpson's taxonomies, learning occurs most effectively when students not only participate in some activity, but also reflect upon the exercise, use analytical skills to derive some useful insight from the experience, and then incorporate their new understanding into their daily lives. This means that the learning process is highly experiential. It also means that it takes a fair amount of time to work through the process and transfer knowledge fully.

> *"By learning, you will teach; by teaching, you will learn."*
>
> – Latin Proverb

Research suggests that learning is most effective when complex information is broken into smaller, logical portions that are then distributed over a period of time. Through consistent, repeated rehearsal, this new information is transformed to long-term memory where it is permanently stored and generally retrievable. Repetition is, therefore, generally good. The irony, however, is that after a certain amount of time dedicated to a particular task, further practice may actually inhibit the ability to pick up a new motor skill.

So, if practice does not always make perfect, what does? A good night's sleep after your practice is actually the key to perfection, according to many researchers. Learning does not occur solely during a training session, it continues for a period of time, even after you quit for the day. The brain continues to learn after practicing stops analyzing, synthesizing, and evaluating knowledge. This process works best during sleep. Consequently, if you want to make the most of your training, you will need to get a full night of uninterrupted sleep afterward.

Student Perspective (by John McNally)

Learning karate has provided me with some unexpected personal challenges. Knowing my personality traits and learning style—physical and mental—has allowed me to make consistent progress in my karate skills.

The goal of a martial artist, at least my goal, is to develop "unconscious competence" that allows me to flow and act without deep thinking. To get to the higher natural state requires passing through a stage of "conscious competence" where I must think about what I am doing before I do it, and then physically control my body to do what I want.

I rely on repetition so that muscle memory kicks in. I know I am getting there, when I say, "Just get me started." Remind me of the first move, and my body goes into automatic mode and takes over the rest of the form, performing the kata *without conscious thought.*

My learning is reinforced with visualization between training sessions, mentally walking through the kata. I feel valuable reinforcement from this visualization. I also use visualization to picture an opponent and a typical application in order to give a sense of purpose to my technique and form.

Sometimes things do not go so well and I feel frustrated and uncoordinated. Sometimes the issue is simply inundation and saturation; there is only so much I can absorb at one time. Sometimes my obstacle is my own pride. There are several things I do to break the cycle.

First is to break away from the activity for a few minutes. I may choose something else or simply stop for a couple of minutes. Intense focus can lock me into a cyclical mode. When I am struggling with something, a temporary break can loosen my focus and I can then act more naturally.

Another technique is to slow down and isolate elements in a technique as much as possible to see and feel the form. I'm a "tactile" guy (kinesthetic learner). I rely on recognizing when it "feels right" and trying to get into forms that repeat the feeling. This builds the basis for muscle memory, and then I go about the process of combining movements and integrating them.

Karate is a system of never-ending refinements. There is always something to correct, improve, or learn. Perfection is never achieved. Learning something new may move me out of my comfort zone. It can be wearing on the ego.

I must quiet the ego when I find myself in this situation. I acknowledge that I have finite bandwidth that limits how much I can absorb or physically control. I strive to consciously turn off the "voice of judgment." To clear my mind, I think of the dojo kun *(virtues or precepts), one of which, for the school at which I train, is, "Give your mind to application." Then I look to the juniors for inspiration.*

The youngest kids are generally self-absorbed and intent upon what they are doing at the moment, oblivious to being watched. As an adult I sometimes need to force myself to emulate that. I acknowledge that improvement requires a process of trial and error and experimentation, and I give myself permission to "work things out."

I am aware that I have a dominant side and a weak side too. To reinforce the physical training, I try to practice techniques on my weak side. I believe that there is positive muscle memory reinforcement by practicing the weak-side physical skills. The left-brain hemisphere controls right-side body functions and vice versa.

I also accept that I have good days and "off" days. My progress is not measured by the advances on the good days, but in skill retention on the not so good ones. Karate competes for energy and attention with other parts of our lives, so I consider that showing up is half the victory. Going through the motions still reinforces muscle memory, minimizing conditioning loss. Viewing technique demonstrations or listening to discussions of application is still adding value.

Understanding how I learn has allowed me to optimize my karate progress. Techniques I use are:

- *Repetition – just do something.*
- *Walk through exercises visually and visualize reasons for the forms.*
- *Interrupt exercises with small breaks when struggling.*
- *Work applications to the weak side.*
- *"Give your mind to application" (remove the voice of judgment).*
- *Show up.*

I am building conscious competence in order to strive for "unconscious competence," but one mental process that I will never turn off is the understanding of how I learn.
– John McNally [28]

Summary

People learn and process information differently. Knowing how you learn and taking best the advantage of that knowledge can facilitate your ability to absorb new information more quickly. Two learning style factors are especially pertinent to mastering martial arts—modality predilections and personality type. Modality predilections refer to the way in which you prefer to receive sensorial information, while personality type refers to the way in which you process information most effectively once you have received it.

Auditory, visual, and kinesthetic learning modes are commonly utilized in martial arts. Knowledge is most effectively communicated when all three of these modes are combined during instruction, yet individual students will be more receptive to certain modes than they are to others. Many people have strong predilections along a single mode for learning, though most tend to have both a primary and a secondary pathway preference for processing new information.

Two character aspects are particularly helpful in understanding learning-style preferences in an actionable wa:, the extraversion-introversion dichotomy and the sensing-intuition continuum. Extraverts direct their attention toward the external world of people and things while introverts direct their energies toward the inner world of concepts and ideas. Sensing personalities directly observe the surrounding tangible reality while intuitive people focus more on impressions and possibilities.

The three learning domains are cognitive (knowledge/thinking), affective (attitude/feeling), and psychomotor (skills/doing). Learning is usually interdependent amongst all three. Researchers have created taxonomies that express performance along these domains hierarchically, facilitating your ability to know how much you have learned. This information can be used not only to track progress, but also to ensure that prerequisite experience is obtained so that missing fundamentals will not inhibit your development.

Mental rehearsal, particularly when it involves imagery, facilitates performance in sports and other physical activities like martial arts. A powerful visualization method is Visuo-Motor Behavior Rehearsal. VMBR involves three phases, relaxing, visualizing, and performing. By repeating this process cyclically, visualization reinforces physical performance which, in turn, enhances your ability to visualize more effectively in a benevolent cycle.

The brain continues to learn after practicing stops, analyzing, synthesizing, and evaluating knowledge. This process works best during sleep. Consequently, if you want to make the most of your training, you will need to get a full night of uninterrupted sleep afterward.

Action Plan

• Understand your modality predilection(s). Look for ways to receive classroom input in a manner that aligns with your preferences, discussing them with your instructor as appropriate. Take additional steps to augment your training outside of the *dojo*, building on the strengths and shoring up the weaknesses of your learning style.

_____

_____

_____

• Understand your personality and its implications for learning. Look for ways to receive classroom input in a manner that aligns with your preferences, discussing them with your instructor as appropriate. Take additional steps to augment your training outside of the *dojo*, building on the strengths and shoring up the weaknesses of your learning style.

_____

_____

_____

• Make use of visualization exercises to facilitate your training regimen and improve your martial arts performance.

_____

_____

_____

• Make every effort to get a good night's rest after each training session so that you can continue to synthesize information while you sleep.

_____

_____

_____

Suggested Reading

Baum, Kenneth and Richard Trubo. *The Mental Edge: Maximize Your Sports Potential with the Mind-Body Connection.* New York, NY: Berkley Publishing Group, 1999.

This book describes a practical program for sharpening physical skills and maximizing sports performance. It covers visualization, performance talk, performance cues, and other methods of identifying and conquering obstacles in your training. An illuminating and actionable perspective, it really can sharpen your mental edge in any martial art.

Kane, Lawrence A. *Martial Arts Instruction: Applying Educational Theory and Communication Techniques in the Dojo.* Boston, MA: YMAA, 2004.

This book offers a unique and holistic approach to teaching and learning martial arts, incorporating elements of educational theory and communication techniques typically overlooked in *budo*. Teachers will improve their abilities to motivate, educate, and retain students, while students interested in the martial arts will develop a better understanding of what instructional methods best suit their needs.

Lawrence, Gordon D. *Looking at Type and Learning Styles.* Gainesville, FL: CAPT, 2004.

Written for both students and teachers, this book helps people discover learning preferences and decide which tools and techniques will give them the best results. It examines strengths, key motivations, and blind spots as they relate to learning or teaching. A bit technical in spots, Lawrence delivers very useful information that is well worth reading.

Recommended Web Sites
Center for Applications of Psychological Type (www.capt.org)
CAPT offers over 400 books and products to help clients understand themselves better in ways that promote personal growth and development, either individually or by working through a trained professional. They also have resources that can help you determine your personality type preferences by taking the MBTI assessment.

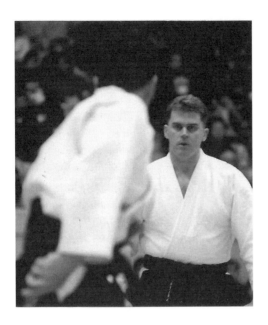

Skill takes focus and confidence.
(Photo courtesy of David Engstrom)

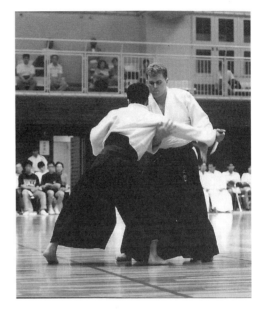

Skill also provides safety for you and your training partner.
(Photo courtesy of David Engstrom)

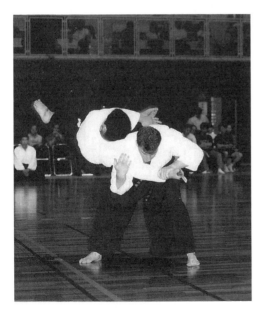

Strength and size will not help a martial artist land safely when he is slammed onto a hardwood floor. Skill is paramount.
(Photo courtesy of David Engstrom)

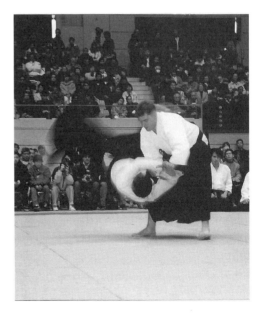

Training and repetition are the keys to gaining skills.
(Photo courtesy of David Engstrom)

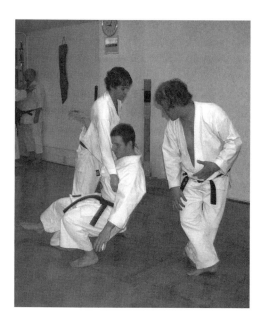

BEGINNING YOUR TRAINING WHILE YOUNG HELPS YOU INTEGRATE SKILLS EARLY, BUT IT IS NEVER TOO LATE TO START TRAINING.

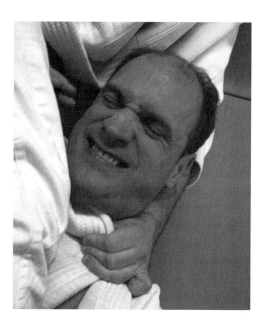

NOTICE THE SMALLER, LESS POWERFUL FINGERS ARE USED TO EXECUTE THIS CHOKING TECHNIQUE. THAT IS SKILL.

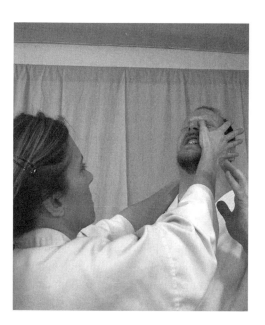

PRECISE STRIKES ARE BORN OF SKILL, EXPLOITING VITAL (WEAK) AREAS OF THE BODY THAT CAN BE DAMAGED EASILY.

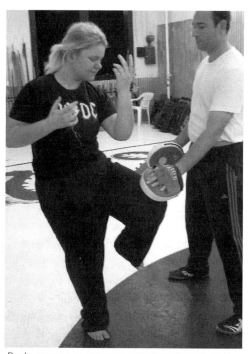

DON'T OVERLOOK THE OPPORTUNITY TO SHARPEN YOUR SKILLS BY HAVING A PARTNER WORK WITH YOU, OBSERVE YOUR TECHNIQUE, AND PROVIDE CONSTRUCTIVE FEEDBACK.

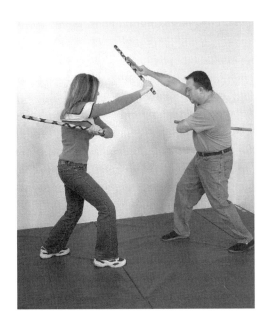

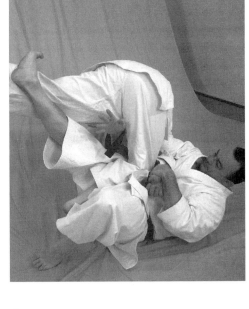

Skill and a weapon are great equalizers when you are mismatched in size and strength.

Complicated movements are rarely based in strength.

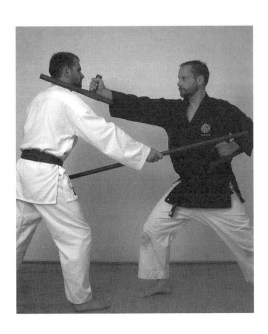

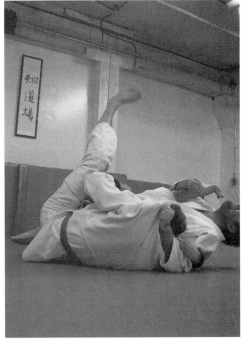

Uncontrolled power or precise technique, which is safer?

The ability to move different parts of your body simultaneously in different directions is developed through consistent, focused training. Over time, complex movements become instinctive.

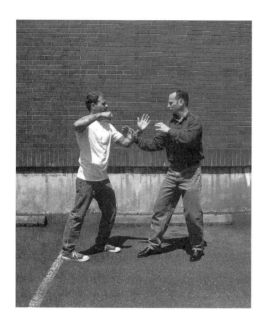

UNDERSTANDING DISTANCE AND TIMING IS NOT BASED IN STRENGTH, BUT RATHER ON LEARNED SKILL.

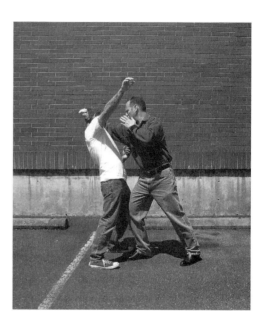

SKILL AND STRENGTH COUPLED TOGETHER BECOME A POTENT COMBINATION.

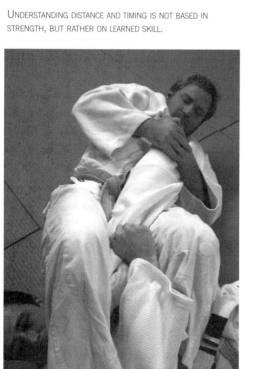

SKILL NOT ONLY MAKES THIS ARMLOCK WORK EFFECTIVELY BUT ALSO PROTECTS THE TRAINING PARTNER'S ARM SO THAT BOTH PRACTITIONERS CAN CONTINUE TO TRAIN DAY AFTER DAY.

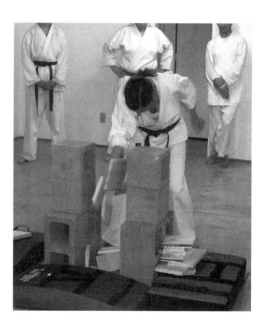

STRENGTH CAN BEAK A BOARD. SKILL KEEPS YOUR HAND INTACT WHEN YOU DO IT.

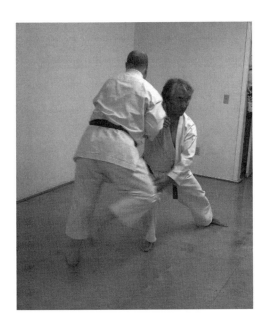

SKILL ALMOST ALWAYS TRUMPS YOUTH AND SIZE.

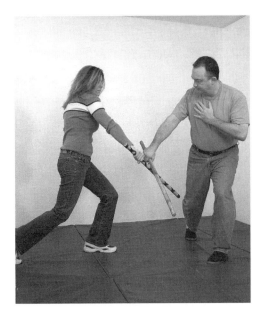

FROM THIS POSITION DO YOU STRIKE OR TRAP? SKILL AND EXPERIENCE FROM DISCIPLINED TRAINING WILL TELL YOU WHAT TO DO.

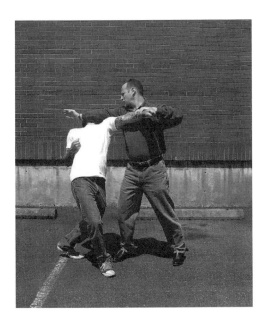

SKILL HELPS YOU KEEP CONTROL OF A CONFLICT. IT NOT ONLY SAFEGUARDS YOUR HEALTH AND WELL-BEING, BUT ALSO HELPS YOU RESPOND WITH A PRUDENT LEVEL OF FORCE THAT CAN KEEP YOU OUT OF JAIL IF YOU HAVE TO USE YOUR MARTIAL ART ON THE STREET.

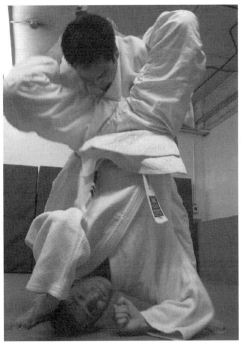

IT LOOKS BAD FOR THE MOMENT, BUT SKILL AND TRAINING MEAN THERE IS NO NEED TO PANIC. SKILL MEANS HAVING THE CONFIDENCE THAT IT IS ALL GOING TO TURN OUT ALRIGHT.

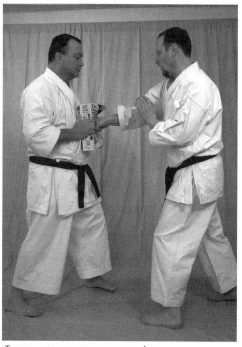

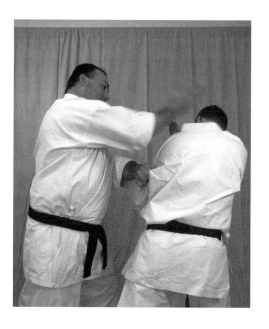

TESTING SKILL WITH THE PHONEBOOK. A PROPERLY THROWN PUNCH WILL TRANSMIT SHOCK THROUGH THE PHONEBOOK WHILE AN IMPROPER ONE WILL MERELY IMPACT ON THE SURFACE. IN THIS FASHION YOU CAN HEAR AND FEEL THE RESULTS, RECEIVE FEEDBACK FROM YOUR TRAINING PARTNER, AND REFINE YOUR TECHNIQUE ACCORDINGLY.

SKILL ALLOWS YOU TO DEVELOP SPEED, RESULTING IN AN OUT-STANDING COMBINATION.

CHAPTER 4

Understand Strength versus Skill

"Beware of the young doctor and the old barber."
– Benjamin Franklin[29]

Introduction (by Phillip Starr)

One of the most misunderstood and controversial subjects concerning the development of real martial arts skill has to do with the development of strength, as opposed to the cultivation of technique. It is important that contemporary martial arts enthusiasts understand that an increase in muscular size and strength does not necessarily imply an equal elevation of martial arts skill. One can be very powerful physically but possess no martial skills whatsoever. On the other hand, one who possesses real expertise in an Oriental martial discipline is also very strong. It is interesting to note that the Chinese character for strength, li, *is actually a pictograph of a tendon. It is not a pictograph of a muscle. Think about that.*

Although it would seem that increasing muscle mass would enhance one's martial arts prowess, the truth is that it can seriously inhibit the development of real technique. Professional athletes know that they should not regularly engage in exercise routines that are not directly related to their particular athletic disciplines. For instance, cross-country runners do not train to develop great upper-body strength and mass; they know that their time is better spent engaging in exercises that will directly affect their ability to run long distances.

The martial arts devotee who focuses heavily on the development of large muscles often has a tendency to overpower his or her techniques due to an over-reliance on excessive muscular force. This results in misalignment of the body, loss of speed, and a subsequent reduction of efficiency.

It is well to remember that the Oriental martial arts instructors of just one generation ago were usually rather small in stature but capable of generating uncanny power. This is because their training emphasizes precision of technique, and the exercises in which they engage are always "technique specific." Every movement, every exercise, is directed towards improvement of technique rather than the development of an eye-appealing physique. As a well-known karate instructor once told his students, "If you want a stronger punch, practice punching!"

– Phillip Starr [30]

Strength and Skill

Understanding your place in life is always a good thing. However, in the world of martial arts sometimes it can be hard to know. In the real world, the employer and employee are clearly defined; parent, child is another example. However, the martial arts are based on skills. A young person with more time on the floor can outrank an older person, in some cases even their own parent.

Ranking in the martial arts is not generally based on age or your position in the business world; your rank is based on a combination of strength and skill. These two worlds of strength and skill must blend within the practitioner giving him or her an ability to use either of these aspects of their training, or most likely a combination.

The adage goes, "old age and craftiness will always overcome youth and skill." While that may not be entirely true in every instance, it is accurate enough in the *dojo*. Experienced practitioners can use their superior skill to overcome younger, stronger individuals. An over-reliance on strength comes at the detriment of skill, leading to plateaus in development and a degradation of prowess as the practitioner ages. Both strength and skill are needed in martial arts, yet knowing how/when to apply them is important in helping you advance more quickly in your training.

To begin, let us go over some fundamental concepts about strength and skill. The following is a rule of thumb concerning strength and skill: Narrow strength always trumps narrow skill; broad skill always trumps broad strength. Below are a few historical and classic examples of this rule of thumb:

Broad strength defeats narrow strength

Late in 1864, as the Civil War raged in the United States, Union General William Tecumseh Sherman began his infamous "March to the Sea." The march carried with it a "Scorched Earth" policy that left everything utterly destroyed in the wake of his army. The minor resistance his troops faced stood no chance against a battle-hardened army that burned crops it did not consume, killed livestock it did not eat or appropriate, and destroyed military and civilian infrastructure alike. This march to the sea was a case of sheer military power moving at full throttle against opponents that had the home terrain advantage, intimately knowing their own battlefields. Their broad strength overwhelmed all resistance.

Broad skill defeats narrow strength

The famous battle of Thermopylae might be considered a skillful victory by 300 Spartan warriors, at least until you take into account the fact that they all died in the process. In 480 BC, King Leonidas and 300 Spartan *hoplites* (foot soldiers) held back the entire Persian army of roughly 250,000 men, defending a narrow pass for several days. The Persians eventually crushed this small force, defeated the Greek army, and sacked Athens, yet the valor of those heroic soldiers is recounted to this day. An epitaph at the battle site reads, "Friend, tell the Spartans that on this hill we lie obedient to them still."

The 300 Spartans who went to Thermopylae were handpicked from thousands of volunteers by the king as a "sire-only" force, those who had already produced male children to carry on their family name (and honor). These warriors never expected to return from the battle. These brave Spartans where successful in holding their ground for seven days, keeping the vast Persian army at bay until a secret mountain pass was revealed to the Persians. With superior numbers, the Persians mounted a second front behind the Spartan lines, using the pass, and cut down the Spartans to a man.

Man-to-man, the Spartans were better trained than their Persian foe. By carefully selecting the battleground, the Spartans were able to utilize that superior fighting skill effectively, holding off forces that outnumbered them over 800 to one. Simply put, overwhelming force when held in check was losing to skill, until the battlefield was changed.

Broad skill trumps broad strength

In 216 BC, a Carthaginian named Hannibal Barca won The Battle of Cannae using skill to overcome a superior numbered Roman army. In the simplest terms, the center of the battle line of Hannibal's army allowed themselves to be driven back, bowing in the middle as the Roman army pressed forward. As the battle progressed, the Carthaginian army formed a crescent and then sealed the crescent into a circle. The Romans in the center of the circle were unable to wield their weapons at the Carthaginian army; only the outer edges of the now encircled Roman army could fight.

Before the day was over 60,000 to 70,000 Romans were killed or captured in a slaughter that still ranks as one of the bloodiest and costliest hand-to-hand battles in terms of human life in the history of Mankind. The skill of the Carthaginians' superior strategy overwhelmed the massive strength of Rome's legions.

Narrow skill trumps broad strength

The Lighting War, or *Blitzkrieg*, employed by the German military during the beginning of World War II used bombardment followed by fast-moving armaments to surprise and prevent an enemy from putting together a sound defense. The

German military used this form of battle against Poland, France, the Netherlands, and the Soviet Union with initial success.

The projection of the Germans' force was based on a narrow thrust moving as quickly as possible to penetrate as deeply as possible into the opponent's home territory. Because they could focus their energy on small portions of the opponent's forces, they were able to avoid becoming mired in a force-on-force battle that they would ultimately lose.

Broad skill trumps narrow skill

The Romans had lost an entire squadron of ships to the naval skills of the Carthaginian navy in 260 BC. A few short months later, however, the Romans were back. At the Battle of Mylae, they handily defeated their Carthaginian foes. What changed between battles? During the interim, the Romans completely reengineered their naval fleet tactics.

The strength of the Romans had historically been in hand-to-hand small group combat, not in naval battle. Consequently, beefing up their naval tactics alone was not enough. They also had their engineers fit the bow of each one of their ships with a *corvus*, a simple gangplank. The Romans then went to battle with intent to redefine the battlefield to favor their strength. The retrofitted *corvus* allowed the powerful Roman military to fight hand-to-hand, boarding the Carthaginian ships where they slaughtered the opposing sailors.

The Romans defeated a superior navy by playing to their strength, turning a naval battle into what effectively became a land battle. A small amount of naval skill plus enormous infantry expertise overcame naval prowess alone.

"Speed in fighting depends not just on your hands and feet in swiftness, but other attributes such as non-telegraphic moves and awareness. Speed in fighting is to hit your foe without yourself being hit."

– Bruce Lee [31]

Broad skill trumps narrow strength

Royce Gracie demonstrated in the early Ultimate Fighting Championships that although lighter than his opponents, he was able to win using skill over raw strength. By using position and wisdom, he was able to take the fights to the ground, his preferred place to fight. He then worked his opponents into a vulnerable position, allowing him to choke or arm lock them into submission. Between 1993 and 1994, he won 11 matches by submission, becoming tournament title holder of the Ultimate Fighting Championship (UFC) 1, UFC 2, and UFC 4. He fought to a draw with Ken Shamrock at UFC 5. Other fighters were so impressed with his skills that many moved toward grappling, cross training, and Mixed Martial Arts for UFC, the PRIDE Fighting Championship, and similar competitions.

Going with What You Know

Every person, whether aware of it or not, will go with what they know, using what has worked in the past. Look at any child. If crying and throwing a fit gets them what they want, they will continue to use that tactic until it does not work anymore. We continue with this pattern of going with what we know throughout our lives. This applies to what you do physically as well as mentally.

Think about how you approach the world for a moment, because the way you move though the world is going to affect how you are going to learn martial arts. Generally, if you are young, for example, you will depend on your physical ability to get by. You will do more sit-ups, more push-ups, more punches, and so on, and do them with greater effort than older members of the class. Moreover, you will most likely get in your own way.

Wilder experienced a good example of this while judging a tournament several years ago. He watched a young man with great intensity slam his head forward as if he was rear-ending a car in front of him every time he punched. While the practitioner undoubtedly felt that he was putting extra effort into each punch making them stronger, he was actually compromising his structure, slowing himself down with extra movement, and punching much weaker than he thought. It could not have been very good for his neck, either. He was going with what he knew, however: youthful vigor—pressing harder, working harder, and relying on strength rather than technique.

In the same way that the Romans pushed forward into the trap the Hannibal had set for them at Cannae, this young man was falling into a training trap that many young people experience. Push harder on what you know and go with what you know. Stepping out of "going with what you know" and building on your strengths is important to learning faster and better. In a classical sense, you will hear this expressed as, "Get out of your own way."

The following tips, broken down by age and gender, will give you a framework to build on your natural strengths and pay attention to your inherent weaknesses.

Observation

Youth is about strength and working hard to achieve your goals. You should work hard, but you should also be aware that unguarded strength can become a weakness. Just like the young guy who bobbed his head while doing his forms thinking his extra effort was making him stronger and the Romans at Cannae who believed they had the Carthaginians on the run only to become trapped, relying purely on strength is not enough. The way to break out of this trap is through observation.

There are two kinds of observation, observation of self and observation of others. These two training techniques are further separated into Youthful Training and

Senior Training. They are not mutually exclusive so you should pay attention to both areas.

Observing others

When observing others, it is best not to be an actual part of the class. If your instructor allows it, make an effort to come to a class that is above your rank. Pick one person to watch. This person should be of the same physical structure as you; if you are tall watch some one who is tall; if you are stocky watch someone with the same build, and so forth.

Once you have selected the person to watch, break it down even further. Choose a body part, say just the hands or waist, and observe how that person moves. Really watch, and then copy the movement. If classes are not separated by rank,

> *"The best strategy is always to be very strong; first in general, and then at the decisive point… There is no higher and simpler law of strategy than that of keeping one's forces concentrated."*
>
> – Carl von Clausewitz [32]

or the teacher does not feel comfortable with your in-class observation, you may be able to work with higher-ranked practitioners outside of regular class hours. Either way, find someone appropriate to observe carefully.

Important tips:
- Find someone with the same body type as yourself and superior skill
- Find someone who is not only a higher rank, but also older than you
- Watch for nuance, subtle movements of small body parts, rather than just taking in the big picture

As you move up the ranks and become more skilled, you can do an interesting variation of this observation method for learning. Use the same observation process, but look for someone who is nothing like you in body type. Watch their favorite techniques are and try to adapt them to your training. This is more difficult than it might seem at first blush and, therefore, is not recommended for newer students. Further down the road of training, you will find this an invaluable means of broadening your skills.

Pay attention not only to physical techniques but also to how the higher-ranked practitioners interact with each other as well. Etiquette and tradition are an important part of *budo*. *Reishiki* (etiquette) comes from two Japanese words. The first is *rei*, which is defined as a bow, salutation, or salute, expressing courtesy, propriety, thanks, and appreciation. The second part of the term is *shiki*, which is defined as a ceremony, rite, or function. Combined, the term *reishiki* can translate as etiquette or manners.

Etiquette is an integral part of *budo*, for without it we would be practicing nothing more than base violence. Watching senior students' behavior during training and in their general actions and interactions in the *dojo* is an excellent way to learn *reishiki* (provided that the senior students themselves have also been observant over the years, of course). The more training a person receives, the calmer, more dignified, and humble that *budoka* should become. Students who practice etiquette ultimately make themselves better people as well as better martial artists.

> *"Small people must be completely familiar with the spirit of large people, and large people must be familiar with the spirit of small people. Whatever your size, do not be misled by the reactions of your own body."*
>
> – Miyamoto Musashi [33]

Observing yourself

Self-observation is best done after observing others. This order of the process gives you a goal and a movement to model. Using a mirror, slowly begin to make the movements you are trying to copy. Observe the smallest part of the technique first. An example of this is if you are working on a punch, begin with the position of the fist in chamber at your side.

Ask yourself, "Is it positioned correctly, rotated correctly, held at the right height?" This breakdown of the technique and the use of a mirror will give you the benefit of training outside of the school (always a good thing) and an opportunity to move at your own pace, which in this instance is very slowly.

Once you have gotten the movement to where you think it ought to be then close your eyes and feel the technique in your body. Ask yourself, how does the correct technique feel in your body, feet, waist, and shoulders? Open your eyes and check your reflection in the mirror on occasion to ensure that you have not inadvertently changed something. This will help you engrain the proper mechanics into your body more swiftly.

Keys to Senior Training

Without a doubt, you are in the minority in your class; most people are younger. They also learn at a different rate than you do, as well as have generally better physical conditioning. Note that you have advantages that they do not have, including a longer attention span, diligence, and experience. Drawing upon these three advantages, you can enjoy a faster and more pleasant path as you pursue your martial arts studies.

Attention span

This is clearly a case where a skill trumps strength. Having a longer attention span allows you to focus on every detail and nuance of what is being taught. Instead of leaping into the action with the "I get it" attitude, stand back for a moment and ask the instructor to "Please show me that again." Patience is a real virtue in learning martial arts where subtle nuances make all the difference between effective and ineffective technique.

"If he is secure at all points, be prepared for him. If he is in superior strength, evade him."

– Sun Tzu [34]

Diligence

Diligence is another attribute that can help you triumph over strength. Having the diligence to repeat a motion over and over until it is exactly correct is essential to good martial arts. This attribute means you do not utter the words, "I'm bored," like your youthful contemporaries. Basic punches, kicks, throws, and grappling applications take on a completely new meaning when you realize that you need to integrate your body to utilize solid technique rather than brute muscle force. Develop the subtlety and understand the nuance necessary to perform any technique "properly" through disciplined, repetitive practice.

It is useful to think of the practice of these basics as an ascending spiral. Each time you repeat a drill, you can incorporate a higher level of understanding, which, in essence, allows you to approach the technique in a completely new way. Theoretically, a technique may be practiced 100 times or 100 techniques may be practiced only once, as each is different and more evolved than the one that came before. Diligence and a long attention span ultimately lead to continuous improvement.

Experience

This is a unique case of skill over strength because it involves wisdom. An important part of knowledge is the recognition of patterns; you only gain that ability through experience. The ability to recognize patterns allows you as an older student to equate one thing to another. Confusing? Think of it this way: when a younger student learns a closed-fist block then later an open-hand block, they appear to be different. To the older student, the two blocks are effectively the same. Experience shows that the structure of the body (e.g., elbow placement, arm angle, tension/contraction) is the same. The only difference is that the hand is open. This experience combined with the recognition of pattern facilitates a more holistic understanding of the art.

Keys to Youthful Training

Most people begin martial arts training as youths or young adults. They tend to learn quickly and are generally in better physical condition than older students. They have an inherent advantage in enthusiasm and endurance. Furthermore, they typically have less outside responsibilities in life so they can devote more time and energy toward training. These attributes help you get good faster.

Enthusiasm

Frankly, youthful enthusiasm goes a very long way when it comes to the martial arts. Enthusiasm draws you to class and gives you the desire to make the extra effort, to do more than just the minimum. Enthusiasm makes you seek additional information from books, magazines, Web sites, and DVDs. It gets you talking with others and practicing after class. Enthusiasm is your strength; use it to keep yourself going, continuously growing, and learning new skills.

Endurance

The youthful body is a gift. It has the ability to go further, faster, and harder than an older person. Simply put, the older you are, the less endurance you have. Go to any grappling class or high school wrestling practice (as these classes are very physical) and you will see endurance at its prime. As a youthful student, you should use this endurance to repeatedly practice the mechanics of your chosen art. Endurance + repetition = better skill x 2. Make the most of it while you can; it will not be there forever.

Life responsibilities

Younger people rarely have the level of life responsibilities that come later on. No mortgage, no children, no home repairs, and so on give you more time to apply to your art. Do not miss this window of opportunity because it will quickly pass. Life moves on and changes occur.

Do not think, however, that we are saying you should forsake these things. We are simply saying that you should know where you are on the life timeline and use that to your advantage. The less life responsibility you have, the more disposable time you get. Use that time well. Above all, enjoy your martial training.

Strength and Skill Training Tips by Age and Gender

No discussion of skill and technique is complete without addressing gender. The bottom line is men are generally stronger than women, while women generally have more stamina. This, of course, is only a general guide. Having been thrown at will by judo instructors several weight divisions below and often older than ourselves, we certainly know that mass, gender, and age are not always the determining factors. Making assumptions about a person's skill level and desire is done at your own risk.

Having said all that, however, there are certain generalities that can prove helpful in focusing your training.

So, how do you get good faster? The following are general guidelines broken out by age and gender. Some items are very similar between the various categories as they apply to more than one. The following are "rules of thumb," not hard and fast conventions:

Younger Men

Be quiet and listen.

Younger practitioners often want to focus more on socializing than they do on learning. It is great to make friends with classmates, but talking or wisecracking during class is inappropriate and a fast way to get nowhere. The adage goes, "God gave you two ears and one mouth because he wants you to listen twice as much as talk." This maxim certainly applies here. While the temptation to chatter may be high, doing so while your instructor is teaching will be done at your own peril. In the *dojo,* we sometimes call this *kuchi waza* (disruptive chatter, literally "mouth technique"). The appropriate behavior is to shut up, pay attention, and train hard! You can talk all you want to outside the *dojo.*

Diligently do as your instructor asks.

Make every effort to do precisely what your instructor asks you to do, and do it with a positive attitude. "Can't" is not a word you use in the *dojo.* You can have a hard time, be challenged by, struggle with, or work on aspects of your training, but the term "can't" does not exist in a serious martial artist's dictionary. By approaching your training in this fashion, you will find you are able to do more, do it better, and learn it in a shorter time. This is because you have a "can do" attitude rather than a defeatist, "can't do" one.

Do not muscle through techniques.

Trying to muscle through techniques is just strength over skill. We learned earlier that broad skill would trump narrow strength. Muscle strength is good, and oftentimes necessary, but using brute force to make a technique work is not good. A skilled opponent will use your strength against you. Even an unskilled opponent will meet you strength-to-strength, again not good. Contrary to what you may think, using too much strength makes you slow. If you want to become stronger, work with your instructor to learn appropriate exercises that will complement your martial skills rather than work against them. Strive for finesse.

Try to understand why it works.

Many younger practitioners simply want to do rather than knowing why. Sparring, for example, is a whole lot of fun but if you are not utilizing solid technique all you are really doing is playing an advanced game of tag. You accomplish very little in the process so your so-called skills will only be effective so long as they

> **Something to think about:**
>
> Muscles get tired; skill never tires.

are used against a weaker, slower, or lesser-skilled opponent. Do not fall into this trap. Look at every technique from a mechanical or technical angle. Search the motion for the most effective way to make it work with the least amount of strength. Look at your body position and your partner's; examine all the angles. Use your mind to see deeper into the mechanics of the technique; this will develop skill. Read books and watch DVDs that can help you understand the deeper aspects of the art (see Chapter 8 for more information).

Younger Women

You are often physically mismatched.

It is just a fact; most martial arts schools have a lot more men in attendance than women. Since men are generally stronger than women, you must understand other avenues of success. Your strength will be found in solid technique rather than in physical force. Do not try to compete on brute physical terms but rather on knowledge and skill. Take advantage of your dexterity and flexibility, too. A combination of quickness and solid technique can put you on par with your male counterparts.

Model other successful women.

You can learn a lot by modeling or copying the more advanced and successful women in your martial arts school. We are not saying that you cannot learn by modeling successful men, yet the women ahead of you have figured out the adaptations you will need to discover too. Look to their wisdom rather than reinventing the wheel for yourself. This will help you develop your skills much faster. The fact is that there are very real differences in physicality between women and men, some of which require subtle changes in the application of certain techniques. If your instructor is male, he may not understand these differences well enough to explain them to you in a way that you will truly understand. Seek what others ahead of you know to supplement this information and help you succeed.

Be first to volunteer.

Be first to volunteer when the instructor needs an assistant. In tandem drills, *tori* means "attacker," the one who initiates a technique, while *uke* means "receiver," the one on whom it is performed. Be the instructor's *uke* whenever you have the opportunity. There is no substitute for feeling a technique as well as watching it. Do not be shy. Younger women tend to be especially hesitant about volunteering in class, yet practice really does make perfect. A good instructor will assure your safety and security, so you do not have to be worried about volunteering.

Whenever you have an opportunity to work with the instructor or senior students take advantage of it.

Learn how to cheat to win

Unlike the mundane educational system, copying other people's work is encouraged in the *dojo*. When you see someone do something that really works, copy it. Furthermore, there is really no such thing as "cheating" in martial arts, at least not in the conventional sense of the term. In self-defense, for example, vital point strikes, pressure point techniques, biting, name calling, hair pulling, misdirecting, and a host of other nasty tricks are all fair game. Understand and utilize these cheats as appropriate. Craftiness can overcome a lack of physical size and strength. Even in sparring or tournament situations, there are some "cheats" that are appropriate.

Older Men

You are not as young as you used to be.

Be aware that you are not twenty years old anymore. You are not as flexible as you once were and you do not heal as quickly. An injury can be a major setback, particularly as you become older and begin to heal slower. The point at which many older men leave training is when they find that the old methods of strength, behaviors left over from youth, no longer work for them. If you take time off because of an injury, your chances of returning to training are roughly 50/50 after just one week, and become practically zero after a month. Do not fall into this trap. Pay attention to your body and do not overdo it. Daily stretching, proper nutrition, and supplemental exercise on your "off days" will be a great help, too (see chapter 8 for more information).

You have life experience.

Simply put, you are experienced. You know how your mind works and how you process new information most effectively. You have life experience you can draw on and say, "Oh, this technique is like water skiing, or this movement is like the one I use in racquet ball." You have the knowledge; use it to make your skills better. Examine how the things you are learning in the martial arts are similar to the things you have learned in other aspects of your life. By observing what is happening and relating it to an experience from the past, you can make quick monumental leaps forward in your training.

Exercise your mind as well as your body

Pay special attention to the non-physical aspects of your martial art, particularly between formal training sessions. Study up on your art, reading books or articles and watching DVDs that can help you learn more about the history, traditions, and strategy to help you truly understand the tactics that you want to master (see Chapter 8 for more information). Practice visualization techniques that help you internalize what you have learned more effectively (see Chapter 3). Supplement your physical experiences in the *dojo* with mental exercises outside it.

The race... is not a race.

The youthful practitioner without a doubt looks at the next belt, or rank. You may too, but you are more inclined to look at martial arts in a broader sense, as a life study, or an enjoyable diversion from your workday. If you look at martial arts in those ways, continue to do so, if not, take time to look at it in that manner. As you have learned in life, the race usually goes to the one that puts one foot in front of the other, not necessarily to the fastest.

Older Women

Seek the subtle side of technique

Omote, which means outer or surface training, is the most common and well understood aspect of any martial art. It is the things you can see, and sometimes feel, when studying a form. *Ura waza*, on the other hand, are the subtle details that make the obvious succeed. Skill is paramount; it can overcome a lack of strength. It is based in *kihon*, the fundamental building blocks of every effective technique. Examine your art from a technical perspective, studying the subtle nuances that make things work or limit their effectiveness and then practice the *kihon* over and over again until it becomes natural and automatic. Women, especially older women, are generally weaker than men yet skill can level the playing field.

Be cautious of declining bone density.

As women age, a major concern is decreasing bone density due to hormonal changes. This can lead to an increased risk for bone breakage, something to be mindful of when training. Weight training and nutritional supplements can help. Check with your physician, a nutritionist, and/or a sports medicine professional to find ways of protecting yourself. Spend time working with other successful female martial artists and understand what has worked for them. Consider studying an art that is not primarily focused on full-contact sparring, board breaking, and other intensely physical activities. There is nothing wrong with engaging in these activities from time to time, but a harsh daily dose of this type of extreme contact may be hazardous to your health.

Balance your commitments.

While both men and women, especially those with families, tend to have a broader range of outside distractions and conflicts than younger practitioners, family-related commitments more often tend to fall upon women than men. While it is important to balance your time wisely, if you cannot make it to class every day there is a tendency to try to attempt to over-train to make up for lost time. That is a good way to get hurt and/or burned out. When you can train, do your best to have fun and learn as much as you can. Work on developing a solo training routine that fits your hectic schedule to supplement your *dojo* time.

Advice for New Students

by Martina Sprague [35]

Old age often carries the stigma of slow reflexes, weak muscles, and low flexibility. But if this is the case, then why are so many older martial artists capable of performing their art with such amazing speed, agility, and power? Two elements go into the equation. The first is training background and experience. A person who starts his or her training at an advanced age will naturally take a little longer to catch up to the older martial artist with forty years under his belt. The second element is the use of correct body mechanics. Posture and body alignment play vital roles in every martial arts technique and allow you to maximize your strength, power, and performance no matter what your age.

The reason many older people in general seem less agile is because when we reach forty, or thereabouts, we start leading sedentary lives. We no longer participate in competitive sports; we no longer go out and play soccer with the kids. We sit for longer hours in front of the television and become armchair athletes instead of real warriors. By the time we reach seventy, we have not done anything physical to speak of in more than thirty years, so how can anyone expect us to be fireballs?

The lesson this bit of knowledge teaches the younger martial artists, those of us who are still naturally energetic and are just beginning our training, is that we cannot quit. Not now. Not twenty years from now. Not ever. Although a person can memorize a series of martial arts moves and still remember those ten years later, strength, power, and agility, along with balance and body alignment, must be maintained over time.

In order to progress toward higher rank and skill, a martial artist needs focus. Note that focus is singular. It is by definition "the central point where everything else converges." If I were to give you a technique goal on which to focus, I would tell you to focus on balance, or more precisely, on the physical balance of your body. All of your martial arts techniques, all of your weapons, are useless when you lack physical balance, no matter how many techniques you have memorized or how many years of training you have under your belt.

You find balance in your stance. Your stance *(dachi)* is your foundation and is determined by the part(s) of your body that is are contact with the ground. When you are standing, your stance is determined by the position of your feet, or just one foot if you are in the process of stepping or kicking. When you are on the ground, your stance is determined by the position of your hands and knees, your feet and elbows, or your belly, back, or side of body depending on what the confrontation calls for. Moreover, your stance is not stationary. It could change consistently throughout any given martial arts technique or physical altercation, not just moving in a particular stance, but changing between various postures as well.

Regardless of what body positions your fighting style demands, the common denominator is that a stance must be stable in order to have value. Your center of gravity must never fall outside of your foundation. When you achieve and can maintain a balanced stance, and so long as you have basic knowledge of technique and a desire to practice the martial arts with intent, power will automatically fall in place. Thus, an older, smaller, or weaker but experienced martial artist can beat a younger, bigger, or stronger fighter.

Never give up.

If you take nothing else from martial arts, use it to keep in shape. An active lifestyle is enormously beneficial as people age, not just to retain strength, flexibility, bone density, and endurance longer, but to maintain mental health as well. If you enjoy martial arts, it can be a fun way of ensuring that you get enough exercise to slow symptoms of the aging process and live better longer.

The Fundamental Importance of Fundamentals

Martial arts, for the most part, are not composed of complicated body postures or advanced, secret applications. They were designed to be successful on the battle-field, in the bar, or in the back alley, relying on relatively simple, straightforward techniques that can work under adverse conditions and adrenaline-charged environments. The trick to using them successfully is *ura waza* (inner ways), a deep understanding of the fundamentals behind the techniques and what makes them function.

Having some understanding of the inner workings of a simple movement sets a practitioner up for success in properly applying it. The secret of martial arts, therefore, can be found in the basics. In Japanese these basics are called *kihon*. *Kihon* covers fundamental building blocks such as stances, spinal alignment, proper breathing, movement, balance, center of gravity, weight transfer, tension versus relaxation, relative angle to an opponent, and a host of other nuances. The way you learn these things is through repetition and constant practice, moving around in foreign stances until they become natural and throwing thousands upon thousands of punches, kicks, and other techniques over a very long period of time.

Once the fundamentals have been mastered, they not only strengthen your ability to perform your chosen art but they can transfer to other arts as well. An excellent example of this is when we hosted a seminar from a very highly skilled Japanese karate practitioner, Yoshitomo Yamashiro *Sensei*. It was his first trip to America so in addition to teaching the seminar, he wanted to do a few things during his visit that were simply not possible in Japan. One was shooting a gun. While common enough in America, firearms of any kind are prohibited for civilians in his native land. He had never touched a gun let alone fired one.

Kane took him to a nearby target range, explained all the safety precautions through a translator, and then demonstrated how to load and fire the weapon. He discussed how to align the sights and explained the importance of proper breathing as well as holding the weapon in a fixed position while the trigger was pulled. Yamashiro *Sensei* adopted a *sanchin dachi* (hourglass stance), took hold of the gun, and promptly placed his first eight shots in the black at about 25 feet, scoring one bulls-eye.

This would seem like a truly amazing accomplishment for someone who had never even touched a gun before, let alone fired one, yet the fundamentals of breath control, stance, and body alignment were so similar to karate that the transition was simple. Once you know the fundamentals, those skills create a foundation of success for almost any martial art, classical or modern.

Student Perspective (by Dan Keith)

For me, I wish I had started younger. My late teens were almost too late. When I first started in the martial arts, it was hard physically to get in shape. Things were pretty confusing. I was told to have faith, go through the motions. At brown-belt level, things started to change for me; it started making sense, it started working. My advice is to pay attention, take it easy, do your best, and practice at home.

There are no shortcuts; hard work and dedication are the shortcuts. I would have gotten my black belt faster if I had been more focused on my forms. When I started, I just wanted to fight, to defend myself. I figured fighting was the only way. Then I was told I needed to work on my forms to improve my fighting. I took the advice and my fighting did get better.

If you are just starting out as an adult, go slow, relax. Pace yourself and you will stay in the martial arts longer. I have changed my fighting style over the years. I fight more defensively now. I'm not so aggressive. I'll wait for my opponent to move and I'll counter so I can get a move in. You must learn to conserve your energy when you are older. Learn how to fire that energy then loosen up to save energy.

To still enjoy the martial arts I teach. Teach someone something they did not know. There is a lot out there to learn. For some people, if they can just learn one during thing each class, they are making progress.

I remember being told, "Once you start, you will always be a martial artist." I always thought about the martial arts even when I was not training. I have been training now for twenty-five years straight.

If you are injured, pace yourself. Some people drop out when they get injured. Others may use the injury as an excuse to drop out. Follow your doctor's advice and give yourself time to heal. Martial arts can be a lot harder for people with physical disabilities. Try not to get frustrated and give up.

– Dan Keith [36]

Summary

Strength and skill are both necessary in the martial arts, but not all practitioners are alike in regards to age or ability. Knowing where you are concerning strength versus skill can be very helpful in your training. Focusing your training based upon your age, gender, and ability can make a critical difference in how successful you are in your training. These tips and tricks regarding your place on the training continuum are time-tested and tried. By using them, you will have more fun and enjoyment over the duration of your training.

Action Plan

• Be clear as to what you want to learn, skill or strength, and when you want to focus on it.

_____

_____

• Make a date to observe an advanced class.

_____

_____

• Be specific in the actions you intend to learn: "I am going to watch _____ and look for _____."

_____

_____

• Keep the training tips appropriate to your age and gender in mind every time practice your martial art. Strive to build on your inherent strengths and shore up your weaknesses.

_____

_____

Suggested Reading

Gendlin, Eugene T., Ph.D. *Focusing*. Bantam Books, New York, NY, USA: 1978.

Focusing gives a pathway to reaching inside yourself and observing what is making you function the way you do in certain situations. A quick read, it provides food for thought you will use for a lifetime. Well written and practical.

Loehr, James E., Ed.D. *The New Toughness Training for Sports, Mental Emotional and Physical Conditioning from One of the World's Premier Sports Psychologists.* Plume/Penguin, New York, NY. USA: 1995.

Loehr takes you through the process that separates raw talent from professional behaviors. This book helps you train your mind to expect the best, shows you how to focus your mind to achieve your goals, and helps you become successful even under the pressure of intense competition. The book is written in a manner that makes sports psychology interesting, understandable, and, most importantly, useable.

Pearl, Bill and Gary T. Moran, Ph.D. *Getting Stronger, Sports Training – General Conditioning – Body Building.* Shelter Publications Inc., Bolinas, CA, USA: 1986.

Dominated by "how to" pictures this book provides weight lifting exercises for men and women. Alternate methods and lifts are shown to provide the changes you need in your routine to stay fresh and motivated. It is a great reference for martial artists and power lifters alike.

Suggested Web Sites

Grapple Arts (http://grapplearts.com/)

This site specializes in Brazilian *jiu-jitsu*, submission grappling, and mixed martial arts (MMA). It provides informative articles, techniques, and information, explaining as well as demonstrating techniques in a manner that incorporates close-ups, "live-speed" sequences, and tournament footage. The site also explores the timing, psychology, and strategy of the techniques shown, which is equally important to the technical explanation. The materials are all thoroughly researched and well thought out.

Steve Pavlina: Personal Development for Smart People (http://www.stevepavlina.com/index.htm)

This site not only helps you make conscious decisions about your personal development but also provides tools to help you follow through on them. This means having the maturity to take 100 percent responsibility for your health, career, finances, relationships, emotions, habits, and spiritual beliefs. It requires taking a hard look at yourself, consciously deciding what kind of person you are on the inside, and then getting your actions to be congruent with your true self. The goal is to help you achieve outstanding effectiveness while maintaining internal balance, where your thoughts, feelings, actions, and skills are all working together to create the life you truly desire. Subjects include time management, motivation, overcoming procrastination, goal setting, courage, work/career balance, wealth and money, momentum (keeping energy/enthusiasm high), problem solving, balance, fulfillment, and consciousness.

Study Guides and Strategies (http://www.studygs.net/)
The Study Guides and Strategies Web site is authored, maintained, and supported by Joe Landsberger and a panel of researchers as an independent educational public service. Collaborative projects are developed across institutional, cultural, and national boundaries. Topics include preparing, learning, studying, classroom participation, learning with others, project management, reading skills, preparing for tests, taking tests, writing basics, writing types, research, math, science and technology, and more. The Web site is an excellent resource for academic and practical information that can help you learn more quickly and more effectively.

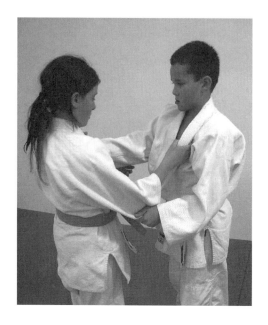

IT CAN BE TOUGH TO MOTIVATE KIDS TO PRACTICE A LITTLE BIT EVERY DAY. MAKE IT FUN AND ADD INCENTIVES. ONCE DAILY PRACTICE BECOMES HABIT, YOU CAN PROGRESS IN LEAPS AND BOUNDS.

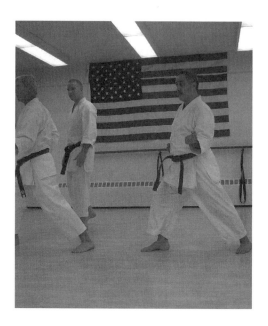

AS AN OLDER STUDENT, IT IS IMPORTANT TO PACE YOURSELF. BREAKING TRAINING INTO SMALLER SECTIONS OVER THE COURSE OF A WEEK CAN BE A GOOD IDEA.

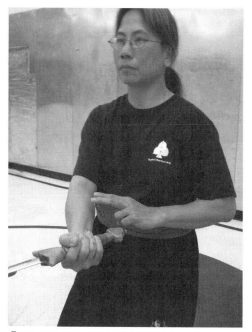

FOCUS, EVEN IF FOR ONLY A FEW MINUTES A DAY, STILL BUILDS FOR THE FUTURE. EVERY PRACTICE SESSION PUTS A DEPOSIT INTO YOUR SKILL BANK.

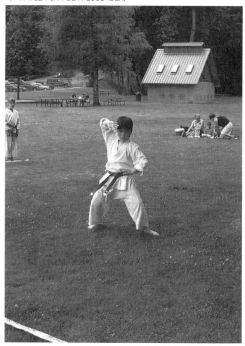

EVERY OPPORTUNITY TO SHOW YOUR ART SERVES AS A LITTLE TRAINING.

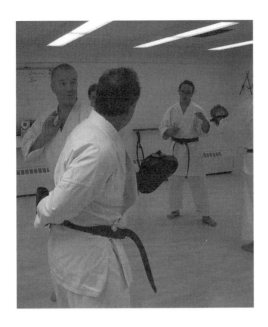

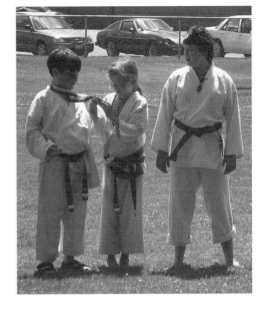

LOOK IN THIS PICTURE AND SEE ALL THE THINGS THAT CAN MAKE PRACTICE ON YOUR OWN MORE FUN. MUSIC? BICYCLE INNER TUBES? WHAT ELSE?

THE REWARDS OF HARD PRACTICE CAN BRING RETURNS FAR BEYOND WHAT YOU MAY HAVE IMAGINED.

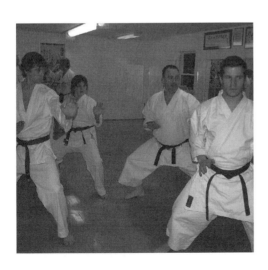

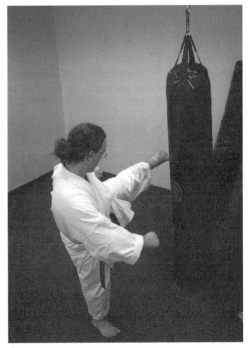

KATA, POOMSE, FORMS, PATTERNS, OR WHATEVER YOUR SYSTEM CALLS THEM ARE IMPORTANT TOOLS TO HELP YOU LEARN. NOT DOING YOUR FORMS LEAVES A HOLE IN YOUR TRAINING.

DIFFERENT TYPES OF BAGS ARE AVAILABLE FOR YOU TO TRAIN WITH. HERE, A BANANA BAG, WHICH REPRESENTS THE HUMAN BODY FROM HEAD TO TOE, IS SHOWN. THIS FULL-LENGTH BAG FACILITATES PUNCHES AND KICKS AT ANY RANGE.

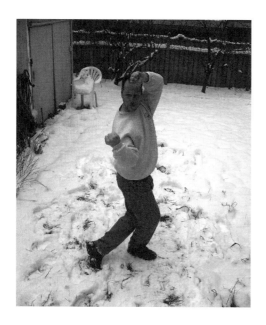

WEATHER CAN EITHER LIMIT YOU OR NOT, THE CHOICE IS ALWAYS YOURS. IF NEITHER RAIN NOR SNOW NOR SLEET NOR HAIL NOR DARK OF NIGHT CAN STOP THE POST OFFICE, WHY SHOULD IT STOP YOU?

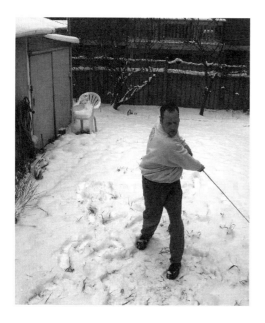

ONE SWIPE OF A TRADITIONAL EDGED WEAPON CAN BE DEADLY. WHEN PRACTICING WITH WEAPONS, MAKE ABSOLUTELY SURE THAT NOBODY ELSE IS IN THE VICINITY, ESPECIALLY SMALL CHILDREN WHO MAY NOT UNDERSTAND THE DANGER OF WHAT IS TAKING PLACE.

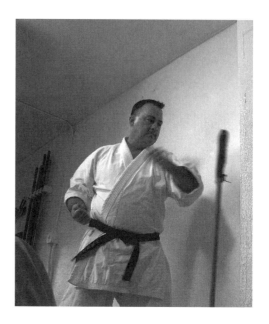

THE LEVEL OF INTENSITY YOU CHOOSE IS UP TO YOU WHEN YOU PRACTICE ON YOUR OWN. SET HIGH EXPECTATIONS FOR YOURSELF. YOUR SOLO WORKOUTS SHOULD BE AT LEAST AS INTENSIVE AS ANYTHING YOU FIND IN CLASS.

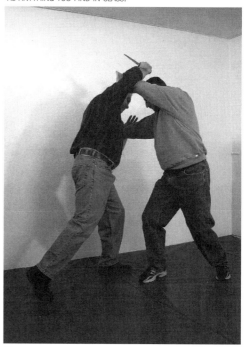

PRACTICING WITH ITEMS NOT NORMALLY UTILIZED IN YOUR CLASS CAN BE FUN, ESPECIALLY WITH A FRIEND FROM THE SAME SCHOOL. MIX THINGS UP A BIT OUTSIDE OF CLASS AND YOU WILL BE SURPRISED WHAT YOU WILL LEARN.

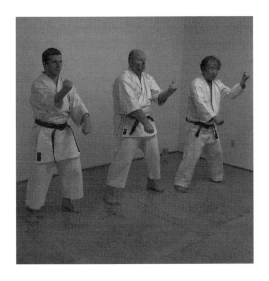

SMALL GROUP PRACTICE UNDER SUPERVISION IS A GREAT MEANS TO GETTING BETTER FASTER.

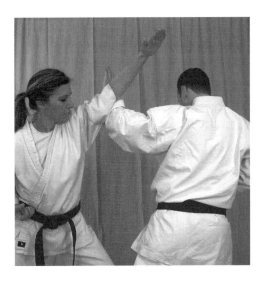

WORKING ONE TECHNIQUE, EVEN FOR ONLY FIVE MINUTES A DAY, QUICKLY ADDS UP.

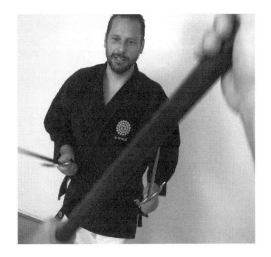

EVEN IN CASUAL PRACTICE THINGS CAN BE LEARNED.

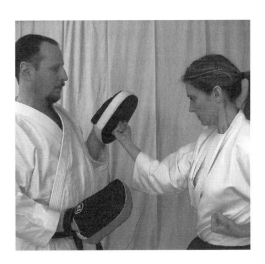

HAVING A FRIEND OR SPOUSE HELP YOU BY JUST HOLDING A PAD FOR FIVE MINUTES CAN BE A GREAT BOOST TO PRACTICING A LITTLE BIT EVERYDAY. SOMETIMES YOU JUST HAVE TO HIT STUFF TO FEEL THE EFFECTIVENESS OF YOUR TECHNIQUE.

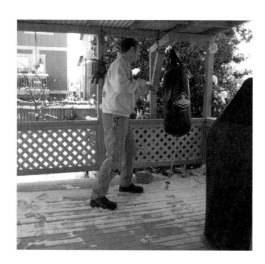

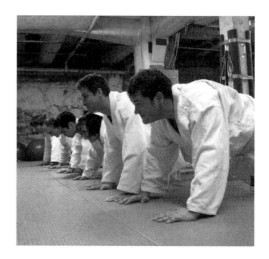

SETTING ASIDE TIME TO TRAIN OUTSIDE THE SCHOOL IS IMPORTANT. PERIOD.

PRACTICE IN A GROUP ATMOSPHERE ALLOWS A BROADER EXPERIENCE. GROUP ENERGY CAN SPUR YOU TO BETTER, STRONGER PERFORMANCE.

CHAPTER 5

Practice A Little Each Day

"A journey of a thousand miles begins with a single step."
– Lao Tzu[37]

Introduction (by Iain Abernethy)

To make consistent progress you need to train on a consistent basis. Consistency in training is undoubtedly more important than any other factor when it comes to making progress.

I was never what you would call a "natural." I was clumsy and uncoordinated as a child and struggled to get my body to do what was requested of it when I first began training. However, I was well and truly bit by the martial bug and trained at every available opportunity. I trained daily and it was not long before things started to come together. Training each day became something I just did. Like sleeping and eating, training became a normal everyday activity. Daily training became a habit: a habit that I still have to this day.

If you can get into the habit of daily training, you are sure to make great progress. On the days when you do not go to the class, you are left in complete charge of your training and can make it specific to your needs. When an area that needs improvement has been identified in the class, you should not wait until the next class to start correcting it. Work on improving a little each day and by the time the next class comes around, your instructor and training partners will notice an improvement. It feels good to know you are making steady progress!

Another great thing about practicing each day is that it gives you the opportunity to introduce a lot of variety into your training. In my own training, I have days where I train with a group, days where I train with a partner, days where I train alone, days where I'll lift weights, days where I'll practice kata, days where I spar, days where I stretch, days where I hit the bag, and so on. If you are only training a couple of times a week, you simply do not have the time for a diverse training program. Training each day means you will become a well-rounded martial artist and the variety that daily training affords you means that training remains fresh and interesting.

Your daily training does not always have to be physical. Indeed, if you train hard every day, you run the risk of overtraining and that can have a negative effect on your progress. There needs to be a balance between the hard physical training and the days where you recuperate. On the non-physical days, you can still train through visualization, watching an instructional DVD, doing some research on the internet, or reading a book such as this one (you are training right now!). Remember that knowledge is power and all martial artists should attempt to expand their knowledge of their art, techniques, and training methods.

It is very important to train every day. Sometimes that training will last a few hours; other times no more than a few minutes. It will all depend upon what you wish to achieve in any given session and your schedule for the reminder of the day. Personally, I love training early in the morning. It is a great way to start the day and it ensures my daily training does not conflict with other areas of my life. Thankfully, many of my training partners feel the same way about early morning training. Back in the days before I became a full-time martial artist and I had a "proper job," I would start work at 6:30 a.m. Having to rise at 5:15 a.m. there was no way I was getting up any earlier to fit training in before I went to work! I would therefore train during my lunch hour if I was going to be busy in the evening. Whatever your schedule or preference, find some time for training each day. You will be glad you did!

Each time you train you will make a little progress. It therefore stands to reason that the more often you train the more progress you will make. It is no coincidence that all the top martial artists that I know train on a daily basis. If you want to be a skilled martial artist, do what the skilled martial artists do: train each day! If you get into the habit of daily training, you will surprise yourself with how much progress you can make.

– Iain Abernethy [38]

Advancement is a Continuous Process

By following a structure of merit, such as a belt system, instructors have a way of monitoring the development and skill progression of their students and can teach them according to set standards. The structure that has been adopted by most martial arts organizations today involves the wearing of colored belts or sashes. As you might recall, it was originally created in the early 1900s by Professor Jigoro Kano. This *dan/kyu* system distinguishes between advanced practitioners and different levels of beginning and intermediate students.

So how does one achieve advancement along this path? For each rank, there is generally a predefined set of competencies you must master in order to advance. Most instructors explain these requirements ahead of time so that you will know what is expected. In order to demonstrate that you have completed all of the necessary pre-requisites and are eligible for a new rank, you must pass an advancement test. Depending on your instructor or organization, this test may be formal or informal.

With formal testing, time is set aside for students to demonstrate required skills under the watchful eye of their instructors and the rest of the class. Typically, one class session every few months is used for this activity. Many schools keep a set schedule, testing once per quarter. A short promotion ceremony follows the testing to advance those who pass all the requirements. This method makes life easier for instructors administratively, but may be a bit scary for students who only have a few chances per year to achieve a higher rank (though make-up sessions are typically made available for practitioners who are sick or injured on the designated test day).

With informal testing, on the other hand, instructors monitor student performance over time and promote them once they have demonstrated the appropriate level of proficiency for each new rank. At the end of a class session, the instructor will hold a spontaneous ceremony to promote those who have successfully achieved advancement. This method can be somewhat more challenging for instructors to keep track of, though it is frequently less intimidating and preferred by certain students.

While testing among the *mudansha* (colored belt) ranks may be either formal or informal, testing in the *yudansha* (black belt) ranks is often formalized, especially at the *shodan* level when a practitioner initially advances into the *dan* ranks. Once again, your instructor will generally set his or her expectations ahead of time, but you can typically expect a formal test to gain your black belt. If your school is part of a large organization, you will likely be tested by a group of *yudansha* in addition to your own *sensei*, in part to assure quality standards and grading consistency throughout the organization.

Advancement is a continuous process. Regardless of the testing schema utilized, your progress is constantly being observed and evaluated as you train. Instructors not only identify strengths and weaknesses in your ability but also in the effectiveness of their teaching. When it comes to awarding new ranks to recognize your skills, your instructor may choose formal or informal testing for any number of reasons. Here is a bit of the thinking behind how he or she might decide which method to pursue:

Formal testing runs the risk of leading practitioners into a "cram-for-finals" mentality where they practice hard right before testing and then slack off afterward. This attitude may work for a short period of time but ultimately leads to failure at the higher levels where criteria become more exacting and expectations more demanding. Many instructors frown on formal testing for this reason. It is, however, much easier to administer.

Informal testing can facilitate a more holistic approach where practitioners are encouraged to do their best each day in each class with advancements awarded whenever appropriate. This approach is arguably more conventional as well. Many instructors dislike this less-structured approach, however, as it is harder to keep track of administratively. Because large organizations can have student populations that run in the hundreds, it may become impractical to use informal testing.

So which method is better? Neither, really; they are simply different. A good analogy might be traveling from one place to another by bus versus car. Like formal testing, the bus follows prescribed routes and stops along the way. If it arrives at one stop too early, it will wait before proceeding. If it is running behind, it will attempt to catch up. The car, on the other hand, can travel by whatever path the driver wishes to follow. While the journey is somewhat different, you reach your destination either way.

Whether your instructor chooses formal or informal testing, it is a very good idea to treat every practice session as if it were an informal advancement test. Regardless of whether you succeed in everything you attempt on any given day or not, if you are trying your hardest your instructor(s) will surely notice. You will not only learn and advance faster, but you will make the most of every opportunity to train. If you are slacking off, on the other hand, your *sensei* will notice that, too. We are a very observant bunch.

Take Things One Step at a Time

All martial arts are both broad and deep. There is so much information to master, in fact, that martial arts can literally be a lifelong pursuit, a wonderful opportunity if you are optimistically inclined, or an overwhelming obstacle if you are cynical. The word *sensei*, which we typically think of as "teacher," literally translates from Japanese as "one who has come before." Your *sensei* may or may not know everything there is to know about your martial art, but he or she most certainly has traveled much further along the path than you have and will continue to progress over time. Consequently, it is useful to think of your instructor as a guide, someone who can help focus your goals and feed you logical blocks of information that will eventually coalesce into a mastery of your chosen art.

This building block concept is very important because you simply cannot take in everything all at once. No one can. When new martial artists begin their training, they find they must relearn basic concepts like breathing, standing, and walking. You will be taught how to breathe through your diaphragm rather than solely with your lungs, introduced to a variety of uncomfortable stances and foreign postures, and shown how to move in unusual new ways. Balance and coordination take on a new meaning. That is just the beginning. There are a huge number of exercises, techniques, forms, applications, drills, and other mental and physical skills to master. Traditional *dojo* emphasize *kata* (forms) and *bunkai* (applications) while other schools may concentrate more on sparring and tournament competition, yet the fundamental building blocks (e.g., punches, kicks, body alignment, quickness, and power) are the same with either approach.

A complete martial artist gains not only solid fighting skills, superior physical conditioning, and improved mental discipline, but also a broad exposure to the history, language, culture, and traditions of his or her chosen art. Traditional (classical) schools often require exploration of the peaceful arts such as *go* (a board game), *shodo* (calligraphy), *kado* (flower arrangement), and *chado* (tea ceremony) in addition to the warrior arts such as *iaido* (way of the sword), *kyudo* (way of the bow), *aikido* (way of harmony), or *karate-do* (way of the empty hand).

> *"It may seem difficult at first, but everything is difficult at first."*
>
> – Miyamoto Musashi [39]

If your style comes from Japan or Okinawa, for example, you will be expected to learn a variety of words and phrases in Japanese. Similarly, if it originated in China, Korea, Thailand, the Philippines, or any other country, you will learn a bit of one of those languages. See Appendix A for an overview of some common martial arts terminology. Foreign language skills not only facilitate your ability to train at nearly any *dojo*, *dojang*, or *kwoon* throughout the world, but they also impart important subtleties that may be difficult to translate from the native vernacular.

For example, many practitioners are led to believe that defensive techniques, called *uke* in Japanese, should be thought of as "blocks." A more accurate translation of the word *uke* would be "receive," a term implying active ownership. Once a practitioner owns an assailant's attack, he or she may redirect it as needed to put an end to the confrontation, frequently disabling the aggressor in the process. Seen in this light, defensive postures can take on an entirely new meaning, so an understanding of the original Japanese terminology is an important aspect to making the most of the art.

You will also pick up a few useful skills like first aid and injury prevention. After all, if you are going to learn how to "break" someone, most instructors will expect you to be able to "fix" them as well, or at least stabilize the victim until medical professionals arrive (see Chapter 7 for more information). The Japanese term for this is *kappo* (resuscitation techniques). You should also learn ways of using your newfound skills wisely, such as gaining a comprehensive understanding of the legal aspects of self-defense. Awareness, avoidance, and verbal de-escalation skills are emphasized in many *dojo*. After all, the only fight you are guaranteed to win is the one you do not get into. Further, the more dangerous you are the less you should feel a need to prove it, and the costlier the consequences if you do.

As you can see, there is a whole lot of important material to cover. Unlike most tests in the traditional education system, you simply cannot cram for your black belt exam. You can expedite the process, of course, but you cannot master the prerequisites overnight. A black belt is earned through steady, consistent training over a long period of time, typically four to eight years depending on what system you study, how naturally talented you are, the quality of instruction you receive, and how effectively you practice.

Do not let it overwhelm you. Just because you are sitting in front of an enormous buffet does not mean that you must fill your plate. Take small bites, set reasonable goals, and make a concerted effort to internalize one new piece of information each day. Perseverance and consistency are crucial. As time progresses, those little pieces always coalesce into a large and powerful new skill set.

Practice and Learn Every Day

Consistent daily training makes all the difference in achieving your rank. Because there is so much to learn and everything builds from *kihon*, it is important to make a commitment to try to learn something new about your martial art, no matter how small, every day. In order to gain that new piece of information, you will need to practice your art form a little bit each day whether there is a formally scheduled class or not.

No matter how many times a strategy, technique, or application is explained by your instructor, there is nothing like experiencing the concept for yourself to truly understand and internalize it. Consequently, you need to make a commitment to practice on your own rather than just working in class with other students. As you struggle to remember movements of a *kata* or define applications for a technique, you can take real ownership of the knowledge you discover and learn confidence from your achievements.

Many new martial arts students are leery of training independently prior to understanding techniques at an intermediate or higher level. The most common fear is that of "learning it wrong" as most assume that once something has been learned incorrectly it becomes difficult, if not impossible, to correct. To help students overcome this concern and facilitate their ability to progress more quickly, many instructors will assign "homework" to individual students. It might be something as simple as watching television for ten minutes while standing in a particular stance, or hitting a punching bag a certain number of times using a particular technique. This homework is always based on something your teacher feels that you know well enough to practice properly, but for which additional improvement is still necessary. If homework is not given to you by your instructor, assign it to yourself.

Once a pattern of independent training has been established, most students incorporate it into their daily habits. Those who do progress much faster than those who do not. If you really want to earn your black belt as expeditiously as possible, you will need to practice continually, but you must do so effectively as well. Your instructor is your first and most effective source of this knowledge; you cannot know what and how to train without spending time in the classroom. Attendance, therefore, must become a priority.

"Read, every day, something no one else is reading. Think, every day, something no one else is thinking. Do, every day, something no one else would be silly enough to do. It is bad for the mind to be always part of unanimity."

– Christopher Morley [40]

Make Attending Class a Priority

Mastery of any martial art comes from subtle nuances, things like holding correct posture and body alignment, maintaining proper breathing, utilizing efficient movement, and taking the most appropriate angle of attack or defense. Even how and where you look at your opponent is important. Because minute adjustments and minor details differentiate effective from ineffective technique, you really need an experienced instructor to show you the way. While books, articles, and DVDs can help, and independent practice is always important, there is nothing like hands-on instruction to learn martial skills expeditiously. Some things must be not only seen, but also felt.

Attending class regularly is extremely important. Most instructors build a curriculum that assures you will pick up essential foundational material before moving on to higher level information. Without these basics, you cannot hope to understand, let alone master intermediate and advanced materials. Because form precedes speed, and both form and speed are necessary to create power, you cannot afford to miss anything along the way. If you truly want to earn your black belt, you must make regular class attendance a priority. Oftentimes, this means missing clubbing, sporting events, movies, poker nights, blogging, and other optional activities.

You must not only make attending class a priority, but also make the most of your time in class. Instructors cannot be everywhere and help everybody all at once. Frequently you will need to rely on senior students or other members of the *dojo* to help you train. In traditional *dojo*, students bow not only to their teacher, but to fellow students as well, demonstrating that we are expected to gain knowledge from everyone. Students learn from teachers, teachers learn from students, and everyone learns from each other.

Make the most of these opportunities. Diverse perspectives will help you gain knowledge more quickly than relying on your instructor alone. On the downside, however, you may find on occasion that something you learn from another student appears to contradict what you were shown by your instructor. Do not let this interfere with your progress. Martial arts instructors are generally very observant. They will not let you train in an unsafe or incorrect manner for long, yet they tend not to want to overwhelm you with information you are not ready to process, either. A rule of thumb that many instructors use for beginning students is to correct no more than three things per day. If something is bothering you that your teacher has not addressed, file the question away and bring it up with your *sensei* at an appropriate time. Regularly attending class will afford you ample opportunities to solidify your understanding.

> *"By nature, men are nearly alike; by practice, they get to be wide apart."*
>
> – Confucius [41]

Show Up Ready to Go

Focused attention and hard work are paramount if you want to achieve success in the *dojo*. Slacking through a training session not only impedes your own progress but that of your fellow students as well. Your training partners will be counting on you to help them learn and vice versa. If you want to make the most out of each training session, you must show up both mentally and physically ready to participate. Let us start with the mental aspect. Your mind must be clear of distraction, focused like a laser beam on the task at hand, whatever it may be.

Many *dojo* begin and end class with a short ceremony that includes a meditation session. This helps to set an appropriate mood, facilitating practitioners' ability to focus on their training without outside distraction. It helps differentiate between "*dojo* time" and "mundane time," too. Once you begin to meditate, emotional baggage, office politics, sibling foibles, and spousal idiosyncrasies can be set aside, at least for the duration of the training session. Meditation at the end of class not only helps you return to your everyday life, but also to internalize what you have learned in class since your mind continues to process information even after you are done consciously thinking about it.

Mushin is a Japanese term meaning "no mind" or "empty mind," a meditative state. When the mind is not fixed on ego, thought, or emotion it becomes open to everything. By emptying your mind of extraneous thoughts, you are more able to devote yourself fully to your training.

Typically, you will sit in *seiza* (kneeling position), close your eyes, and empty your mind, focusing only on your breathing. Silently breathe in through your nose and out through your mouth. If your instructor does not set time aside for this activity, it may be prudent to do it on your own anyway. Clearing your head before class helps you achieve the appropriate mental state for optimal learning. If you feel uncomfortable doing so in public, spend a few minutes meditating in your car or in the *dojo* locker room before and after class. Either way it will help clear your head and put you in the mood to train.

Now to the physical side: Just as your head must be focused on your training, your body needs to be ready to go, too. After the introductory ceremony, many instructors begin class with a warm-up session that includes stretching and basic calisthenics, though some expect you to arrive early and limber up on your own before instruction begins. Either way, it is good to work a little before class in the *dojo*, or even at home if space is not available, to ensure that you are fully warmed up and ready to go at full speed once the class begins.

Give yourself a physical once-over before heading to class, too. If you have any injuries that may be aggravated by strenuous physical activity, take appropriate precautions and/or limit what you will do in class. Remove any jewelry that might cause damage to yourself or others who may come in contact with it. Things like watches, rings, necklaces, and earrings are hazardous in class. Keep your fingernails and toenails trimmed short so that they cannot accidentally scratch or be torn by anyone. If you have long hair, either cut it short or tie it back so that it cannot easily be entangled and cause injury. Bring appropriate safety equipment, assuring that it is functional and in good repair before you leave. If shoes are allowed, be sure that they are clean and free of rocks, dirt, and other debris that can damage the training room floor or fly into someone's face.

Take care of your physical needs such as diet, exercise, and sleep. If you show up to class with the best of intentions mentally but your physical body is just not able to perform, your training will be suboptimal at best. This generally means maintaining a nutritionally balanced diet, minimizing consumption of alcoholic beverages, and staying away from cigarettes and illicit drugs (see the section titled *Ensure That Your Nutritional Needs Are Met* in Chapter 8 for more information)

Solo Training is an Essential Complement to the Classroom

If you really want to progress as rapidly as possible, you need to be able to effectively train alone. Most practitioners think that training in the *dojo* is fun. Conversely, many feel that training alone is not so good. Not only is there no one around to help you when you are working alone, there is also no one around to help motivate you either. Nevertheless, some techniques are best practiced outside of formal class, especially where you need to focus on improving deficiencies that may not be shared with the rest of the group. Solo practice is an excellent way to reinforce the techniques you are good at as well, not only for making improvement on those areas where you might need more work.

There are a variety of drills and exercises you can easily work on your own. Examples include *kihon*, *kata*, speed training, flow drills, and strength/conditioning exercises. *Kihon* is fundamental for mastering any martial art so that is an especially good aspect to practice at home. *Kata* is the foundation of traditional systems, yet it takes many repetitions to perform these forms smoothly. This is another area that makes a great deal of sense to practice on your own. A few tips for making the most of your independent training time include:

When working *kihon*, you can punch or kick a *makiwara* (striking post), heavy bag, or even perform techniques in the air in front of a mirror. Try techniques like *seiken tsuki* (fore fist), *tate tsuki* (standing fist), *shuto uchi* (sword hand), *shotei uchi* (palm heel), *tetsui uchi* (hammerfist), *uraken tsuki* (backfist), *koken tsuki* (wrist strike), *furi uchi* (swing strike), *hiji ate* (elbow strike), *hiza geri* (knee strike), *mae geri* (front kick), *yoko geri* (side kick), *ushiro geri* (back kick), *mikazuki geri* (hook kick), *mawashe geri* (wheel kick), and so on. Work both your strong side and your weak side. Unless you are ambidextrous, it is a good idea to practice two to three times as many repetitions on your weak side as you do on your dominant side since it will be less coordinated.

Blocks work much like strikes in real-life street fighting, imbalancing and frequently incapacitating an adversary. If you have access to a *muk yang jong* (wooden dummy), you can practice a variety of blocks against a stable target, building power while simultaneously conditioning your arms and legs. Like punches and kicks, defensive techniques can also be performed on a *makiwara*, heavy bag, or in the air. Be sure to work a wide variety of closed- and open-hand applications such as *jodan uke* (head block), *chudan uke* (chest block), *gedan uke* (down block), *harai uke* (sweeping block), *sukui uke* (scooping block), *koken uke* (wrist block), *kakai uke* (hooking block), *hiki uke* (pulling/grasping block), *osae uke* (pressing block), *mawashe uke* (circular or wheel block), *ude uke* (wing block), *hiji uke* (elbow block), *uchi uke* (inside forearm block), *ashi uke* (leg block), *hiza uke* (knee block), *yama uke* (mountain block), *wa uke* (valley block), and so on.

Stances are an essential component of *kihon*. Being able to move and turn while maintaining stance integrity and balance is essential, though not always particularly fun. To spice it up a little you might want to try practicing your punching and kicking techniques from a variety of different stances such as s*anchin dachi* (hourglass stance), *shiko dachi* (sumo stance), *zenkutsu dachi* (front stance), *kiba dachi* (horse stance), and *neko ashi dachi* (cat leg stance), among others. Try it both statically as well as moving. Be sure to use everything you find in your system (typically what you find in your *kata* if your art utilizes them). You can also shadowbox to work on flow or train in front of a mirror to perfect your form as well. Working on stances in ocean surf, swimming pools, and on hilly terrain is beneficial, challenging, and fun.

Maintain your mental focus, performing each technique with perfect form. Ten techniques executed with all your skill are better than a hundred performed haphazardly. Not only are you more likely to become injured with sloppy form, but you will also be reinforcing poor technique. What you do in training will heavily influence what you will do during tournament competitions as well as on the street. If you practice haphazardly, you may well be setting yourself up to lose or become injured when you try to implement your applications against an opponent or training partner.

Working in front of a mirror is an excellent way to learn not to telegraph your blows. Each strike should suddenly explode from chamber at your side (or wherever your starting point is) into your target as fast as possible with no warning. Avoid cocking your arm back; taking a sudden breath; tensing your neck, shoulders, or arms; widening your eyes; grinning; grimacing; or making any other inappropriate movement before each blow. Videotaping your workout can help you identify and avoid these mistakes as well. The best martial artists develop a very effective "poker face" that disguises what they are intending to do when they fight, adding an extra edge in competition and on the street.

Kata are built from *kihon*, logical patterns of movements containing a series of offensive and defensive techniques that are performed in a particular order. The ancient masters hid the secrets of their unique fighting systems within these dance-like movements. Almost all Asian martial systems have *kata* of one type or another, from *arnis* to kung fu, karate to judo, and *taekwondo* to *taijiquan*. While *kata* practice is fundamental to mastering any traditional martial art, it remains a great vehicle for working logical combinations of techniques and movement at mixed-martial-art or tournament-focused schools as well.

For a variety of historical reasons, practical applications and sophisticated techniques remain hidden from the casual observer. There is so much packed into these forms that it is critical to perform them with as much precision as possible. If you study at a traditional *dojo,* you will learn how to decipher combat applications over time. Once you learn how to read your *kata*, you will find that there are almost unlimited applications or *bunkai* hidden within each movement. Applications can even be found *between* the movements of a *kata*. Consequently, you should not limit yourself to practicing only the physical movements of *kata* on your own, but also work on deciphering combat applications.

Practice Any Time, Anywhere

While training starts in the *dojo*, it is never restricted to the *dojo*. In real life you are not likely to be attacked in a wide-open, obstacle-free area while you are already warmed up and wearing your *gi*. Practicing outside the *dojo* on occasion can, therefore, help you realistically prepare for street confrontations. It is very important to understand how you might interpret applications should you be fighting on a hill, around furniture or other obstacles, in a stairwell, under water, in a crowd, or in any other unusual situation. While you need to be able to perform your techniques wearing a traditional loose-fitting *gi*, you must also know the restrictions of your street clothes as well.

You can practice elements of your art just about anywhere. Having said that, however, it is prudent to avoid doing anything in public that might inadvertently provoke a fight, get you arrested, scare your neighbors, or cause other forms of trouble. Wearing your uniform and belt on the street, for example, could certainly invite confrontations. Practicing swordsmanship in a public park is less advisable than doing so in a secluded backyard where you will not appear threatening to anyone. Working *kata* in an empty gym at your health club will generally go over much better than performing the same movements in other venues.

Do not limit yourself solely to physical practice. You can think about your art throughout the day, particularly when you are stuck in traffic, sitting on hold (on the phone), or otherwise not engaged in important activities. Visualize techniques, analyze applications, and walk through exercises in your mind. Think about strategies and tactics for succeeding in self-defense scenarios and tournament situations.

Training should never be restricted to the obvious either. You can practice stances and balance in moving transportation (e.g., airplane aisles, boats, trains, buses), do breathing exercises in the shower, perform calisthenics in front of the TV, or practice *kata* in your living room. Think up creative ways and places to train. The possibilities are nearly endless. Varying your routine will help you stay focused and motivated to learn.

"Once a form has been learned, it must be practiced repeatedly until it can be applied in an emergency, for knowledge of just the sequence of a form in karate is useless."

– Gichin Funakoshi [42]

Take Advantage of Every Opportunity to Learn

Just because someone has earned a black belt does not necessarily guarantee that person will be any good at teaching. Furthermore, even if your *sensei* is a fabulous instructor that fact alone does not necessarily guarantee that he or she can teach your learning style and meet all your educational needs more effectively than everyone else in the world. Take advantage of every opportunity to learn from everyone in your class, not just your instructor.

Ask others how they see things. Because people learn and process information in a variety of different ways, the odds are good that you can find someone in your class who has unique insight into resolving whatever challenges you are currently experiencing or difficulties you are about to encounter. Diverse perspectives can be valuable. We have stumbled across epiphanies in our training simply by talking about issues and practicing techniques with a variety of knowledgeable people.

Tandem drills (e.g., *bunkai, kumite, randori*) are nearly impossible to perform on your own, so soliciting a training partner to work with outside of class can be very helpful. Work one-on-one with classmates or instructors, and participate in extra focus sessions whenever they become available. On the street, sane individuals simply do not pick fights with people they are convinced they cannot beat. Consequently, it is extremely important to train with partners who are bigger, stronger, and/or more skilled than you are whenever you have the opportunity. Working with practitioners who are taller, shorter, older, younger, or stronger than you are helps you train for any real-life possibility. Unlike tournament competitions, street combatants are not segregated by size, weight, age, gender, or rank.

On occasion, look for opportunities to take seminars, participate in tournaments, and work with folks outside your *dojo*. These opportunities can help round out your training, but be sure to check with your *sensei* beforehand to understand the etiquette for handling these situations. Your teacher will help ensure that you are capable and prepared before attending.

Another excellent learning opportunity is the chance to teach. You clearly cannot teach effectively without in-depth knowledge of your subject matter, so preparing to teach others helps you internalize the material and develop a deeper understanding of the techniques you will instruct. *Sensei* frequently ask

"The principal basis for karate's world-wide popularity is the 'anytime, anywhere, anyone' principle. Simply put, the practice of karate knows no limitations; there are no time, place, age, or gender restrictions. One can train any time, any place, with anyone, or even by one-self. Moreover, one can practice for fitness, self-defense, recreation, competition, character development, or personal discovery."

– Shoshin Nagamine [43]

Advice for New Students

by Wim Demeere [44]

If there is one key attribute you need to achieve your black belt, it is consistency. Depending on which art you train in, getting to the black belt exam can take from two or three up to seven or eight years. In some systems, it takes even longer than that. How regularly you train throughout those years determines the outcome of that exam because, unlike school exams, you cannot cram for a black belt test.

Performing complex physical motor skills, applying techniques against an opponent, learning forms so well you know them by heart, and so much more are in the curriculum of virtually any martial art. Getting these things right is a never-ending process, one you must work at all the time with progress coming slowly but surely throughout the years. Sure, you can be a slacker for years and train several hours every day a month or two before the big test. You will surely be a better martial artist than before if you take this approach yet, whatever skill you get that way pales in comparison to training consistently for years and then increasing your training regimen to prepare for the big test.

Training consistently also makes the test easier. By the time you must take the test, you have ingrained the techniques in your subconscious mind so much that they are more likely to come out under the stress you invariably feel during such a test. Because you trained them regularly over the years, the techniques and forms have become like old friends; you know them and their specific traits inside and out. Without consistent training, they remain mere acquaintances you perhaps know up to a certain point but a large part of them remains a mystery. Chances are high that finding out about these mysterious parts during the test leads to embarrassing or even painful results. Instead, make them old friends by the time you step on the mat to get your black belt. Just like real-life old and dear friends, they will be there for you when you need them.

higher-ranking students to lead portions of a class (e.g., *daruma*, *kata*, *kiso kumite*, or *kata bunkai*). Additionally, senior students are usually required to practice with their juniors from time to time, helping them advance their skills. This also helps instructors ensure a productive classroom environment by accommodating a variety of skill levels simultaneously, making efficient use of class time, and optimizing the amount of personal attention that the instructor has with each student.

Do Not Overdo It

We have spent this entire chapter telling you to train every day, even if only for five minutes at a time. While every bit of this aforementioned advice is valid, it is equally important to remember that you are striving to earn a black belt, not to join a monastery, shave your head, and become a *Shaolin* monk. Unless you are dedicating your whole life to martial arts, it is critical to balance work, family, religious, and social commitments along with your training. Frankly, it is simply not healthy to live in the *dojo* every waking hour of the day. Overtraining can be just as detrimental as undertraining. Commit yourself to daily practice but not at the expense of your work or school, your health, your family, or your friends.

"Every day you may make progress. Every step may be fruitful. Yet there will stretch out before you an ever-lengthening, ever-ascending, ever-improving path. You know you will never get to the end of the journey. But this, so far from discouraging, only adds to the joy and glory of the climb."

– Sir Winston Churchill [45]

Student Perspective (by Irene Doane)

I began looking over four years ago, and was fortunate to find a school where the instructor's goal was not to make black belts, but to teach karate. I did not understand the importance or even the difference then, but this played an important role in forming the foundation of my study. Another piece of good fortune was that there were many high-ranking students in the class who willingly shared their knowledge and workout time with new students. Their unselfishness was invaluable to my growth and progress.

I observe a lot. Much learning, perhaps most, is gained by careful observation of what is going on in the dojo. *When high ranks do* kata, *I watch them. I select one specific thing (e.g., foot movement) to focus on. It is amazing how much I learn and correct by doing this. I observe the best students—what are they doing? They watch, they practice, they listen, and they hardly speak. I watch other students during* bunkai *to determine why a technique works or not. Is it body placement, timing, distance, etc.? By seeing and understanding why things work, it helped me see where I needed to make my own corrections.*

I made several rules for myself early in my training, all of which I still employ:

- *Never speak when higher ranks instruct*
- *Always take others' corrections as my own*
- *Emulate the best students*
- *Train hard*
- *Practice* kata *daily*

When something particular seems not quite right, I work on it at home until it improves. I make it a point to do each kata *at least once every day, and oftentimes I employ a drill which requires me to begin and end on the same point, and must do it three times in a row before I proceed to the next* kata. *By breaking down the movements, I see exactly where my stances are off. I also envision real opponents when I do* kata, *a great mental drill. It is the easiest and most thorough way to learn the "official" interpretation, rather than "cramming" before a promotion test.*

As I have progressed, I now teach several classes. Teaching provides yet another facet to learning. One cannot effectively teach without knowing your subject, and there is nothing like teaching to identify those areas in which you fall short. It is in the basics which lays the foundation and strength of any art.

My sensei *has told me, "I empty myself of all that I have (to my students) that I continually grow to be full." This teaches me not to hold back, but rather it forces me to challenge myself to understand more, seek out more, practice more.*

– Irene Doane [46]

Summary

Martial arts are both broad and deep, covering far more information than anyone can learn at one time. Mastery occurs slowly, building highly complex knowledge, skills, and abilities from fundamental building blocks and foundational materials. These building blocks are laid out logically in a predefined set of competencies that must be mastered at each stage of development so that practitioners can advance from rank to rank.

Consistent daily training makes all the difference in achieving new ranks expeditiously. It is important to make a commitment to practice your art daily, trying to learn something new, no matter how small, with each practice session. This training begins in class, but should never be restricted to the *dojo*. Solo practice, seminars, and other opportunities to train and teach can help practitioners learn and advance more quickly. Do not limit yourself solely to physical practice. You can also think about your art throughout the day, visualize applications, and exercise your mind.

Something to think about:

Practice should never be limited solely to physical training. Think about your art throughout the day, particularly when you are stuck in traffic, waiting on hold, standing in line, or otherwise not engaged in important activities. Visualize techniques, analyze applications, and walk through exercises in your mind. Think about strategies and tactics for succeeding in self-defense scenarios and tournament situations.

Action Plan

• Make a commitment to attend regularly scheduled classes in the *dojo*. Show up on time, mentally and physically prepared to participate and learn.

_____

_____

_____

• Know your advancement requirements, setting reasonable goals for internalizing this material. Make a concerted effort to learn one new piece of information, no matter how small, each day.

_____

_____

_____

• Develop a solo training routine to supplement your classroom instruction. A variable, interesting routine will help you stay focused and motivated to learn. Even when you cannot physically practice, think about your art throughout the day when your mind is not otherwise engaged in important issues.

_____

_____

_____

• Look for additional chances to learn, taking advantage of focus sessions, training partners, seminars, tournaments, and similar opportunities. Training with a diverse set of practitioners can provide valuable insight into all aspects of your art.

_____

_____

_____

• As you advance into the higher *kyu* ranks, look for opportunities to teach. Preparing to teach others helps you internalize the material and develop a deeper understanding of the techniques you will instruct.

_____

_____

_____

• Take care of yourself. Eat a healthy diet, exercise regularly, and get enough sleep. Minimize alcohol consumption and stay away from cigarettes and illicit drugs.

_____

_____

_____

Suggested Reading

Christensen, Loren. *Fighter's Fact Book: Over 400 Concepts, Principles, and Drills to Make You a Better Fighter.* Wethersfield, CT: Turtle Press, 2000.

This book is an all-encompassing collection of useful training information. The drills, principles, concepts, and exercises will improve your martial skills no matter what style you practice. There are quick and innovative ways to improve your punching, kicking, sparring, and self-defense skills along with dozens of tips to work fundamental areas like speed, power, and flexibility.

Christensen, Loren. *Solo Training: The Martial Artist's Guide to Training Alone.* Wethersfield, CT: Turtle Press, 2001.

If you really want to progress as rapidly as possible, you need to be able to effectively train alone. This excellent book provides numerous tips, techniques, and exercises to get the most out of your solo training. It is chock-full of useful tips you can implement right away to improve your performance in any martial art.

Christensen, Loren. *Solo Training 2: The Martial Artist's Guide to Building the Core for Stronger, Faster and More Effective Grappling, Kicking and Punching.* Wethersfield, CT: Turtle Press, 2005.

This book offers an outstanding follow-up to *Solo Training*, sort of an advanced solo training manual. It is even better than its predecessor is, though there is very little overlap so it is useful to own both books. There are exercises to develop functional fighting strength in every part of your body. Most of these can be done alone though some require a partner. Some require training aids (e.g., weights, Body Opponent Bag) while others do not. There are some useful icons throughout that call your attention to cautions (i.e., extra care items), workout tips (i.e., critical information), important information (i.e., reasons behind the drills), partner drills, and training tips (i.e., techniques you can focus on for maximum impact). These icons make it easy to reference important information after you read it the first time.

Kane, Lawrence and Kris Wilder. *The Way of Kata: A Comprehensive Guide to Deciphering Martial Applications.* Boston, MA: YMAA Publication Center, 2005.

The ancient masters developed *kata* as fault-tolerant methods to preserve their unique, combat-proven fighting systems. Unfortunately, while the basic movements of *kata* are widely known, the principles and rules for deciphering advanced practical applications and sophisticated techniques are largely unknown. Once a great mystery revealed only to trusted disciples of the ancient masters in order to protect the secrets of their systems, the theory of deciphering *kata* applications (*kaisai no genri*) is illuminated in this groundbreaking book. The site unveils these methods, not only teaching you how to analyze your *kata* to understand what it is trying to tell you, but also helping you to utilize your fighting techniques more effectively—both in self-defense and in tournament applications.

Recommended Web Sites

Iain Abernethy's Web site (www.iainabernethy.com)

A content-rich site for anyone looking to understand practical applications of *kata bunkai*, this information is very useful for all traditional practitioners, regardless of style. It includes some excellent free content such as articles and an interactive community forum, as well as books and DVDs for sale. The forum is an excellent resource to discuss training tips, drills, techniques, principles, and other martial arts fundamentals with knowledgeable practitioners throughout the world. Abernethy publishes audio and video podcasts and an interesting blog too.

Loren Christensen's Web site (www.lwcbooks.com)

LWC Books is a distributor of hard-to-find, unique books and videos for martial artists, people concerned about their personal safety, military personnel, and law enforcement officers. You can find free articles and dumb crook stories as well as purchase books and DVDs by a variety of martial artists, including *Sensei* Christensen himself.

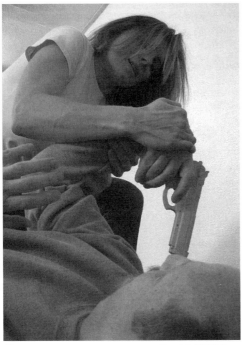

THE STRATEGY OF THE GUN IS THE ABILITY TO AVOID CONTACT WITH A VICTIM, STRIKING FROM A DISTANCE. HERE, THE TABLES ARE TURNED.

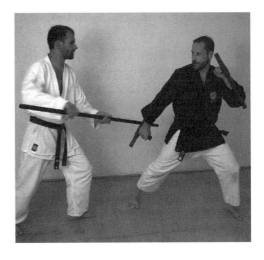

THE *BO* (STAFF) WORKS BEST IN LONG-RANGE WHILE THE *TONFA* IS SHORT RANGE WEAPON. ONE SAYS, "STAY AWAY FROM ME," WHILE THE OTHER SAYS, "I MUST CLOSE THE DISTANCE." THESE BASIC STRATEGIES DICTATE THE TACTICS OF EACH.

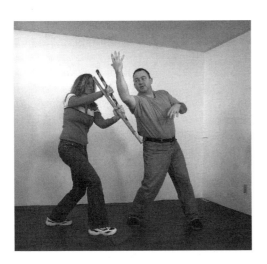

STRATEGY; HIT WITH THE STICK, AND NOW SHE HAS TWO. THE GUY IS CLEARLY AT A DISADVANTAGE, UNLESS HE CHANGES HIS STRATEGY.

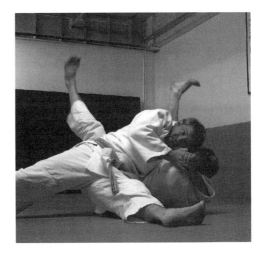

"TO THE GROUND AND UNCONSCIOUS" IS THE STRATEGY. THE TACTICS ARE HOW THAT HAPPENS. IN THIS INSTANCE, A HIP THROW AND A CHOKE CAN GET THE JOB DONE.

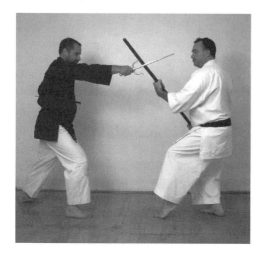

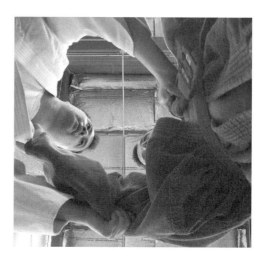

METAL VS. WOOD/SHORT RANGE VS. LONG RANGE. EACH HAS INHERENT ADVANTAGES AND DISADVANTAGES.

TO THROW SOMEONE TO THE GROUND WITH IMPETUS, YOU MUST CONTROL DISTANCE AND DISRUPT BALANCE WITH PERFECT TIMING. GRIPS HELP DETERMINE THE TYPE OF THROW THAT MAY SUCCEED.

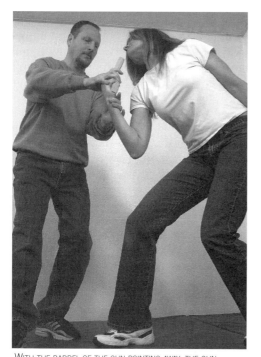

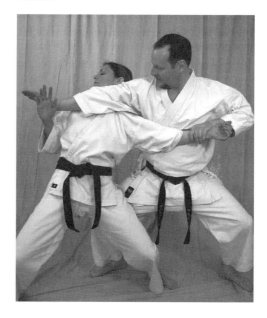

WITH THE BARREL OF THE GUN POINTING AWAY, THE GUN BECOMES VIRTUALLY USELESS. HOWEVER, A FEW INCHES ONE WAY OR THE OTHER AND THE GUN REMAINS A DEADLY THREAT.

GETING CLOSE AND THROWING YOUR OPPONENT TO THE GROUND IS ONE TYPE OF STRATEGY. STANDING OFF AND STRIKING FROM A DISTANCE IS ANOTHER. IF THE TACTICS AND STRATEGY ARE MISALIGNED THE APPLICATION WON'T WORK. WHEN THEY COME TOGETHER IN HARMONY, HOWEVER, THE EFFECTS CAN BE DEVASTATING.

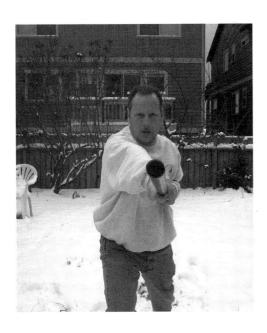

LIKE A PREDATOR ANIMAL, THE END OF A *BO* (STAFF) IS VERY HARD TO SEE. A THRUST FROM THE *BO* COVERS A LONG DISTANCE VERY FAST. STEALTH AND SPEED ARE A POWERFUL COMBINATION.

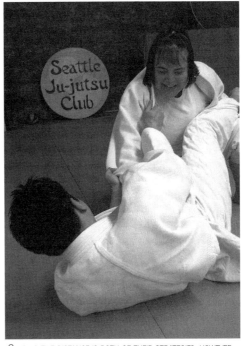

CLOSING THE DISTANCE IS BOTH OF THEIR STRATEGIES; HOWEVER, ONLY ON THEIR OWN TERMS. HE IS FIGHTING FOR ADVANTAGE AND SHE IS FIGHTING TO CLOSE.

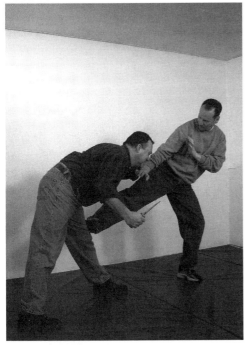

KNIFE! GET AWAY! GET DISTANCE, AND DO IT FAST.

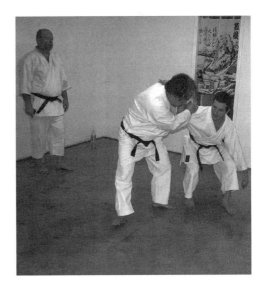

A BROKEN ARM, SEPARATED SHOULDER, AND A FAST COMING FACE-PLANT INTO THE GROUND. THIS IS AN EXAMPLE OF NOT AFFORDING THE OPPONENT ANY OPPORTUNITY TO MAINTAIN CONTROL.

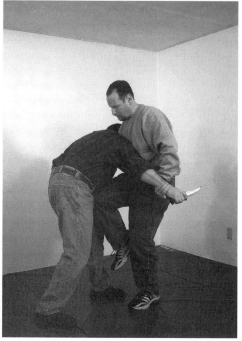

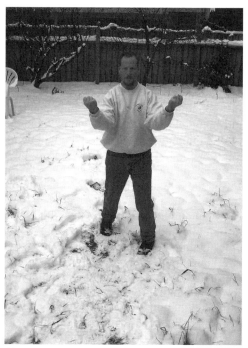

GET HIM DOWN, NOW! TAKING ON AN ARMED ASSAILANT WITH-OUT A WEAPON IS PROBLEMATIC AT BEST. PRACTICING WITH A RUBBER WEAPON AND A PADDED FLOOR HELPS PRACTITIONERS FIGURE OUT WAYS TO DISABLE AND DISENGAGE AS QUICKLY AND SAFELY AS POSSIBLE.

UNDERSTANDING THE *SANCHIN* BODY MECHANICS LEADS ONE TO UNDERSTAND THE MOTIONS OF THE SYSTEM. WHAT TYPE OF BODY DOES YOUR ART REQUIRE OF YOU?

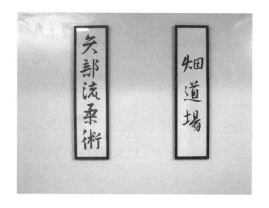

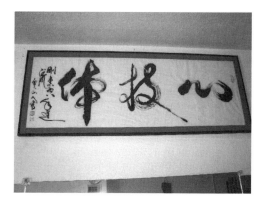

THE NAME OF A SCHOOL AND/OR SYSTEM IS FREQUENTLY DIS-PLAYED IN A TRAINING HALL. TRADITIONAL STYLES CARRY FORWARD A RICH HISTORY THAT, ONCE STUDIED, CAN HELP YOU UNDERSTAND THE STRATEGY AND EVOLUTION OF THE STYLE.

FROM A TRADITIONAL KARATE, THE *KANJI* (JAPANESE CHARACTERS READ, *SHIN GI TAI*, WHICH TRANSLATES AS "TO HAVE A FIRM OR TAUGHT BODY."

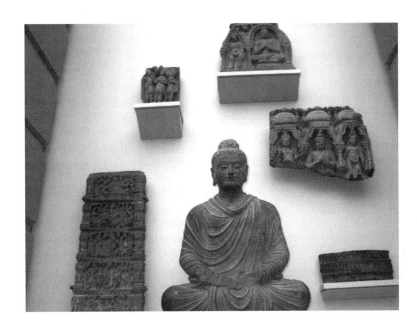

MANY EASTERN MARTIAL ARTS LAY SOME CLAIM TO A LONGSTANDING
PHILOSOPHICAL BACKGROUND. THIS HELPS CREATE A WELL-ROUNDED PRACTITIONER.

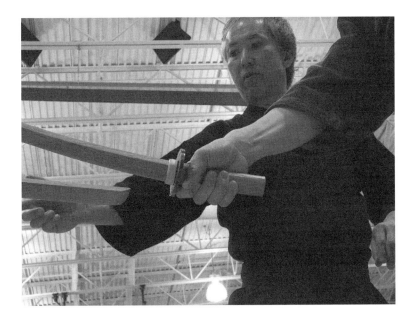

GRIPS, TIPS, SLASHES AND THRUSTS ALL COME INTO PLAY WITH A SWORD NO MATTER ITS CULTURE OF ORIGIN.

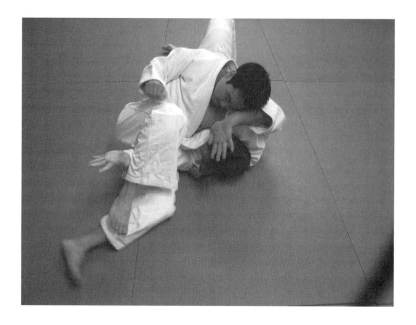

SLOWLY GAINING THE ADVANTAGE PIECE BY PIECE LIMB BY LIMB. PATIENCE
AND PERSEVERANCE ARE IMPORTANT FOR CONTROLLING AN OPPONENT.

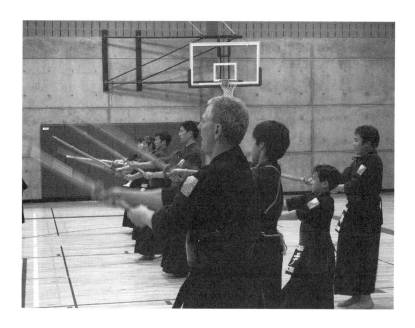

MIYAMOTO MUSASHI, ARGUABLY THE GREATEST SWORDSMAN WHO EVER LIVED, SAID THAT THERE IS A DIFFERENCE BETWEEN A CUT AND
SLASH AND THAT ONE NEEDS TO KNOW THE DIFFERENCE. INTENT IS AN IMPORTANT PART OF STRATEGY AND TACTICS.

CHAPTER 6

Understand the Strategy to Master the Tactics

"When you truly understand the Way, you can take any form that you want to. It is almost as if you had developed miraculous powers. You can become as light as a feather, as fluid as water, or as stiff as a board. Regardless of the form you take, once you have understood my strategy you cannot be beaten by one man or ten thousand. Once you have understood my strategy you will be a warrior to be reckoned with."
– Miyamoto Musashi [47]

Introduction (by Rory Miller)

Like most martial artists, my first art was a matter of luck. Without any real idea beyond books and movies of what a martial art was, I joined the first martial arts class I found, the judo club at Oregon State University (OSU). It was a very lucky choice. Wolfgang Dill, a professor at OSU, was a former member of the German National Team. Mike Moore, who taught the day-to-day classes, was a former junior national champion. These were guys who lived for judo, they ate it like it was candy and they formed me into one of them—a martial arts addict. We had a running joke that you could take out the whole OSU judo team if you just waited to catch us after practice when we were too tired to stand without help.

This was martial arts, baby! As I grew and expanded, judo was always my foundation. When I discovered jujutsu, *that art became my core. Nine-and-a-half years after my first judo class, when I walked into a Maximum Security jail on a new career path as a corrections officer, my core and my foundation served me very well. I knew how to move a body. I knew how to put a bigger man on the ground. I did not need much room or space and did not panic at being grabbed. Standing, rolling around on the concrete, or flying through the air was all the same to me. To stumble upon a school with excellent instructors where the skills were applicable to a position I would find myself in a decade later was nothing but blind luck.*

Like too many beginning martial artists, I would not have recognized a quality instructor or real fight experience if it had bit me on the ass. Steeped in movies and books, anyone with a twelve-dollar strip of black cloth around their waist could have told me or taught me anything and I would have believed it. Because I was lucky, I started with quality instructors who taught me how to recognize other good instructors.

Forward another seven years—a new sergeant, teaching officers how to stay alive and leading a tactical team. All our sergeants are required to be trained in the Incident Command System (ICS), the universal template for emergency response. ICS is based on a strategic "goals backward" model of problem solving: What needs to be done? What do you need to get it done? Gather what you need, then get it done. The model contrasted greatly with the "resources forward" model that I saw everywhere else.

It seemed that everyone approached problems and life and martial arts thinking, "What do I have and how can I use this to solve problems?" For instance: "I can kick really well and punch. What do I do if someone comes at me with a knife?" "I'm a good grappler and can throw. What do I do if someone comes at me with a knife?"

The strategic template is different. When someone comes at you with a knife, how do they do it? From where? How close? How much warning? What do I need to survive that? Then you go and learn the skills you need.

As I learn more about violence, that knowledge becomes the driving force in my training. It is less and less attractive to collect techniques and try to fit them in or figure them out later. My world is simplified because I know precisely what I am training for.

– Rory Miller [48]

Strategy versus Tactics

Every martial system contains both a strategy, which may be hidden, as well as tactics that can readily be found in *kata* or *bunkai*. Strategy is a plan of action. In martial arts as in war, it is what you do to prepare for engagement with an enemy long before the fight begins. Tactics, on the other hand, are expedient means of achieving an end, in this case defeating an adversary. Tactics are the applications that you see (or decipher), while strategy is the overarching plan that ties them together into a cohesive whole.

Looking at how frequently techniques come up in the various core *kata* of a system can be a good way to ascertain its strategy. Look for patterns that are repeated within and between the various *kata*. Tactics are selected during the heat of battle. Like a house without a solid foundation, tactics without strategy will ultimately fail. The tactics of every combat art were developed within a strategic framework that allows them to work effectively.

Tactical thinking is based around the concept of "if"—"if he does this, I will do that." The challenge is that you simply cannot think of enough ifs to anticipate every conceivable situation. When faced with an unexpected movement during actual combat, your brain will freeze, if only for a brief moment, rendering you temporarily defenseless and vulnerable. If the strategic foundation is strong, on the other

> **Something to think about:**
>
> A strategy is a long-term plan of action designed to achieve a particular goal. It comes from the Greek word *strategos*, a title reserved for military commanders in the Athenian army. Tactics, on the other hand, are expedient means of achieving an end. Everything from stances to breathing, including movement, striking, kicking, grappling, and defensive postures are all directly tied to a system's strategy. Like a house without a solid foundation, tactics without strategy will ultimately fail.

hand, appropriate tactics can be employed automatically without conscious thought, letting you react appropriately to most any situation without hesitating.

A deep understanding of strategy, therefore, is a necessary prerequisite for being able to make the most of any martial art. There are simply too many techniques to apply without knowing the context in which they work most effectively. While most arts cover the entire gambit of punching, kicking, throwing, choking, pressure points, and whatnot to some degree, every art excels at certain areas to the detriment of others. You simply cannot be the best at everything. Karate, for example, is primarily a striking art while judo is primarily a grappling style. Both are effective and both share many of the same tactics, yet their strategies are different.

To appreciate fully how an in-depth understanding of your art's strategy and tactics are vital in a physical confrontation, it is useful to delve a bit into the OODA loop, otherwise known as Boyd's Law.

Boyd's Law

The OODA (Observation, Orientation, Decision, and Action) loop, oftentimes referred to as Boyd's Law for military strategist Colonel John R. Boyd who codified it, is a way of quantifying reaction times in combat. Here is how the OODA loop works. Each party to a physical confrontation (be it on the street or in the tournament ring) begins by observing themselves, their physical surroundings, and their adversary. This takes a quantifiable amount of time which delays immediate action, even if only by milliseconds.

Next each combatant must orient themselves by making a mental image of the tactical situation, building on past experiences to interpolate the current environment before deciding how best to respond. Because it is impossible to process information as quickly as we perceive it, there is also an orientation delay that precedes any action a person chooses to take.

Once a combatant has observed and oriented on the tactical situation he or she can decide what to do to defend him or herself. This decision ultimately takes into account the various factors present at the time of the orientation.

Upon deciding an appropriate response, there is another delay between thought and action. Once again, this delay may only last a few milliseconds yet the cumulative hesitation between each step of the OODA loop can add up. Consequently, a person who can consistently cycle through the OODA loop faster than his or her opponent gains a tremendous advantage.

By the time the slower person reacts, the faster one may already be doing something different so the defensive action is less effective than anticipated. With each cycle, the effectiveness of the slower party's action becomes more and more diminished. Boyd's Law dictates that the aggregate resolution of these cyclic episodes will eventually determine the outcome of a conflict. In other words, he who moves through the OODA loop fastest, wins. Consequently, it is important to find ways of minimizing how long it takes to go from observing your adversary to acting in a manner that thwarts his or her aims.

Hick's Law

Hick's Law states that response times increase in proportion to the logarithm of the number of potential stimulus-response alternatives. That is a fancy way of saying that the more choices you have available, the longer it takes to make a decision. That may seem rather self-evident at face value, but it is a point that many martial artists only learn the hard, painful way after getting beat (or beat down). While you may know and even practice hundreds of techniques in your martial training, a limited subset is required in self-defense or tournament situations.

This goes back to the value of deeply understanding your art's strategy. During the OODA loop, the orientation and decision flow time will be adversely affected if you think too much, ultimately leading to disaster. When the strategic context is strong, however, you eliminate the propensity to over-think. Once you understand your chosen art's strategy and discover that it is sound, it is imperative that you follow it. Because all tactics are built around this strategy, failure to follow it will almost certainly lead to failure in practical application.

The Decision Stick

So, if the combatant who cycles through the OODA loop the fastest has the best chance to win, and if the more choices you have the longer it takes to make a decision, it makes sense to focus on a minimal set of fault-tolerant techniques that can be adapted to almost any situation. That is where the power of knowing your martial art's strategy comes in. Once you truly understand the strategy, the tactics become much easier to implement and you are more likely to do so successfully.

Rory Miller, who wrote the introduction to this section, has been personally involved in more violent encounters than most people can conceive of, significantly over 300 documented altercations. He leads an Emergency Response Team in a corrections facility, kind of like a S.W.A.T. team to handle situations where inmates get out of control. When asked about how he has survived so many encounters unscathed, he talks about having a "decision stick."

So what is a decision stick? Let us start by defining what it is not: Those who work in the business world are probably familiar with the "decision tree." Decision trees are excellent tools for making financial or number-based decisions where much complex information needs to be taken into account. They provide an effective structure in which alternative decisions and the implications of taking those decisions can be laid down and evaluated. They also help analysts and mangers form accurate, balanced pictures of the risks and rewards that can result from a particular choice.

The decision tree is a tool that helps map problem resolution processes. Each action one proposes to take follows a different branch of the tree until the problem is resolved. While it may be a good analytical tool, the decision tree is not really designed for quick action. A decision tree creates a complex matrix that involves (metaphorically) time, space, height, and width with every branch on the tree. It works only when you have time to map out decisions before you make them.

In a fight, you do not have that luxury. Decisions—often life-or-death ones—must be made in an instant. If you do not have time to use a decision tree, you must use a decision stick. This "stick" represents a limited set of choices or preferred techniques that you can apply in self-defense situations. Compared to a decision tree, of course, the decision stick offers an extremely narrow set of choices. That is exactly what you need in the heat of battle. You must be engaged in the moment of now.

Part of the success of using the decision stick theory is to choose an appropriate application and let your opponent do what he or she will. That is how Rory has survived so many violent encounters without harm. Proper techniques do not rely on specific actions from your opponent. A good head block, for example, works just as well against a left-hand punch as it does versus a right-hand one. In one case such as right arm to right arm contact, it might close down your opponent, redirect his or her energy, and set you up to counterstrike. In the other such as a right arm to left arm scenario, it might work like a counter in and of itself, as you can get inside the opponent's blow, opening him/her up, and strike his or her head with your forearm. Either way, you successfully defend yourself from harm.

These techniques do not try to second-guess what an enemy will do. They do, however, anticipate expected physiological reactions (e.g., turning the head away from a poke to the eye) as you progress from one technique to another. Stick with your art form's strategic framework, selecting applications that naturally fit your style and physical abilities.

Strategy and Tactics in Action

Almost all of the martial arts we might choose to learn today have been around for a very long time. They have been tested in actual combat throughout the ages. Consequently, if you apply them correctly they are very fault tolerant. It is not just the modern martial styles that work this way. Warrior arts throughout history have been built around solid strategic foundations. Here is an example: by the height of their empire, Rome's legions (*legio*) had conquered much of the known world. A large reason for their amazing success was a solid strategy on which everything else was built. The core of that strategy was, at its most basic level, based on discipline and unity.

Professional foot soldiers formed the vast majority of the Roman army at that time. These soldiers trained specifically for close-quarters combat. Though the exact formation and structure of the legions varied depending upon the time period one examines, each division of soldiers—*century* (about 80 men), *cohort* (about 480 men), and *legion* (about 5,240 men)—had its own battle standard. Though used primarily to facilitate command and communication, battle standards also helped to preserve the cohesiveness and pride of each unit, as they represented a concrete symbol of that unit's achievements and were also used in various religious rituals designed to promote unity. The most important standard in each legion was the legionary eagle made of a precious metal (usually silver), a potent symbol of the power of Rome and the honor of the legion. In wartime, officers called standard-bearers (*signifer*) held these battle standards. These individuals stood out from other soldiers by the animal-head skins they wore on their heads.

> *"A man who does not plan long ahead will find trouble right at his door."*
>
> – Confucius [49]

Just as the military structure of the legion was designed to promote discipline and unity, so too was the equipment the troops were issued and tactics they deployed. Each foot soldier was given a very short thrusting sword (*gladius*), a large shield (*scutum*), a couple of javelins (*pila*), and at least minimal armor (covering much of the head, torso, forearms, and shins). When fighting, they threw their *pila* to disrupt an enemy, picking off easy targets, and then closed ranks to engage in carefully orchestrated hand-to-hand combat. In close-quarters range, they were trained to attack the nearest enemy soldier diagonally across from them, thrusting through the small gaps between their interlocked shields. Roman soldiers almost never aimed for an enemy combatant directly in front of them, relying instead on their fellow warriors to handle that threat.

> *"Wing Chun's* origins are in the cramped, tight alleyways of Hong Kong where side-to-side mobility was significantly hampered. This art excels under those conditions. The larger movements and low stances of many northern Chinese styles are designed to work in wide-open, more mountainous areas where movement is not as restricted, but footwork can be treacherous and uneven. Whereas, the low crab-like movements of *Hari Mau Silat* are extremely effective in the slick, muddy terrain that occurs during Indonesia's monsoon seasons. Each art evolved to operate with radically different environmental conditions and how they fight reflects that. If you are willing to do a little research you will begin to see the wide scope of the factors that affect the art you study. In the same way that a species evolves for existing in particular conditions, so too will a fighting style."
>
> *— Marc MacYoung* [50]

These short swords and interlocking shields forced the Romans to work together as a unit, each protecting the other. Individual fighting ability counted far less than organization and coordination. They methodically moved forward as a disciplined unit, decimating and trampling their less organized opponents. In this manner, everything in the military structure, equipment, training, and tactics all reinforced the Romans' overall strategy.

Strategy works the same way in the martial arts. Everything from stances to breathing, including movement, striking, kicking, grappling, and defensive postures, are all directly tied to a system's strategy. It is holistic, self-contained, and unique to every art. We will look at some brief examples from both striking and grappling arts to demonstrate in a little more depth how this works.

The Striking Arts

The striking arts are typified by karate, kung fu, and boxing (yes, boxing really is a martial art). The strategy of these forms is to stop an attack as fast as possible by physiologically incapacitating the opponent. In the boxing ring, this would be by delivering a knockout blow. The competitor's strategy, therefore, is to win as quickly as possible to sustain minimal damage in return from his or her opponent. This is not accomplished by hitting the opponent in the arms until they cannot continue to punch back; that would obviously take too long, leaving the competitor vulnerable in return. A more prudent strategy would be to strike the opponent's head, or another vital or vulnerable area, hard enough to make his or her brain stop functioning for a moment.

Put another way, boxing is about going directly to the command center of the opponent's body and pulling the power switch to the "off" position. Watching some of the early fights by former Heavyweight Champion "Iron" Mike Tyson, you can see how a powerful blow to the head ends a fight very quickly, even when competitors are wearing padded boxing gloves. For example, on June 27, 1988 Tyson fought Michael Spinks, the first Light Heavyweight Champion to capture the Heavyweight title, knocking him out at 1:31 of the first round. This fight is often regarded as the pinnacle of Tyson's career. Body blows can work too, of course, but not nearly as expeditiously, hence not the primary target of attack.

The sport of boxing was not always as civilized as you might find your local Golden Gloves tournament. It was, in fact, a martial (warlike) art, retaining much of its violent origins today. The Marquess of Queensberry Rules, established in 1867, have made significant progress in establishing a fair and equal stand-up fight, one that is more or less safe and sane for the competitors. Among other things, it created three-minute rounds with one minute of rest in between, banned wrestling or grappling, outlawed seconds (interference by a third party), and prohibited blows to a fighter who was incapacitated, hanging from the ropes, or down on one knee.

Despite these advancements, some major international medical associations have called for abolition of the sport because of its damaging nature to the body and most significantly the brain. Many boxers experience diminished mental capacity in later years because of damage they received during competition. This state is sometimes called "punch drunk," because the former boxer appears to have many of the symptoms of drunkenness such as slurred speech, slowed reaction time, and the inability to perform everyday tasks (particularly mental ones) successfully.

Karate is similar. As a striking art, its goal is to end a confrontation as quickly as possible for the same reasons that boxers want to end things quickly. The longer a confrontation lasts, in the ring or on the street, the higher your chances are of getting hurt. To paraphrase Bruce Lee, "No fight should last more than three seconds." Bruce Lee created the art of *Jeet Kune Do*, building upon his earlier training in *Wing Chun Kung Fu*. These were both striking arts.

The origins of modern karate can be traced to the island of Okinawa. Sometimes called a "peasant art" because it did not use the swords and other high-end weapons of the era, karate was developed as a means of protection for the average person. Although karate is classified as a striking art, it also uses grappling applications such as joint dislocations, sweeps, and throws. Keeping true to its strategy, however, these grappling techniques are generally followed immediately by a hand or foot strike to finish off the opponent.*

At the most basic level, the strategy and tactics of striking arts can be defined as follows:

- Strategy of striking arts: End a confrontation as quickly as possible.
- Tactics of striking arts: Use concussive force to incapacitate the adversary physiologically (e.g., punches, kicks).

---

* Be cognizant of the legal issues surrounding self-defense and countervailing force before doing something like that on the street though.

The Strategy and Tactics of *Goju Ryu*

To delve a little deeper still, the strategy of *Goju Ryu*, a style of karate, is to (1) close distance, (2) imbalance, and (3) physiologically incapacitate the opponent. Closing distance is a brilliant strategy for unarmed combat. It allows the practitioner to bring all of his or her "weapons" on line, leaving nothing out. In striking range, practitioners are able to punch, kick, or grab. When they move just slightly closer, they can perform a throw, choke, arm bar, or hold. Further, closing distance invades an opponent's personal space, a strategy that can be quite disruptive to those who are not familiar with it.

Happo no kuzushi, the eight directions of imbalance, are utilized by most martial systems to undermine an opponent's stance integrity and body alignment, rendering the adversary momentarily defenseless. Imbalance goes beyond just the body structure, however. Vision, breathing, and movement can be attacked as well. In fact, if any two of the three can be incapacitated, the fight is already won. Further, imbalance can also apply to any of the five senses. Strikes to the eyes, nose, and ears are fairly common. It is very challenging to fight what you cannot see. Moreover, anyone who has experienced a severe ear infection (or even a really bad head cold) knows how hard it is to maintain one's equilibrium when your ears do not work correctly.

Adrenaline rushes through your system in combat, supercharging the body for a short period of time. It increases pulse rate and blood pressure while simultaneously making a person faster, meaner, and more impervious to pain than ever before. Unfortunately it works the same way for both the attacker and defender as well. Consequently, strikes to non-vital areas generally have very little effect. Strikes or grabs to an attacker's vital (anatomically weak) areas, on the other hand can elicit pain, temporary paralysis, dislocation of a joint, knockout, or even death.

Looking at how frequently techniques come up in the various core *kata* of a traditional fighting system can be a good way to ascertain its strategy. These individual techniques are, of course, the tactics that support that strategy. In the twelve core *kata* of *Goju Ryu*, *te waza* (hand techniques) appear about 70 percent of the time. This reinforces the idea that *Goju Ryu* is fundamentally a striking art. Here is how the techniques sort out:

- Hands (*te waza*) ~ 70 percent
- Feet (*ashi waza*) ~ 20 percent
- Throws (*tachi waza*) ~ 5 percent
- Groundwork (*ne waza*) ~ 5 percent

If you drill down through the tactics of *Goju Ryu*, you will find strikes from hands, elbows, knees, or feet to anatomical weak points, attacks to joints (e.g., locks, separations), throws, nerve attacks, and chokes. Each of these tactics supports the fundamental *Goju Ryu* strategy of closing distance, unbalancing, and using physiological damage to incapacitate an opponent.

The Grappling Arts

The grappling arts are typified by judo, *jujitsu*, and wrestling (yes, wrestling is a martial art too). These arts are based on the strategy where both opponents are going to wind up on the ground. From there the battle will be settled by choking, suffocation, submission, or breaking an arm or a leg.

The art of *jujitsu* has its roots with the *samurai* in feudal Japan. As a *samurai* warrior, if you lost your sword on the battlefield, it was important to take your opponent to the ground as fast as possible because to stand in front of an armed opponent with no weapon of your own was an instantaneous ticket to the afterlife. Putting a fully armored Japanese warrior on the ground, on the other hand, quickly leveled the playing field, in essence removing the long-range weapons such as swords and spears from the situation. Dislocations of joints such as the elbow and shoulders while standing or on the ground were favored. The art of *jujitsu* began to grow in popularity as the *samurai* fell from favor during the *Meiji* Restoration. Teaching the grappling arts was a means for an out-of-work warrior with no other skills with which to go on making a living.

Economy of energy, balance, and grace were the outstanding hallmarks of the good *jujitsu* practitioner. Unlike many hard styles, the *jujutsu* fighter was expected to be soft and pliable, winning by appearing to yield. Judo grew out of *jujitsu*, founded by Jigoro Kano in 1882. By removing some of the more lethal or potentially crippling techniques, Kano was able to introduce judo into the police academies and school systems, thus ensuring its survival as both a martial art and a sport. It is even found in the Olympic Games today. Judo follows the same strategic principles as its predecessor *jujitsu*.*

At the most basic level, the strategy and tactics of grappling arts can be defined as follows:

• Strategy of grappling arts: Close with an opponent and take him or her to the ground

• Tactics of grappling arts: Cause the opponent to submit through control techniques (e.g., pins, locks, chokes)

---

* There are some interesting tactical differences, however. For example, classical *jujitsu* generally favors pinning an opponent face down so that he or she can be dispatched as quickly as possible, whereas judo requires competitors be pinned face up so that they might have an opportunity to continue to fight.

To delve a step further, the strategy of judo is to throw the opponent to the ground with impetus, to make him or her submit. This requires closing distance, imbalancing, and controlling an opponent. The rules of the sport of judo assign partial points to falls that require follow-up techniques such as a pin, choke, or arm-lock to complete the submission. If you can execute a full throw, placing the adversary on his or her back while maintaining control of your opponent, you earn a full point, ending the match with your victory.

To achieve this goal, the practitioner needs to initially create or take advantage of imbalance within the opponent. There are many tactics to create imbalance but it is probably best explained in the words of the system's founder: "When the enemy comes welcome him, when he goes, send him on his way." You can think of it this way: when the opponent pushes, you pull; when he pulls, you push. Then using a technique such as a trip or throw, you can use this imbalance to assure the opponent forcefully falls to the ground. The tactics of judo include a huge variety of throws, trips, sweeps, takedowns, joint locks, chokes, strangulations, and holds, among other things.

This strategy and associated tactics can work equally well on the street. Judo champion Kenji Yamada* often says, "The ground hits harder than the fist."

Linkage between Strategy and Training

Because a style's strategy and tactics are inexorably linked, it makes sense that you consider how this might affect other aspects of your training. For example, let us assume for a moment that you have decided to learn *taekwondo*. The name *taekwondo* is composed of three words: *tae* meaning "to strike or smash with the foot," *kwon* meaning "to strike or smash with the hand," and *do* meaning "way" or "path." Loosely translated, the form can be thought of as "the way of the foot and the fist."

It is interesting to note that the word "foot" is called out first; the style has a predilection for foot techniques (as opposed to most karate forms that have a propensity of hand techniques). *Taekwondo* practitioners deliver powerful kicks to defeat opponents, typically from a longer range than many other martial forms. Common applications include *ap chagi* (front kick), *yop chagi* (side kick), *dollyo chagi* (roundhouse or turning kick) *ap hurya chagi* (hook kick), *naeryo chagi* (axe kick), *chiki chagi* (crescent kick), *dwet chagi* (spin kick), and *twimyo chagi* (jumping kick), among others.

In order to be successful in performing the various kicks promulgated by this style, you need to build leg strength while maintaining flexibility. Consequently, your training regimen must focus on stretches that keep you limber as well as exercises that enhance kicking power. As you can see by this example, the strategy of your art affects all aspects of your training.

---

* Yamada *Sensei* began studying judo when he was 13 years old. An active competitor until the late 1960s he won many competitions, including two U.S. national championships. Among his many accomplishments, he received the "Best Technique Award" for his *uchimata* in the All-U.S. Championships in California in 1963. Since his retirement from competition, Yamada *Sensei* has been dedicated to teaching judo at the Seattle *Dojo*, and he continues to share his vast knowledge and experience with his students to this day. He is an 8th *dan* black belt. Wilder earned his judo black belt from Yamada *Sensei* and Kane has taken lessons from him.

Advice for New Students

by Michael Thue [51]

As I have matured as a martial artist, I have come to appreciate that, first and foremost, a committed study of the martial arts is about accumulating the attitude and protection skills necessary to prevail in interpersonal combat. This does not mean that one needs to participate in numerous street fights or no-holds-barred competitions to study the martial arts. Nor is this comment meant to overlook the numerous other non-combative benefits of training.

In his book *Living the Martial Way*, Forrest Morgan wrote, "Where the *bujutsu* practitioner is concerned first and foremost with learning how to prevail in combat, the true *budo* aspirant devotes himself to a system of physical, mental, and spiritual discipline through which he attempts to elevate himself in search of perfection." A common line of thinking I encounter among martial artists is to create an artificial and unnecessary divide between the ideas (as expressed in the Japanese martial arts) of *do*, or "ethical martial ways," and *jutsu*, or "combat" methods.

This disassociation has the unfortunate result that *do* is often mistakenly opposed to *jutsu* in an either/or manner, and not seen more correctly as its complement in true *In/Yo* (or *Yin/Yang*) fashion. Thus, many self-proclaimed "pragmatic" or "reality-based" martial artists believe that one cannot possibly learn anything about practical self-protection in a system using traditional methods or with moral, spiritual, theoretic, or philosophical underpinnings. Likewise, many "classical" or "traditional" martial artists believe that systems focused primarily on combat effectiveness are somehow "just fighting" in a pejorative sense.

As a mature practitioner, I have come to realize that neither perspective could be further from my own experience, or less helpful to the growth of an intermediate martial artist. Instead, what has been more useful in my own growth is to see the ideas of *do* and *jutsu* as inextricably linked, analogous to the integral (yet different) sides of the same coin, the twinned aspects of day and night, or the complementary revolution of the pedals of a bicycle. *Do* is not opposed to *jutsu*; rather, *do* is revealed through a serious and committed study of *jutsu*. If I have realized one thing as a mature practitioner, it is that the philosophical "way" of martial arts lies through combat.

The observant reader will note that I have not said that martial arts are about the accumulation of fighting skills, and at first glance, this distinction may seem contradictory when compared to an insistence upon the combative core of the martial arts. However, my own experience and observation of the so-called "real" thing, has been that most fights are avoidable altercations having more to do with bruised egos and refusal to retreat than actual life or death situations.

Clearly, lifestyle choices, personal associations, and environment are contributory factors that influence a person's chance of experiencing violence, as are numerous other situational specifics left to the reader's intelligence. However, in spite of what you frequently see sensationalized in media, I believe that if a person is truly intent on avoiding violence and is willing to occasionally swallow his or her pride in order to do so, this objective is typically achievable in most civilian situations.

As a practitioner matures, he or she also tends to see fighting skills as a less important dimension of overall training, despite the fact that with competent instruction and hard work, both technical ability and personal understanding continue to increase relatively unabated. Eventually we come to realize (through maturity or experience) that human interpersonal violence is not so much schoolyard fighting, but ugly, potentially deadly, and rife with medical and legal consequences. When this knowledge is combined with a subsequent comprehension of the very real limitations of one's own fighting skills, a thoughtful practitioner will gravitate almost naturally toward developing the "soft" skills like awareness, negotiation, and conflict avoidance that actually provide the real backbone of self-protection.

At a certain point in one's experience, a mature practitioner realizes that no matter how much he or she trains, all fighting skills are extremely fallible, fraught with opportunity for miscalculation and error, and in fact almost certain not to proceed according to plan. Technical fighting skills are therefore correctly categorized by veteran practitioner Iain Abernethy as "what come into play when you are making a complete hash of protecting yourself."

The realization that no amount of martial arts training provides a mythic silver bullet, but instead only increases a practitioner's chances of survival therefore causes an advanced practitioner to approach training with renewed seriousness and self-criticism. A mature practitioner "trains as if his or her life depends on it," because he or she fully comprehends that someday, it might. Training becomes (or should become) focused with pinpoint clarity on the discovery, practice, and habituation of fighting techniques that are above all things effective, regardless of style, instructor, source, or rule.

That fighting skills must be effective to have value in self-protection may seem a bit obvious. However, I am often struck by the naïvely accepting and unquestioning nature of many martial artists I encounter, and the extant parallels between organized martial arts and organized religion. By contrast, the operating paradigm of the mature practitioner becomes instead: question and personally test everything.

This statement should not be seen by developing martial artists as an endorsement to disrespect an instructor or *sensei*, far from it! In fact, just the opposite typically occurs, in that the mature practitioner realizes he or she learns a great deal about what does work by critically studying much of what does not. However, a serious combat orientation to martial training, an accompanying questioning mindset, and a willingness to view instruction critically can only lead a practitioner to eventually conclude that a great many techniques do not work "as advertised"; only work for certain body types; or only work in certain situations for which they are designed, many of which are highly contrived.

It is through such an introspective process of open-minded testing and evaluation that the mature practitioner comes to understand that all styles are artificial constructs attempting to delineate the more universal problem of human combat. Recognizing the combative core of the martial arts is much more than the simple acknowledgement that "there are no superior martial arts," a fact which almost all practitioners arrive at eventually. Instead, coming to the more holistic conclusion that all martial arts—traditional, sporting, and combative—are merely limited individual vantage points from which to consider the larger and more total subject of human combat is an important step in a student's growth and an indicator of developing maturity. Reaching this point of development begins to take the student outside of style and toward the fundamental bedrock of the martial arts.

In order to perceive the overarching combative dimension of martial study, a student must first recognize the overall human dimension of that study. Due to the inherent limitations of the body (in terms of available natural weapons, targets, and physiological reactions), an objective consideration of human combat reveals that there is often much more in common between dissimilar styles and systems than there are differences.* Such a perspective eventually leads an advanced practitioner to a point where an understanding of the underlying principles common to all martial arts begins to synthesize and emerge. It is realized that the "bedrock" of the martial arts is how the human body acts, moves, and reacts—both your own body as well as your opponent's.

Along these lines, I have found two things to be helpful in my own development. First, in the words of Tadashi Yamashita:[†] "*Budo* is always two." At a basic level, this maxim can be seen to mean there is always an omnipresent relationship between a student and his or her instructor. However, at an advanced level, this concept can also be seen as supporting the idea that martial arts—the study of human combat and human motion in combat—cannot be undertaken in personal isolation or through a study of forms alone. Instead, it requires at least one committed training partner, or better, a group of partners that allows the pressure testing and cross-pollination necessary to the development of an advanced martial artist. I have found developing such a peer group of committed training partners to be an indispensable asset in my growth.

Second, and related to this, is the idea that at an advanced level a mature practitioner should begin to "look outside the box" of his or her base style. At an advanced level, studying outside your base allows one to better perceive recurring patterns in human attack; that there are only certain ways that a particular joint or limb can move without injury; or that certain techniques are designed to produce or capitalize on a particular physiological reaction common to the species. It is therefore understood that ultimately, there may be a "correct" method to execute technique X within system Y, but ultimately, another system utilizes a nearly identical body mechanic in a related and equally effective manner to counter the same recurring human self-protection problem. The only "correct" method, therefore, becomes the effective application of that body mechanic in neutralizing or escaping a threat, and the study of individual style (judo, *jujitsu*, karate, *aikido*, and so on) comes to be seen as simply an individual on-ramp to what amounts in the end to a much larger road.

A level of autonomous self-awareness is eventually reached, with the practitioner realizing two critical points: First, that it is ultimately they who are responsible for the effectiveness of their own training and development, not their *sensei, sifu*, or coaches; and second, that ultimately, it is they who are the object of study. When martial arts are understood to be a fundamentally human study at their core, the inherent limitations of any single individual viewpoint become increasingly clear. Because all systems are artificial constructs, the student eventually comes to understand that ultimately, they are the system.

---

* For further discussion of the human principles and similarities between multiple arts, particularly those of Southeast Asia, see Dan Inosanto's *New World of Martial Arts* VHS video tape, available from the Inosanto Academy, Los Angeles, California, 310-578-7773.
† Tadashi Yamashita *Sensei* is a 9th *dan* black belt in *Shorin-Ryu* karate and the founder of *Suikendo*.

Jutsu and *Do*

When trying to find a martial art that fits your goals, you may find significant insight in the name of the art, particularly those arts of Japanese origin. In general, there are two important suffixes that may be attached to the name of the art, *jutsu* or *do*. *Jutsu* is the Japanese term for "technique" or "method," implying that you will learn a combat skill from such study. Examples include *kenjutsu* (methods of swordsmanship), *ninjutsu* (stealth or secrecy techniques), *taijutsu* (methods of body striking), and *battojutsu* (sword cutting techniques).

Do, on the other hand, is the Japanese term for "way" or "path," oftentimes translated as the "ethical ways." It is used as a suffix for a variety of martial and civil arts, or ways, implying that they are not merely a collection of techniques but also contain spiritual elements as well. For example, the martial arts of *aikido* (the way of unified energy), judo (the gentle way), *kendo* (the way of the sword), and *karate-do* (empty hand way) or the civil arts of *chado* (the way of tea ceremony) and *kado* (the way of flower arrangement) all use the suffix "*do*." This convention can found in Korean martial arts as well (e.g., *taekwondo*).

We can readily see how the perspective and beliefs of *do* influence a martial art by examining the development of judo, a relatively modern style that finds its roots in *jujutsu*. Kano *Sensei* added a strict code of ethics and a humanitarian philosophy to his newly created system specifically to transform it from a martial art (*jutsu*) to a martial way (*do*). Instructors and students in his *Kodokan Dojo* were expected to be outstanding examples of good character and honest conduct. Any hand-to-hand combat outside of the *dojo*, public demonstrations for profit, or any behavior that might bring shame to the school could lead to suspension or expulsion from the *Kodokan*.

Martial styles with *jutsu* or *do* are not necessarily polar opposites, but rather might be best considered different sides of the same coin with somewhat divergent focus areas. A practitioner who studies *jutsu* may be looking for pragmatic, street-worthy fighting techniques and find them through his or her art. While etiquette and tradition are not stressed to the same degree as you would find with *do*, that does not necessarily imply that the practitioner will become a thug or bully. Likewise, a practitioner of *do* will also find combative techniques. Because this aspect is not the sole focus of the art, however, it may take a bit longer to acquire the same level of fighting skill as someone who primarily studies *jutsu*. Either way, you will typically find both aspects covered to a greater or lesser degree.

Student Perspective (by Mark Swarthout)

I do not think anyone below first-degree black belt (shodan), or perhaps brown belt (1st or 2nd kyu), really knows what a particular style has to offer. Once you have developed sufficient knowledge and skill to really understand a specific style, then you can start to see what the flaws are in it. Too often I see someone flitting from style to style, trying to take whatever they think is of value. To me, that shows a lack of patience and a lack of true understanding.

Many of us could fix a leaking faucet. Some of us could re-seat a toilet or replace a water tank. But few of us could actually put in all the plumbing in a house. It is not just a physical thing. Any of us has the physical ability to do it. It is an issue of understanding the entire system, and all the rules and laws associated with it and being able to confidently deal with the strange and unusual circumstances. If you stick only to the normal or simple things, you will never learn in depth what it truly takes to be a master plumber. If you flit from the plumber to the electrician to the carpenter and then to the tile-layer after a stop at the cabinetmakers trying to learn all they have to offer, you will never reach your full potential.

I think the same thing is true of a martial artist. You learn how to handle the usual, common, and general situations. But when they get truly unusual and out of the norm, it takes a deeper background then a few bits and pieces learned at a dozen different schools. That is not to say that it is not possible to become both a master plumber and a master electrician. But it is not really likely to happen in the real world.

In my mind, I will always be an apprentice, learning from my master. Perhaps I will become a Journeyman some day, but I do not ever expect to be a Master. I have found my "profession" and will stick to it, hoping to unlock my full potential as a martial artist. Just another reason to see what I can learn about my art from others who practice it...
– Mark "Blackwood" Swarthout [52]

Summary

A deep understanding of strategy and tactics is a necessary prerequisite for being able to make the most of any martial art. There are simply too many techniques to apply without knowing the context in which they work most effectively. Strategy is a plan of action while tactics are expedient means of achieving an end, in this case defeating an adversary.

A practitioner who cycles through the OODA (Observer-Orient-Decide-Act) loop faster than his or her opponent will ultimately prevail in combat. Further, the more choices a person has to make during a fight, the longer it will take to make any decision. Consequently, it makes sense to focus on a minimal set of fault-tolerant techniques that can be adapted to almost any situation. That is where the power of knowing your martial art's strategy comes in. Once you truly understand the strategy, the tactics become much easier to implement and you are more likely to do so successfully.

It is imperative to understand your martial art's strategy in order to use its tactics effectively. For example, at the simplest level the strategy of a striking art such as karate might be to end a confrontation as quickly as possible. Tactics might include concussive force such as punches or kicks that can physiologically incapacitate the adversary.

"Perception is strong and sight weak. In strategy it is important to see distant things as if they were close and to take a distanced view of close things."

– Miyamoto Musashi [53]

Action Plan

• Spend some time researching your martial art. Read up on the art's strategy, history, tactics, and traditions.

_____

_____

_____

• Look for integration between your art's strategy and other aspects of your training such as your strength and conditioning regimen.

_____

_____

_____

• Look for the common glue that puts your tactics in perspective, building toward a "decision stick" that helps you utilize your art on the street or in the tournament ring successfully.

_____

_____

_____

• Do you study a martial art or a martial way? Examine how the philosophical background of your style influences its techniques and traditions. The better you understand your art the better you can utilize it.

_____

_____

_____

Suggested Reading

Christensen, Loren. *Fighter's Fact Book 2: Street Fighting Essentials.* Wethersfield, CT: Turtle Press, 2007.

You will fight how you train, which is the theme of this book; setting you up for success should you ever have to defend yourself in some of the most desperate situations imaginable. Nearly a dozen veteran instructors of street-oriented martial arts have come together with Loren Christensen to teach you how to defend yourself against multiple attackers, violent dogs, knives, close quarter attacks, and attackers impervious to pain. Then they show you how to make your street techniques fast and explosive, and help you prepare yourself mentally to use extreme force should it ever be warranted. Kane and Wilder both contributed chapters to *Fighter's Fact Book 2*, as did many of the guest writers of this book.

Clausewitz, Carl von and J. J. Graham (translator). *On War.* New York, NY: Penguin Books, Ltd., 1968.

Writing at the time of Napoleon's campaigns, Prussian soldier Carl von Clausewitz developed this landmark treatise on the art and philosophy of warfare. Distinguishing between war and politics, he describes not only when war is appropriate but how to assure victory as well.

Lovret, Fredrick, J. *The Way and the Power: Secrets of Japanese Strategy.* Boulder, CO: Paladin Enterprises, Inc., 1987.

This insightful book reveals Japanese strategy in depth, applying examples to both the world of military and business ventures. Each chapter presents a particular strategy, describing the philosophical basis and detailing a number of specific, tactical applications. The topics addressed include such subjects as distancing, timing, centering, momentum, appearances, and initiative, among many others.

Kaufman, Stephen F. *The Art of War: The Definitive Interpretation of Sun Tzu's Classic Book of Strategy.* North Clarendon, VT: Tuttle Publishing, 1996.

Sun Tzu's *Art of War* is perhaps the best-known and highly regarded treatise on strategy ever written. Although its wisdom is thousands of years old, its principles are still relevant for both the boardroom and the battlefield. Thirteen sections present insightful stratagems for large-scale engagements, from how to treat your subordinates to assessing an enemy's strengths/weaknesses to the use of espionage and subversion.

Rosenbaum, Michael. ***Kata and the Transmission of Knowledge: In Traditional Martial Arts.*** Boston, MA: YMAA Publication Center, 2004.

This brilliantly researched tome provides important insight into the history and development of martial arts—both military and civilian. It is more of a textbook than a light afternoon read, yet it provides fantastic insight into the views and ethics of societies that created the fighting forms that many of us practice today.

Thompson, Geoff. ***Dead or Alive, the Choice is Yours: the Definitive Self-Protection Handbook.*** Boulder, CO: Paladin Enterprises, Inc., 1997.

Classically trained in karate, and with years of experience as one of Britain's top bouncers and coolers, Thompson gives you the background and techniques that can make the difference when it comes to fists and feet. The book is first and foremost about how to avoid violent situations. Should you find yourself in one, however, it will also show you how to control yourself and your emotions so you can function on a physical level to defend yourself.

Wiley, Mark V. ***Filipino Martial Culture.*** North Clarendon, VT: Tuttle Publishing, 1997.

The author's thorough examination of the ancient and modern Filipino martial culture is ground breaking, exemplary, and extremely well researched (there are 175 books referenced in the Bibliography). This book is well written and very informative, covering the martial history of the Philippines; the ethos and worldview of the Filipino warrior; structure, rites, and symbols of the indigenous martial arts; typology of weapons; and more. Eighteen masters of the Filipino arts are interviewed, covering *arnis, escrima, kali,* and a variety of lesser-known arts (e.g., *hagibis, sikaran, sagasa,* and *kuntaw lima-lima*). There are some wonderful pictures as well. In 1521, Filipino natives killed the famous explorer Magellan. Learn about the fighting spirit, weapons, strategies, and tactics of these fierce warriors, ancient and modern.

Wilson, Scott William. ***The Lone Samurai: The Life of Miyamoto Musashi.*** New York, NY: Kodansha International, Ltd., 2004.

The author spends the first half of the book chronicling the extraordinary life of Miyamoto Musashi, arguably the best swordsman who ever lived. This portion is intriguing, insightful, and very well researched. The second half covers Musashi's famous *Go Rin No Sho* (*Book of Five Rings*), the strategy he spent the final days of his life writing. One of the best books on the strategy of individual combat ever written, the *Book of Five Rings* is a must read for every martial artist.

Recommended Web Sites

The Clausewitz Homepage (www.clausewitz.com)

The Clausewitz Homepage is edited by National War College professor Christopher Bassford. This fascinating site is designed to help anyone seeking to know more about the life, works, ideas, and impact of Prussian soldier and influential strategic theorist Carl von Clausewitz (1780 – 1831). It includes images, links, bibliographies in several languages, online bookstores, articles, academic papers, military manuals, complete books, and indices to Clausewitz's book, *On War*. Research links can tie you into related historical Web sites, books, and academic studies. This is an excellent resource for military personnel, martial artists, academic researchers, and businesspeople.

The Art of War (www.chinapage.com/sunzi-e.html)

This Web site provides free online access to Sun Tzu's remarkable *The Art of War* in both English and Chinese. The English was translated by Lionel Giles. This is a straight translation without commentary or graphics.

The Book of Five Rings (http://www.samurai.com/5rings)

This Web site provides free online access to Miyamoto Mushashi's outstanding *Go Rin No Sho*. The English was translated by Victor Harris. This is a straight translation without graphics although it does include some commentary and reference links.

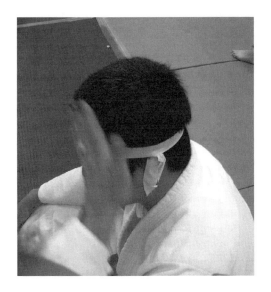

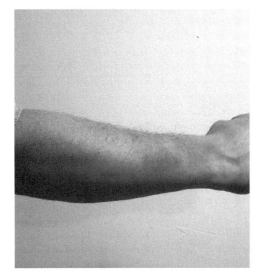

DON'T LET AN INJURY BECOME YOUR EXCUSE TO DROP OUT, BUT RATHER USE IT AS AN IMPETUS TO DO MORE ONCE YOU HAVE RECOVERED.

BRUISES CAN RESULT FROM INTENSE TRAINING.

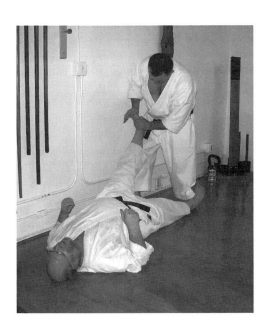

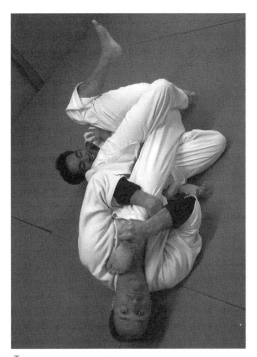

CRAMPING CAN BE PAINFUL. MARTIAL ARTS INSTRUCTORS ARE TYPICALLY TRAINED IN FIRST AID AND RESUSCITATION TECHNIQUES. THEY ARE NOT ONLY RESPONSIBLE FOR ENSURING A SAFE TRAINING ENVIRONMENT, BUT ALSO A FIRST LINE OF DEFENSE WHEN THINGS GO AWRY.

THE KNEES CAN BE VERY STRONG, YET ALSO VERY VULNERABLE IF STRUCK FROM THE PROPER ANGLES. KNEE INJURIES CAN BE EXTREMELY SERIOUS, PERHAPS EVEN PERMANENTLY DEBILITATING, SO IT IS VERY IMPORTANT TO USE CAUTION WHEN MANIPULATING THE KNEE JOINT.

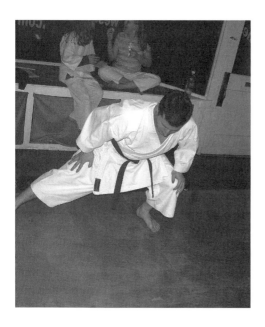

STRETCHING IS AN IMPORTANT PART OF ANY WARM-UP TO AID IN INJURY PREVENTION.

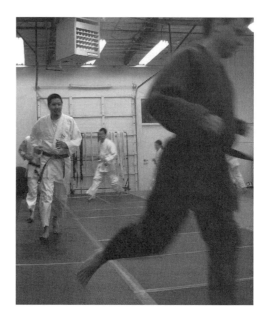

RUNNING IS A GOOD WAY TO WARM-UP, ELEVATING THE HEART RATE AND GETTING CIRCULATION MOVING THROUGHOUT THE BODY.

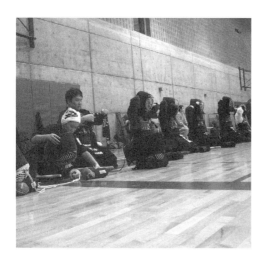

VITAL AREAS OF THE BODY ARE PROTECTED WITH A FACEMASK, CHEST GUARD, GROIN PROTECTOR, AND PADDED GLOVES.

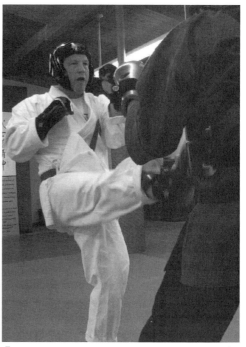

FULL CONTACT SPARRING REQUIRES EXTRA SAFETY PRECAUTIONS. A CHEST PROTECTOR DISSIPATES SOME OF THE FORCE FROM THIS KICK.

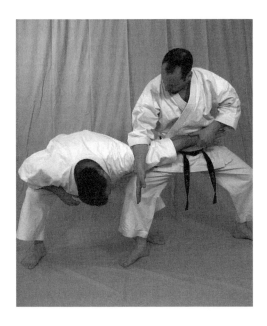

While working a joint technique, you can see the attacker looking for response from the other person. This vigilant attitude makes for good training and keeps everybody healthy.

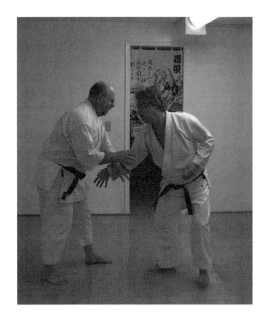

Black belts can work at their own level during self-study, as hopefully, a deeper understanding of technique allows for intensity and safety.

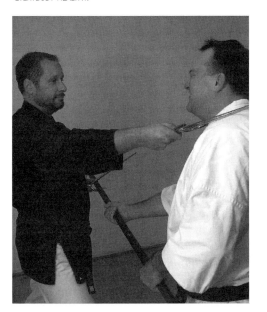

When working one-on-one, especially with weapons, trust is important. These two practitioners have known each other for more than twenty-five years and are confident in each other's skills.

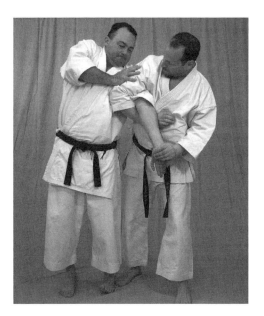

Martial artists often "stress test" the effectiveness of their techniques with a partner. Tapping repeatedly (with the hand or foot) is the international signal for, "Stop." Your partner has yielded; stop immediately before you hurt him.

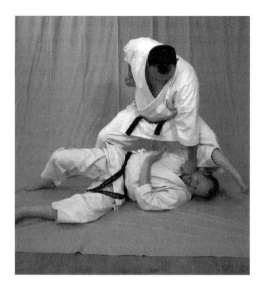

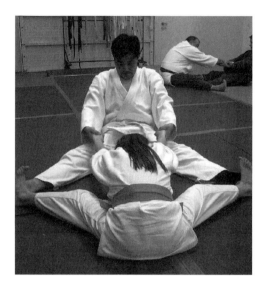

As good as this punch may appear, look again, and see the attacker breaking his fist on his jaw of the opponent with a poorly oriented fist. The strike should have landed with the first two knuckles. Even the smallest things can result in unintended injury.

You may need a special stretch if you are recuperating from a specific injury. A partner can be of great assistance when addressing injury.

CHAPTER 7

Know How to Work Through Injuries

"Healing is a matter of time, but it is sometimes also a matter of opportunity."
– Hippocrates [54]

Introduction (by Wim Demeere)

I had been training for only a few years when Stefan came to my class. He was ex-military and had been turned away by numerous other teachers in his search for a martial arts school. It had been a childhood dream of his to become a martial artist but he had never had the time for it. Now he had plenty of time, but there was just one problem: a tank had run over him during his service, making amputation at the knees the only solution to save his life. Because of his handicap, nobody wanted him in their class except my teacher. Stefan made it clear from the start that he expected to be treated like everybody else, no pampering or watering things down. That meant doing all the forms, techniques, and sparring full contact against his classmates (which included getting axe-or side-kicked by myself and the other students). He trained hard and became a competent martial artist over time, an inspiration to all.

Whenever I have an injury or feel some pain in training, I think of him and how he made his dream come true. Life dealt him a bad hand but he stayed in the game just the same. He found a way to overcome his physical limitations through sheer courage and determination. If a man without legs can do that, I'm sure you can do the same when you sprain your wrist or have a black eye.

On your road to the black belt test, there are many obstacles. Some of the most diffi-cult to overcome are injuries. From bumps and bruises to broken bones and joints, there is a wide range of painful conditions you can encounter in your training. A select few of them invariably mean the end of your martial training. But the vast majority either heal completely or go away or you can find a way to work around them. Dealing with injuries takes a three-part strategy: You need prevention, common sense, and creativity.

Prevention
The best kind of injury is, without a doubt, the one you manage to avoid. In martial arts where you punch, kick, throw, or lock joints on your partner, it is near to impossible

to avoid injuries completely. But you should try to lower the odds of them happening. Here are a few things you can do to that effect:

- *Always do a good warm up and end every training session with a cooling down period. This prevents injuries during the session and helps recovery.*
- *Maintain your flexibility with regular stretching. Having sufficient ranges of motion in all your limbs makes it not only easier to perform the techniques but also prevents injuries.*
- *Get enough sleep, at least eight hours a day, to recover from your grueling workouts. Rest is a key factor in performance so get plenty of it. That includes at least one day off from all forms of physical activity a week.*
- *Eat healthy foods and drink plenty of water. You need to fuel the machine if you want to become a competent martial artist and perform at your best. As sweating is an integral part of training, do not forget to replenish the fluids you lose.*

Though the previous points go a long way in preventing overtraining, you can do even better. It is important to train your techniques over and over to increase your skill. But you should not train them the exact same way every time. Mindless repetitions of straight punches in a horse stance are not enough to develop that punch. Find all sorts of variations to keep it fun. Use different sorts of footwork, work on a different timing, rhythm or speed with it, even try slow-motion, but just keep mixing things up. You then not only perform your techniques better, you avoid overtraining. It is not necessary to do the same repetitions the same way year after year. It is, in fact, counterproductive and leads to overtraining injuries. Instead, challenge yourself to train your techniques and forms slightly (or a lot) differently than the last time you did them.

Common Sense

Pain is a signal that something is wrong. If you become injured during practice, your first priority is to listen to this signal and assess the damage. You must differentiate between a light injury and one requiring medical attention. In short, you must learn when to go see a doctor.

This might not be as easy as it sounds, though. Martial artists are notorious for "toughing things out" and often keep on going when they should not. There is no set of rules that tell you when exactly you should go visit a doctor and when you can get rid of the injury with just a few day's rest. For the most part, you must use common sense. Obviously, when there is blood spurting out of an arm or leg, you need immediate treatment. With other injuries, it might not be so cut and dried when you feel some pain but not that much. Or it mostly goes away after a few days and then lingers for weeks. Interpreting the pain is an ongoing learning process of trial and error.

As you receive small and larger injuries throughout the years, you learn what they feel like. Remember how you treated them last time and what the result of that treatment was. When you have an injury similar to a previous one, you compare them and determine a course of action. For example, you might get punched or kicked in the ribs during sparring. When the pain goes away after training, or it is just a tender spot where the punch or kick landed, chances are you will be fine. But when your partner thumps a good one right into your floating ribs and you feel as if you were hit by a truck and fall down unable to breathe and feel a stabbing pain—there is a good chance he busted one of your ribs. It is time for you to go to the hospital. These examples are perhaps a bit extreme but the point is that it is a matter of degrees and sometimes hard to tell. As a rule of thumb, if you are not sure what to do play it safe and go to the doctor. If it is nothing, there is no problem. If it is, you will be happy you went.

If the injury is not an emergency, you are usually better served by going to a doctor specializing in sports medicine than seeing a general practitioner. Sports medicine has a different goal than general medicine: it wants the patient/athlete to heal while staying in the best possible physical condition for his or her sport. Where a general practitioner is likely to say you need two weeks' rest and pop some pills, a sports doctor looks for options that allow you to continue training yet let the injury hea, or at the very least, give you alternative training methods that keep you in shape until you are fit to resume martial arts training. Perhaps you can strength train with free weights or machines to stay active. Or if you must avoid impacts on your joints, you can go swimming to maintain strength and aerobic conditioning. Just ask the doctor what you can and cannot do until the injury is gone and set up a strategy with him or her for a training schedule until then.

Creativity

Even though injuries are probably unavoidable for the martial artist, there is virtually always a way to train around them. The only thing it takes is putting your mind to finding creative solutions to whatever limitations your body forces upon you. Sometimes this can even lead to amazing growth in your skills. When I was in my late teens, I had some minor neck surgery. Nothing really important but the wounds meant I could not twist my neck to the left. That made it impossible to train in my usual left-lead fighting stance.

I found two solutions to this problem: First, I trained myself to work from a right lead. This was difficult at first but I got used to it quickly and my right punches and kicks improved tremendously. The second thing I tried was throwing the techniques with my left side without turning my head. I targeted the heavy bag using only peripheral vision or flat out not seeing it and guessing where it was. This increased my control and accuracy on the left side. When I was allowed to train from a left-lead again, I had gained skills on both sides. The added benefit was that I now found it easy to spar from both leads and used that versatility to confuse classmates and my opponents in competitions.

The point of this story is that an injury can be a blessing in disguise. But only if you make it so by being creative in finding answers to whatever problem the injury causes. Here are some ideas to get you started:

Opposites. *If you cannot move one arm, work with the other one. If you cannot use your arms at all without pain, focus on kicking techniques. And vice versa, work your arms when your legs are injured. Even if the injury limits you to just one technique, train it as much as you can, making it a powerful weapon for you once you are done healing and back to normal training.*

Go slow. *Some injuries do not limit mobility as much but prohibit explosive movements. So make this a benefit by performing your techniques and forms slowly but with perfect execution. Get every detail right: the punches and kicks follow the correct angle, they come in at the right height, your guarding hand is correctly placed, and every stance is perfect and so on. Go slow but aim for a flawless performance. If you like an extra challenge, try to do everything slow but close your eyes as well.*

Every now and then, you might be forced to stop all physical activity. This is as bad as it gets but it still does not mean you get to quit training. Instead, focus on aspects of your training you might otherwise neglect: deep breathing, meditation, relaxation, and anything else you can think of. Here are some ideas to get you started:

Mental imagery. *Scientific studies have shown that when you watch yourself perform on TV, your body reacts similarly than when you are actually doing the techniques you see on the screen: Your heart rate goes up, adrenaline is dumped into your system, you can even "zone out" and totally forget everything around you. Mental imagery takes this a step further: Sit in a comfortable chair or lie in bed if you must and do some deep breathing to calm your mind. In your mind's eye, see yourself standing in the* dojo, *ready to perform a form. Make yourself do it ever so slowly at first, imagining every detail you can remember without moving your body. Do this until you can go through the whole form without interruption. When you can resume training, you will notice a distinct improvement in concentration when you do that form.*

Study. *When you cannot train your body, train your mind. Brush up on the theory of your art by reading books or watching tapes and DVDs. The goal is not simply to learn more about how to turn your hips in a kick or any other practical aspect of a technique. You can do that in the mental imagery mentioned before. Now, you focus on learning as much about the history, principles, and theory of your art. Look for answers to questions like:*

- *Who founded my art? In which country and in what era? How does this affect the art?*
- *What is the preferred fight strategy of my art? Striking? Grappling?*
- *How do we accomplish this? Which strategies and tactics do we use?*

> **Something to think about:**
>
> Pain is a signal that something has gone wrong. If you are injured, your first priority must be to listen to this signal and assess the damage. Martial artists are notorious for toughing things out, often continuing on going far longer than they should, yet professional football players whose livelihood depends on their ability to make plays have learned to stop immediately and wait for the trainer's or a doctor's examination before risking further damage.

- *What are the weaknesses and strengths of my art? How would I go about defeating myself?*
- *How do other teachers from a similar art answer all these questions? For instance, if you do* Shotokan *karate, how do* Shito-Ryu *players view all this? How do other arts (Japanese, Chinese, Indonesian, etc.) answer them?*
- *What are their strengths and weaknesses? How would you defeat them?*

The goal is to use your "down time" as efficiently as possible. A competent martial artist knows both theory and practice. If practicing is not an option, work on your theory. Being injured is never fun; it always seems like a waste of precious training time. But once an injury presents itself, you must deal with it. It is my firm belief you can turn such a situation around to your benefit. Sure, if you could actually train that would benefit you even more. But sadly you are limited by whatever damage your body sustained until the healing process is finished. However, with some effort and by trying out the ideas listed above, you can still practice martial arts while your body gets back in perfect condition.

– Wim Demeere [55]

Impact of Injuries

A physical injury is often a watershed moment in a martial artist's training, especially at two points: the beginning of their training and later in life. In the beginning of one's training, you are not into the ritual of the process, that is to say that the martial arts have not become something that is part of who you are, it is merely part of what you do. To know that you have crossed from "what I do" to "part of who I am" is when you choose martial arts over something else that would normally compete for that spot on your schedule like watching a football game on television, something that can be swapped out with no sense of loss.

On the other end of the training spectrum, you have the person who has been training for many years and is older. Training has become ingrained in them. While it may be physically more difficult to practice martial arts, the ritual of training has become as deep-rooted as brushing their teeth. The trade-off between training and watching television is not even considered.

These two attitudes have much to do with injury in the martial arts and how severely your training is affected by it. Simply put, an injury to you as the student at the beginning of your training is the event that allows people to quit. For longer-term practitioners, this is rarely a problem.

"Allows people to quit," sounds odd but look at it this way: few if any students ever walk up to their instructor and simply say, "I am going to quit training, I do not owe you an explanation, it is my choice, good-bye." The conversation goes more like, "I am going to take a break right now, the doctor says I need to stay off this for a month, and so that is what I am going to do." Then the student is rarely, if ever, seen again.

The injury provides the "out," the vehicle of simply drifting away with no real effort. As we know, the time that used to be filled with training and learning soon becomes filled with other things, some meaningful and others not so meaningful. Do not let an injury become your excuse to drop out, but rather use it as an impetus to do more once you have recovered.

This is the point, the watershed moment. If you truly want to earn a black belt, you cannot let any injury, no matter how severe, hold you back. There are ways of working through just about anything. As the old saying goes: "What does not kill you makes you stronger."

There is always pain of one sort or another to work through in martial arts, everything from minor bruises and strained muscles to the occasional serious injury. Back in his younger days, when he entered tournament competitions on a regular basis, Kane eventually needed surgery on both knees (at different times) due to cartilage damage. It would have been very easy to quit after a surgery, and even easier after two, but he worked his way back and now has stronger, more pain-free knees than he did before he got hurt.

He has also been stabbed, sliced, abraded, bruised, contused, and concussed, and suffered a wide range of injuries from martial arts training, physical confrontations, a hunting accident, and a few run-ins with wayward power tools (he is a bit of a klutz at times it seems…). He passed his *nidan* (second-degree black belt) test just a few weeks after being stabbed in the thigh, before the injury had completely healed. While this ⅞" wide by 1¾" deep wound limited his ability to perform certain techniques, he refused to let it keep him from performing as best as he was physically able. Learning to deal with pain and recover from injuries not only builds character but can also help you survive a real-life confrontation should you ever find yourself in the unenviable position of utilizing your martial arts skills on the street.

How the Body Responds to Injury

We have all heard the stories of someone becoming severely injured and commenting later on that he or she did not really feel the injury too much. The person knew that he or she was injured badly but they were not in much, if any pain. This is nature's way of addressing injury. Pain clearly exists every time a significant injury occurs, of course, but our biology provides natural morphine-like chemicals to get us through tough times. Think of it this way: In some instances the body says, "This is real bad, you know it and I know it, but losing is not going to get us help. We must be cool about this." At that point, the body takes over.

While this can occur with any type of injury, it is particularly true in physical altercations. The injury with a closer proximity to violence oftentimes invokes a greater reaction than a similar injury that is clearly an accident. For example, while a broken leg suffered in a climbing accident causes the same damage as one initiated by a thug's baseball bat, the latter is almost always more traumatic.

Once a confrontation escalates into combat, adrenaline rushes through your system. This dramatically increases your pain tolerance and helps you survive in fighting mode. This "fight or flight" reaction instantly supercharges your body for a short period of time, increasing pulse rate and blood pressure, while making you faster, meaner, and more impervious to pain than ever before.

Your heart rate can jump from 60 or 70 beats per minute (BPM) to well over 200 BPM in less than half a second during a violent encounter. Here is how combat stress (accelerated heart rates) can affect you:

- For people whose resting heart rate is around 60 to 70 BPM, at around 115 BPM, many people begin to lose fine motor skills such as finger dexterity, making it difficult to dial a phone, open a lock, or aim a weapon. While martial techniques requiring fine motor skills become less effective, those involving gross motor skills remain unaffected.

- Around 145 BPM, most people begin to lose their complex motor skills such as hand-eye coordination, precise tracking movements, or exact timing, making complicated techniques very challenging if not impossible to

> **Something to think about:**
>
> If your body says, "do not walk on that foot," then do not walk on it. If you body says, "I just need a minute," give it a minute. You are the judge of you body and its tolerances. Listen to what it is telling you and respond accordingly. There is perseverance and there is stupidity. Know the difference.

perform. Simple, straightforward applications, especially those involving pre-programmed muscle reflex actions, are quite feasible. Trained martial artists can operate very effectively in this range.

- Around 175 BPM, most people begin to lose depth perception, experience tunnel vision, and sometimes even suffer temporary memory loss. It is very challenging to think logically at this point, yet conditioned gross motor responses are still effective.

- Around 185–220 BPM, many people experience hyper-vigilance, loss of rational thought, and inability to consciously move or react. Without prior training, most people cannot function at this stress level. Even highly trained practitioners tend to experience degraded performance.

Combatants operating under adrenal stress can take tremendous damage without realizing it. You often find this phenomenon in the sparring ring too, though to a lesser degree. Because you may not realize the significance of your injury, it is prudent to evaluate the cause of any pain as soon as possible. To do otherwise risks exacerbating the damage.

Genuine Injury vs. Superficial Injury

Injuries should not be trifled with. Wilder's high school football coach once said, "In my day if you got injured, you died in the huddle." In other words, be tough, be macho, walk it off. Well, those days are gone; watch any sporting event at the professional level and absolutely no one will try to carry on without having an injury addressed. Have your injury assessed before you carry on.

Assessment prevents further injury and aggravation. It is that simple. If your body says, "do not walk on that foot," then do not walk on it. If your body says, "I just need a minute," give it a minute. You are the judge of your body and its tolerances. Listen to what it is telling you and respond accordingly.

A genuine injury is not necessarily identified by size or severity. Swelling, redness, and motion restriction are all small nagging forms of injury and very real. Bleeding and painful motion are two examples of gross and genuine injury as well, so do not be fooled by appearance. Injury is injury—it is the extent of the injury that needs to be measured.

Even superficial injuries can turn severe. A cut can be small and of minor consequence, but add bacteria combined with a macho "I do not need to see a doctor" attitude and you may wind up with a very serious infection. For example, Wilder chose to ignore a spider bite on his little finger as a young man because, "It was just a spider bite," until a grandmotherly lady he worked with pointed out that the infection was streaking up his hand. The doctor let him know that he was a day or two away from losing his finger when he finally got around to having it examined. A superficial injury he chose to ignore, even with a swollen finger that he was unable to bend, was within a day or two of amputation. You need not overreact to injury, but you do need an honest assessment. That assessment responsibility initially lies with you.

Even simple injuries can become complicated as they can ripple throughout the body, affecting surrounding areas beyond the point of initial damage. For example, if you sprain your right ankle you will generally favor your left side until you can put weight evenly on both legs. Imbalanced walking can strain muscles, pull your spine out of alignment, and cause a host of other problems that spread beyond the damaged area.

There are two kinds of sports-related injuries: acute and chronic. Acute injuries occur suddenly when participating in physical activities. Sprains, strains, and broken bones are examples of acute injuries. Signs of acute injuries may include sudden, severe pain, swelling, inability to flex a joint, or a bone or joint that is visibly out of place. Chronic injuries occur when you perform a physical activity over a long period of time. Signs of a chronic injury may include pain during physical activity, dull aches when at rest, or longer-term swelling or tenderness not associated with any particular event.

Acute injuries may require immediate medical attention while chronic injuries may require rest, physical therapy, or possibly even surgery. You cannot ignore either type of damage.

First Aid Basics

Many martial arts students must receive first aid certification as part of their advancement testing requirements, typically somewhere in the upper *kyu* (colored belt) ranks. The Red Cross (or Red Crescent) provides relatively inexpensive, comprehensive first aid and CPR classes throughout the world so access to quality training is rarely a problem. We wholeheartedly approve of this approach. If you have learned how to break someone, you ought to know how to fix him or her as well. Traditional *kappo* (resuscitation techniques) are often taught in the *dojo* as well.

Once you have received training, it is a good idea to carry a first aid kit in your vehicle. Be sure to include rubber gloves to protect yourself from blood-borne pathogens (e.g., hepatitis B, hepatitis C, or HIV/AIDS) if you must treat others as well. Most *dojo* have first aid kits on site, of course, but injuries do not occur solely on the training floor.

Martial artists frequently suffer minor bruises or contusions during training, but other common injuries can include concussions, hyperextended joints, or broken bones. While open-hand training can be somewhat safer than weapons forms when it comes to the potential of major injuries, you can become seriously injured from any martial art if things go awry. It is a rare occurrence in a properly supervised environment yet common enough that you need to know what to do.

If you or a training partner has been seriously injured, you may have to take care of yourself or someone else until professional help can arrive. Some martial arts such as *arnis*, *iaido*, or *kobudo* are primarily based on weapons forms and many others incorporate them into the training. When you are playing with three feet of razor sharp steel (e.g., *katana*) or six feet of solid hardwood (e.g., *bo* staff), accidents can and do happen. Your attitude plays a large part in your ability to survive a significant injury such as a crushing blow, stab wound, or a gunshot. While the latter is highly unlikely in the *dojo*, the former do happen on occasion.

"We live in a time when the words impossible and unsolvable are no longer part of the scientific community's vocabulary. Each day we move closer to trials that will not just minimize the symptoms of disease and injury but eliminate them."

– Christopher Reeve [56]

Control your breathing. Try to stay calm and rational when you are injured or caring for someone else who is. If you are the victim, panic will not do anything but kill you faster as it raises your blood pressure, increasing the impact of shock and hemorrhaging. The adrenaline rush from your fight-or-flight reflex can significantly dampen pain, so take advantage of this time to call for help and begin treating your wounds. If you are the responder, you may lose your ability to rationally assess the situation and provide appropriate care. Like anything else, this can be overcome by training and experience.

The American Red Cross recommends a check, call, care approach. Discern the safety of the scene and the condition of the victim(s) first then call 9-1-1 (or the local emergency number), notifying them of the emergency so that they can dispatch an ambulance and professional help. The faster the paramedics arrive, the better the victim's chances of survival. Only after these first two steps have been completed do you begin to care for the victim.

After training for a while, you should be able to differentiate between the normal bumps and bruises inherent with martial arts and "real" injuries about which you need to be concerned. Never try to "work through" the pain of an injury, at least not until you have assessed its severity. Unless you are engaged in a fight for your life, immediately stop physical activity and examine the source of the pain. Failure to do so may increase the level of harm. Some injuries should be seen by a doctor right away, while others you can safely treat yourself.

Call a medical professional immediately if the injury damages an eye, causes severe pain, swelling, or numbness, eliminates your ability to put any weight on the area, or causes a joint to move in an unusual manner or feel unstable. It is better to be safe than sorry. Also, pay attention to old injuries that act up, aching, swelling, or recurring in some fashion. In most cases, you should not have to deal with acute injuries for any significant period of time without the help of professionals such as paramedics or doctors. Nevertheless, certain injuries such as arterial bleeding can prove fatal in mere minutes so it is important to know what to do until help arrives. Here are some common injuries and triage methods:

Severe bleeding

Heavy bleeding is controlled first through direct, firm pressure on the injury site, preferably through a gauze pad or sterile dressing. If it is a limb, it will bleed less if it is elevated so that the wound is above the heart. If hemorrhage persists, use pressure points. Only in the worst cases when emergency services will not be available for an extended period of time should you consider use of a tourniquet, which if improperly used could cause gangrene or death. The Red Cross has dropped tourniquet techniques from their curriculum, as they are rarely needed and dangerous to apply.

One of the most street-proven trauma dressings is a sanitary napkin or a box of tissues (e.g., Kleenex), something that ought to be in your first aid kit in addition to regular gauze pads and bandages. Key first aid methods for stopping heavy bleeding include:

Cover the wound with a sterile dressing such as a gauze pad. If the dressing becomes soaked with blood, apply additional layers over the top of it without removing the original dressing.

Apply direct pressure to the wound. If bleeding does not stop through a combination of dressings and pressure, you may have to apply direct pressure to a nearby artery to slow the flow of blood. On the arm, the best point is along the inside of the upper arm between the shoulder and elbow. On the leg, the best point is at the crease at the front of the hip in the groin area.

Elevate the wound above the level of the heart, if possible. If you suspect head, neck, or back injuries or broken bones, however, it may be prudent to remain in place. Moving may increase severity of the damage.

Imbedded objects should never be removed before you arrive at the hospital. Doing so may increase hemorrhaging and severely reduce your chances of survival. Bulky dressings should be placed around the object and bandaged in place to support it.

Severed body parts, if any, should be wrapped in a sterile dressing, placed in a plastic bag, and covered with ice or cold water sufficient to keep the part cool without freezing. Limbs preserved in this manner can frequently be reattached at the hospital. On the other hand, freezing the severed part will cause irreversible damage.

Head, neck, and back injuries

Head, neck, and back injuries can be very serious. Do not move the victim unless absolutely necessary. If you do need to move the person, be careful to support the injured area, avoiding any twisting, bending, or other contortions that could cause additional damage. If the person becomes unconscious, you will need to maintain a clear airway and possibly perform rescue breathing or cardio pulmonary resuscitation until medical help arrives.

Concussions

The brain is extraordinarily delicate yet it is protected by a rigid skull and cushioned with cerebrospinal fluid. Trauma to the head can cause the brain to bounce against the skull, however. This force may damage the brain's function. There is very little extra room within this cavity, so any resulting swelling or bleeding can quickly become life-threatening. In general, a blow to the front of the head is less dangerous than one on the side or back of the head.

Symptoms of a concussion can include severe headache, dizziness, nausea, vomiting, ringing in the ears, mismatched pupil size (left vs. right), seizures, or slurred speech. The person may also seem restless, agitated, or irritable. Often, the victim experiences temporary memory loss. These symptoms may last from hours to weeks, depending on the seriousness of the injury.

Any loss of consciousness or memory resulting from a head injury must be promptly evaluated by a medical professional. As the brain tissue swells, the person may feel increasingly drowsy or confused. If the victim has difficulty staying awake, experiences persistent vomiting, develops seizures, or loses consciousness, medical attention should be sought right away.

Watch the person closely for any changes in level of consciousness until medical help arrives. The victim may need to stay in the hospital for close observation. The standard test to assess post-concussion damage is a computerized tomography (CT) scan. Surgery is not frequently required but may become necessary if swelling persists.

Recovery from a traumatic brain injury can be very slow. Sometimes several days can go by without seeing any major visible change. Post-concussion syndrome may also occur in some people. This syndrome generally consists of a persistent headache, dizziness, irritability, emotional instability, memory changes, depression, or vision changes. Symptoms may begin weeks or even months after the initial injury.

Although the symptoms generally go away over time, some victims will need a rehabilitation specialist to oversee a program for their recovery. People who have had a severe concussion also double their risk of developing epilepsy within the first five years after the injury. There also is evidence that people who have had multiple concussions over the course of their lives suffer cumulative neurological damage. A link between concussions and the eventual development of Alzheimer's disease also has been suggested.

Rest is generally the best recovery technique since healing a concussion takes time. For headaches, acetaminophen (e.g., Tylenol) or ibuprofen (e.g., Motrin) can usually be used but it is best to avoid aspirin as it can increase the risk of internal bleeding. Check with your doctor before administering medications. Bumps and contusions can be treated with ice packs. Wrap ice in a damp cloth rather than placing it directly against the skin.

Eye injuries

Do not attempt to treat severe blunt trauma or penetrating injuries to the eye yourself; medical assistance is required in such instances. Tape a paper or Styrofoam cup over the injured area to protect it until proper care can be obtained. If there is an imbedded object, do not attempt to remove it.

In the case of a blow to the eye such as a finger rake, jab, or gouge, do not automatically assume that the injury is minor even if you can see properly afterward. An ophthalmologist should examine the eye thoroughly because vision-threatening damage such as a detached retina could be hidden. Immediately apply an ice compress or bag of frozen vegetables (e.g., peas, corn) to the eye to reduce pain and swelling. If you experience pain, blurred vision, floaters (black spots that move around), starbursts (firework-like bursts of color or light), or any possibility of eye damage, see your ophthalmologist or emergency room physician immediately.

While not really an issue in martial arts, the most common type of eye injury is a chemical burn so we will go ahead and address it briefly here too. Alkaline materials (such as lye, plasters, cements, and ammonia), solvents, acids, and detergents can be very harmful to your eyes. If you are exposed to these types of chemicals, the eyes should be flushed liberally with water immediately. If sterile solutions are readily available, use them to flush the affected eye. If not, go to the nearest sink, shower or hose and begin washing the eye with large amounts of water. If the eye has been exposed to an alkaline agent, it is important to flush the eye for ten minutes or more. Make sure water is getting under both the upper and lower eyelids.

Chest wounds

Large chest wounds can cause a lung to collapse, a dangerous situation. Cover the wound with a sterile dressing or clean cloth and bandage it in place. If bubbles begin forming around a wound of significant size (open area that is greater than about an inch in diameter), cover that area with plastic or similar material that does not allow air to pass through. Tape the dressing in place, leaving one corner open to allow air to escape with exhalation.

Most normal stab and bullet injuries will not cause a sucking chest wound because the hole from the wound is smaller than the opening in the trachea. Consequently, it will not cause negative pressure that inhibits breathing. If you seal a wound that does not need it, you run the risk of tension pneumothorax, which can cause a complete cardio respiratory arrest and subsequent death. If advanced medical care is readily available, it is generally more important transport the victim to the hospital quickly than it is to seal off the wound with anything more than a breathable sterile dressing.

Abdominal injuries

For abdominal injuries, try to keep the victim lying down with his or her knees bent, if possible. If organs are exposed, do not apply pressure to the organs or push them back inside. Remove any clothing from around the wound. Apply a moist, sterile dressing or clean cloth loosely over the wound. Keep the dressing moist with clean, warm water. Place a cloth over the dressing to keep the organs warm.

Joint injuries

While it may be challenging to tell the difference between a sprain, strain, dislocation, hyperextension, or fracture, you really do not need to diagnose the injury precisely in order to treat it until it can be looked at by a doctor. Common symptoms include pain, bruising, and swelling. Be sure to call medical professionals if a snap or pop was heard at the time of the injury, if it feels or sounds like bones are rubbing together when the joint is moved, if you cannot move or use the affected area, or if the injured area becomes cold and numb. Immobilize the injured part to keep it from moving until help arrives.

Broken bones

Broken bones should usually be splinted to keep the injured part from moving and increasing the damage. If medical personnel will quickly arrive on the scene, you may be best off simply comforting the victim while keeping him or her stable. If you do need to make a splint, there are a variety of ways to create an effective one. The method you choose will be based in part on what materials you have available, the position in which you find the injury, its location on the body, and a variety of other factors. The most important initial treatment is to pad and immobilize the injury to the extent possible until help arrives.

Anatomic splints affix the injured body part to a convenient uninjured one such as tying one leg to the other. A soft splint can be made from a towel, blanket, jacket, or similar material. A rigid splint can be made from boards, tightly rolled magazines, and similar materials.

Shock

Shock can occur whenever there is severe injury to the body or the nervous system. Because shock can cause inadequate blood flow to the tissues and organs, all bodily processes can be affected. Vital functions slow down to dangerous levels. In the early stages, the body compensates for a decreased blood flow to the tissues by constricting blood vessels in the skin, soft tissues, and muscles. This causes the victim to have cold, clammy, or pale skin; weakness and nausea; rapid, labored breathing; increased pulse rate; and decreased blood pressure. As shock progresses, the victim will become apathetic, relatively unresponsive, and eventually lapse into unconsciousness.

Keep the victim lying down, legs slightly elevated, and cover with a blanket or coat to prevent loss of body heat. If possible, treat any major injuries such as bleeding or broken bones to help ameliorate the source of the shock. Check airway, breathing, and circulation on a regular basis until medical help arrives. It is not advisable to give liquids to shock victims.

Infection

If you have been injured by anything that breaks the skin, infection is a possibility even after medical treatment. If the wound area becomes red or swollen, throbs with pain, discharges pus, or develops red streaks, contact medical personnel immediately. If you begin to develop a fever, it may also be a sign of infection. Seek direction from your physician as to how to bandage your injury, how frequently to change the dressing, and how best to clean the wound to minimize the chances of infection.

Rest, ice, compression, and elevation

If you do not have any of signs of significant injury, it may be safe to take care of things by yourself at home. Nevertheless, if the pain or other symptoms become worse, you should call your doctor. A common self-treatment method involves rest, ice, compression, and elevation or RICE for short. It is a good idea to follow these four steps right after the injury and continue them for at least 24 to 48 hours afterward:

Rest: Reduce your regular activities. If you have injured your leg (knee, ankle, or foot), take steps to keep your full weight off of it. A cane or crutch can help when necessary. Support the opposite side of the injury with the cane; if your right leg is injured, support the left side and vice versa.

Ice: For bruising or swelling, apply an ice pack (or bag of crushed ice or frozen vegetables) to the injured area for 20 minutes at a time, four to eight times a day. Do not apply ice directly to the skin, but rather wrap the ice pack in a towel to avoid overcooling the injury.

Compression: Put even pressure on the injured area to help reduce swelling. You can purchase an elastic bandage or neoprene brace from most pharmacies and some sporting goods stores or may receive a medical device such as an air splint or boot from your doctor.

Elevation: Put the injured area on a pillow, at a level above your heart, to help reduce swelling. This step can be combined with ice and/or compression.

Seeing a Doctor

If you think you need to see a doctor, do it. If someone else tells you to see a doctor, then you should give his or her advice strong consideration. The old saying goes, "An ounce of prevention is worth a pound of cure." Today, the most advanced forms of medicine known to humankind. Consequently, there are few legitimate reasons not to take advantage of a doctor when addressing injury.

Your general practitioner will be able to take care of most immediate or short-term problems although you may need to see a specialist for surgery or long-term rehabilitation. It is important to choose someone who understands sports medicine. Athletes often have different needs and issues than the general patient population. You will want someone who not only expedites your recovery but also helps you understand the limits of what you can and cannot safely do as you heal. This may include a physical therapist or sports medicine professional.

Sports medicine is not a single specialty, but rather an area that involves a wide variety of disciplines, including cardiology, psychology, orthopedics, and biomechanics. It is not only curative and rehabilitative, but also preventative. These physicians obtain additional training through accredited fellowship programs.

The best way to find a sports medicine physician, orthopedic surgeon, or any other type of doctor for that matter, is to seek referrals. Ask your personal physician, *sensei*, training partners, friends, or co-workers for personal recommendations. If you know other athletes, trainers, or coaches, regardless of sport, this is another excellent source of referrals. It is important to choose a doctor who treats athletes (not all orthopedic surgeons do), so you need to ask questions.

Your local university may also have a sports medicine program that includes a clinic available to the general population, so call or look online for their information. You can also search through online database listings, including the American Medical Association, the American College of Sports Medicine, the American Orthopedic Society for Sports Medicine, and other specialty groups.

Medicine is an art as well as a science. While a qualified, experienced professional will offer well-founded recommendations and advice, the treatment approach for certain injuries is simply not all that clear. You may have several options from which to choose such as rehabilitation versus surgery, for example. You should try to develop a partnership relationship with your doctor, working together to find the best path for you.

It is important to feel comfortable with your doctor's communication style and personality. While this is not always the best indication of a qualified physician, it does help you feel more comfortable if you have concerns or questions. Get a second opinion if you are not satisfied or comfortable with your physician's approach to treating your injury. It is your body after all; you should want the best possible care that you can find for it. At times, alternative approaches such as naturopathic medicine, chiropractic manipulation, acupuncture, or massage therapy are appropriate, so you may wish to look into those areas as well.

Gender Differences and Injuries

Despite efforts to treat all martial artists alike, there are certain physical and psychological differences between how men and women train that can lead to differences in how they are most likely to become injured. While there are exceptions to almost every rule, it is valuable to understand these differences and avoid falling into common age- or gender-related pitfalls, or both.

Injury During Training – Male

Enthusiasm is the initial earmark of beginning training in the martial arts. It is no doubt something you have thought of over sometime and the moment is right, and suddenly you find yourself on the floor or the mat. The uniform, the ritual, the entire event is new and exciting, and it should be.

Unfortunately, injury during this period is common. Although generally not borne out of malice, the injuries that happen at this time of training are often a result of the enthusiasm one has during this time. Several things can contribute to this injury rate, all of them stemming from the excitement of a new experience. A common one among young men is being macho, ignoring the pain of a technique in attempt to really "feel it" or, "see if it works." This is not a condemnation of young males, merely an acknowledgment of the nature of young men. Engaging in machismo or the "see if it works" attitude is a dangerous place to work from because the injury that may occur is not just to one's body but to one's ego as well.

> **Something to think about:**
>
> The two deadly "F's" of martial arts are fatigue and frustration. These two factors almost always lead to injury. They can cause a vicious circle of injury, leading to fatigue and frustration and more injury.

For example, many high school wrestlers try judo. Wilder has experienced many instances when they come into the *dojo* and attempt wrestling techniques and timing on the upper ranks, as all students work together. They were there to prove that their training and technique were at the least as good as the *judoka* standing across from them. Their conditioning and wrestling might have been superior, but the rules of the game were different. Without exception, the wrestler's failure to adapt to those rules resulted in loss after loss to the judo practitioners.

As frustration sets in, machismo arises and injury often results. Not deliberate injury, but rather those occurring from a combination of the two deadly "F's" of martial arts—fatigue and frustration. The two "F's" are a "path killer," a vicious circle of injury, leading to fatigue and frustration, and more injury. These two "F's" end training prematurely for many promising practitioners. This is a mentality that creates a roadblock to truly understanding the art and ultimately yourself.

So, young men, this one is specifically for you. Understand it is your nature to find injury by way of the two "F's." Train hard, train smart, and you will not have injury cut your training short, and kill the path to black belt. Simply put, do not let injury serve as the vehicle for you leaving your training.

Injury During Training – Female

Injury is injury. It knows no boundaries of gender, yet women face different challenges regarding injury than men do. Most often, a martial arts school is populated primarily by men. The downside of being a woman and training in a school that is dominated by men is that often, but not always, the physicality of the men is superior to the women. On the other side of the coin, women generally do not engage in the same kind of macho behavior that often clouds men's minds to the potential of injury.

A woman at Wilder's judo *dojo* was tough. She took no quarter from anybody. Male or female, it made no difference. She fought all comers at her rank or above and did it with enthusiasm and smarts. Often outweighed and frequently outranked, she was light, fast, and aggressive. She used her lightness to her advantage in that she was hard to "feel." Opponents rarely felt her technique coming. She was fast because of genetics and size, and she was aggressive. She took whatever anyone offered and more.

In all the time Wilder saw her train, he never saw her injured. He did see her tap out, surrendering before damage could occur. He also saw her stop techniques that, while they would inevitably allow her to win, would risk injury. She was smart. She knew her limitations. She understood that pushing through or being macho would ultimately lead to injury, and injury would lead to downtime, so she played it smart.

Oftentimes, as a woman, you are in a man's world at a martial arts class. Knowing your limits should come easier for you than it sometimes does for your male counterparts. Use this to your benefit to avoid injury. Continue training and as a result get better with less downtime.

Injury Prevention

Many injuries can be prevented simply by exercising some modicum of common sense. Always begin with a good warm up to loosen and strengthen your muscles. Learn to perform your martial art correctly, using good body mechanics and proper form to reduce the risk of strains, sprains, and overuse injuries. Whether you practice a couple of days a week or solely on the weekends, do not be a "weekend warrior." Do not try to cram a week's worth of activity into a day or two. Use safety gear where appropriate.

Know your body's limits. Build up your fitness level gradually. Strive for a total body workout of cardiovascular, strength, and flexibility exercises. Use braces, supports, and/or nutritional supplements as necessary to protect your joints.

Stretching is always important, both before and after your workout. It is one of the most important things you can do to avoid athletic injury. In some martial systems, flexibility beyond the normal ranges of motion you find in everyday people is essential. *Taekwondo* and Brazilian *jiu-jitsu* are two examples of martial arts that require extreme flexibility for top performance.

Taekwondo practitioners must be flexible in their hips, legs, and groin to facilitate high kicking techniques. Brazilian *jiu-jitsu* needs similar flexibility to be able to move legs and arms into odd positions to gain a grappling advantage. Some Okinawan karate systems or Filipino martial arts systems are not all that concerned with flexibility for the sake of technique. To these systems, it is more about injury prevention and not necessarily ranges of motion.

These factors should be taken into consideration as you choose a school for training. Examine your physical state in regards to stretching and flexibility. It takes time to develop ranges of motion to which your body is not accustomed. To rush the process is a sure path to injury. Because tendons do not have the same circulation as muscles and other organs, healing takes more time if you overstress them.

Stretching can prevent injuries to tendons, ligaments, and muscles by improving your muscular elasticity. Whenever you want to stretch, it is very important to warm up properly before you get started. You should then proceed to stretch your joints first and then move your tendons and muscles. If you begin stretching cold, you may injure yourself. Further, when stretching joints or tendons, it is best to begin working from the ground up so that you do not miss anything (e.g., ankles, then knees, and then hips, and so on).

A special note to the under thirty practitioner

The greatest piece of advice that can be given to a younger practitioner, one under thirty, is simply, "Do not lose your flexibility." By maintaining your flexibility, you will push back nagging injuries. This time in life is a great period to establish a level of flexibility you may very well carry with you the rest of your life. Flexibility, or more importantly suppleness, of the body is a huge benefit to your quality of life and your martial arts. Muscle pulls, strains, and aches can be staved off simply by stretching regularly.

A special note the over-thirty practitioner

As a rule of thumb, you are entering

"Stretching is invaluable in preventing pulled or torn muscles. In the early 1970s, the Pittsburgh Steelers were the first professional football team to have its players emulate gymnasts by stretching regularly. The thought was that gymnasts, who are super flexible, did not pull muscles often. If football players could stretch their heavy muscles, maybe they too would be less likely to pull them. The theory proved to be correct. Lengthening muscles led to fewer muscle pulls among football players. Within two years, every team was following the Steelers' example."

– Dr. Allan Levy [57]

into a new phase of life. Reduction of flexibility is one of the earmarks of this phase. Retaining or even gaining in flexibility is one means of pushing back the living rigor mortis* many people just accept as a part of aging. This living rigor mortis slowly restricts the ranges of motion. Unless you make a deliberate effort to increase your ranges of motion, the body slowly but surely becomes more set in its ways, and before you know it your flexibility and ranges of motion are severely decreased.

This living rigor mortis can be staved off through preparation and a little effort on a regular basis. Today people do not use their bodies with the same physicality as in the past. Attempting to move from a sedentary lifestyle to stepping on the floor of a martial arts school is leaving one way of life and moving to another. You must be mindful of the change in context. Being aware of this change and keeping it in context will aid in preventing injury and in not impeding your goal to becoming a black belt. Older people need to spend more time warming up and pay closer attention to stretching than younger ones do.

---

* Rigor mortis is the phase a body goes through shortly after death where chemical changes in the muscles cause it to become stiff and immobile. At mild temperatures, rigor usually sets in about 3 to 4 hours after clinical death, with full rigor being in effect at about 12 hours, and eventually subsiding to relaxation at about 36 hours. "Living rigor mortis" is our way of saying that as we age, our ranges of motion decreases over time unless we actively work to maintain it.

Liniments and *Jow*

Dit da jow is an external liniment that can be used to heal damage to the body such as bruises, muscle aches, and bone injuries. Originally applied by martial artists who practice Iron Palm to aid in the healing and conditioning of their hands, it is not restricted to that particular style or that part of the body. *Jow* is made up of formulas that oftentimes reflect the region of origin due to ingredient availability. A plant that grows in one part of China may not grow in another part so a plant that produces comparable results will be used as replacement.

These formulas were often held secret and passed on from master to student yet they are all fundamentally the same in the way they work, stimulating the affected area to increase blood flow, which aids in healing, while simultaneously acting as a skin conditioner. Many products are available over the counter that can provide similar results as traditional *dit da jow*, such as Ben Gay, Tiger Balm, or Icy Hot to relieve strains and muscle pulls, though many martial artists feel that the traditional recipe is superior for treating bruises and bone injuries.

Some schools apply two applications of *dit da jow*, one prior to and another immediately after training, while others just does it once before or after each session. Each school has its reasons for the form and methods of application they recommend. Your *sensei* or *sifu* should be able to hook you up with a source of this liniment as well as tell you when it is appropriate to apply it. Proper application of traditional or modern remedies is much the same. Do not apply to broken or torn skin and be cautious to avoid too much heat build-up if the affected area is covered or wrapped.

Using *dit da jow* or any modern product requires common sense and reason. It can be purchased just about any martial arts magazine or catalog. On occasion, the quality and quantity of integral ingredients can be suspect. As with any purchase, a little research can go a long way in finding the best product available. Some instructors sell commercially available preparations at their schools and others prepare their own private recipes and make it available to their students.

Hydration

A significant fraction of the human body is made of water. This liquid is distributed in different compartments in the body such that lean muscle tissue contains about 75 percent water, blood is about 83 percent water, body fat contains about 25 percent water, and bone is about 22 percent water. In adults of average weight, build, and musculature, males have roughly 72 percent of their total body mass comprised of water (total body water percentage). This value is about 68 percent in women due to a normally higher proportion of body fat.

Advice for New Students

by Dr. Jeffery Cooper [58]

Many would claim that nothing sets back martial training more than an injury. However, I would claim that not training at all sets one back the most. So, I would like to discuss training despite injury.

One of the great things about martial training is the wide variety of emphasis areas that can be trained. Punching, kicking, grappling, speed, power, flexibility, tactics, strategy, spirit, focus, accuracy; all of these are subjects that can be highlighted. This allows one to concentrate on certain areas when others areas are impaired by injury. My judo teacher, for example, learned to throw left sided *uchimata* (inner thigh throw) due to a right foot injury. This ended up becoming his "signature" technique.

Training with an injury can change one's stance, forcing one to develop better balance and proprioception. The injury may force one to go slow and work on grace and flow, or to focus on form rather than speed and power. Make being injured an opportunity for improvement.

One must be cautious about training with an injury. Overuse syndromes such as tendonitis are easily encountered, and one must avoid stressing the injured area that can lead to instability and scar tissue build up. This can lead to delayed healing and poorer long-term outcomes. However, there are many medical benefits to continued training as well: maintaining ranges of motion and flexibility, keeping up strength and muscle mass, ameliorating spasm and reflex sympathetic dystrophy, and improving proprioception, stability, and rehabilitation.

More important benefits of training with an injury deal with the mind and spirit more than the body. Training through a painful condition builds fighting spirit and discipline. It motivates and sets a brave example for others. It demonstrates sincerity and seriousness of intent to one's teachers. There is a tremendous sense of accomplishment in facing the adversity of injury and refusing to quit.

Training through injury ameliorates what would otherwise be a training set back. It allows one to find the silver lining in the black cloud. Remember, Bruce Lee did much of his best thinking and writing while recovering from what was supposed to be an incapacitating injury.

Making sure you have enough water in your body, being hydrated, is extraordinarily important in injury prevention. When the water level is low in the body, it can adversely affect the brain. Because the brain is the driver of the body, a fatigued mind (via dehydration) can set you up for injury or even death. If you are drinking water because you are thirsty, you are already behind the curve. It will take time to raise your fluid level up to an amount that allows for optimum athletic performance. You need to drink regularly throughout the day whether you feel you need to or not.

Hydration should take place at least an hour prior to training and should continue throughout and shortly after your training. For seminars, tournaments, or other intensive efforts, you should begin taking extra water at least a week ahead of time. Sports drinks are okay, but they are often composed of things like artificial flavorings, watered-down juice, and salt. Electrolytes in these drinks can be very beneficial, but you are usually best off drinking at least two or three times as much water as sports drink when you exercise. You can either water down your sports drinks or alternate between water and the sports drink. Either way is fine so long as you consume mostly water. Caffeinated beverages, on the other hand, run counter to hydration, because they are diuretics; they make you discharge water and are consequently counterproductive.

Dehydration symptoms generally become noticeable after two percent of your normal water volume has been lost. Initially, you may experience thirst or discomfort, possibly along with loss of appetite and dry skin. You will begin to suffer degraded performance, experiencing low endurance, rapid heart rate, elevated body temperature, and fatigue.

Symptoms of mild dehydration include thirst, decreased urine volume, urine that is darker than usual, unexplained tiredness, headache, dry mouth, and dizziness. In moderate to severe dehydration, there may be no urine output at all. Other symptoms in these states include lethargy, fainting, or seizures. The symptoms become increasingly severe with greater water loss. Heart and respiration rates increase to compensate for decreased plasma volume and blood pressure, while body temperature may rise because of decreased sweating. With severe dehydration, muscles may become spastic, skin may shrivel and wrinkle, vision may dim, and delirium may begin.

The best treatment for minor dehydration is water. Most sports drinks actually leach water from your system in order to be adequately absorbed in the stomach. You must either significantly dilute them with water or stick to water alone. For severe cases of dehydration where fainting, unconsciousness, or any other severely debilitating symptoms are experienced, immediate medical attention is required. Fluids to rehydrate and restore electrolyte counts are typically administered intravenously in these cases as it can no longer be absorbed through the stomach.

Bottom line: Drink lots of water. Do it before, during, and after each training session.

Fitness and Muscle Tone

Jumping onto the floor of a martial arts school without taking into consideration your physical condition is a fool's game. The outcome is almost certainly going to result in the subject of this chapter—injury. The older you are, the slower you need to go at the beginning. The younger you are, the less prone you are to injury, yet you

---

Something to think about:

Hydration is extremely important. If you are feeling thirsty, you are already behind the curve. It will take time to raise your fluid level to a level that allows for optimum athletic performance. Drink lots of water. Do it before, during, and after each training session.

---

still need to move slowly at first. Remember our goals are to gain experience and become better; downtime from injury is no way to get there.

Consider whether or not you have been participating in some sort of regular physical activity or if you have been living a sedentary lifestyle and are trying to do something to change it. Your age, body type, family history, and the amount of time you will have to devote to the arts will all play a factor as well. Even if you are very physically fit, participation in martial arts will undoubtedly stress your body in ways it is not already used to.

Wilder remembers that his first day of judo was spent simply learning to do a back fall. Sitting on the *dojo* floor with feet and hands extended, he simply fell backward, slapped the mat, and rolled back up into the sitting position. After a few minutes, the instructor came over and told him to take a break, to relax and sit out for a moment, but he felt fine. So over the course of a half an hour he fell backward, slapped and sat up, ignoring the cautionary comments of the *sensei*. He thought, "Why would I?" Clearly, he had more repetitions in him, so if a couple of repetitions were good, well, many would be better... The rest of class went fine and all was good until he tried to get out of bed the next morning. He wanted to sit up but his stomach had a different idea. He was a wreck. Day 2 was even worse.

Even if you are in generally good physical condition as Wilder had been when he started judo, the movements you are performing will be very different from what you normally do. Consequently, it may be much easier to overdo it than you might think. Listen to your instructor.

Nutrition

There are those that choose to eat only natural foods, become vegetarians, or take supplements ranging from vitamins to meal replacement powders in order to augment their health. You need to make the choices that are best for your body. Edgar Martinez, one of the greatest Designated Hitters ever to play baseball and a certain inductee into the Baseball Hall of Fame, tried different diets to increase his performance, especially later on in his career as age began to catch up with him. After some experimentation with high protein diets, ultimately he returned to his previous diet of foods he was familiar with, and in some instances eaten, since his childhood in Puerto Rico. Upon resuming his original diet, he commented that he not only felt better, but also played better that year, increasing his hitting percentage.

Understanding your nutritional needs is important. We all know that eating a diet of fast food composed of sugar-laden drinks and fatty meats is not something on which to build a strong body. Your nutrition should help your body, not fight against it. One student of Wilder's never learned the fundamentals of proper nutrition. His mother did not understand it and his father lived fifteen hundred miles away. His idea of a good meal was whatever filled his stomach. When he was suddenly faced with a congenital, life-threatening illness, his eating habits had to change or the doctors simply would not perform the operation he needed to live. The doctor's attitude here was not one of insensitivity, but rather a very real assessment of a person's lifestyle and its affect on his health and longevity. He simply was not going to perform an operation, life saving as it was, on a person who treated his body so poorly until he made the required changes in habit.

You might want to ask yourself if faced with the same assessment by you doctors how you would fare. It is an old saying that, "Food is the fuel of the body." What kind of fuel you put into your body largely determines the ability of it to perform well. Gaining this ability allows you to both increase your enjoyment of your martial arts training and prevent injury. Individuals with high body-fat percentages, for example, cannot become as fast, flexible, or agile as similarly experienced practitioners with lower body-fat percentages. Proper nutrition is the foundation to good physical movement and good physical movement helps prevent injury. Less injury equals faster progression. See *Ensure That Your Nutritional Needs Are Met* in Chapter 8 for more information.

How to Train Through Injury

In the early 1980s, Wilder was involved in a very rough-and-tumble karate school. He remembers watching in amazement during one promotion test when a high-ranking black belt squared off against a brown belt. In one motion so swift that Wilder could hardly track it, the black belt flashed forward and struck the brown belt's nose. The brown belt then staggered backward, turned, and took a knee. The instructor who was watching this match swiftly jumped in between the two competitors, placing a hand on the black belt's chest to keep him from laying more punishment onto the kneeling brown belt.

The black belt turned and went back to his initial spot on the *dojo* floor. The instructor then leaned down and spoke firmly to the brown belt. Wilder cannot recall his precise words, but they were something along the lines of, "Are you going to quit or are you going to go on? I need to know now."

The brown belt got back up onto his feet, was given a torn paper towel, which he shoved into his bleeding nose, and took his spot opposite the black belt. "You ready?" asked the instructor. A curt nod from the brown belt as he lifted his hands into fighting position demonstrated that he was ready to continue.

"Fight!" yelled the instructor and, once again, the black belt flashed forward in a movement difficult to see. The brown belt went down. This time his nose was not just bloodied, but broken.

Within three months of this incident, Wilder also suffered a variety of injuries, including a dislocated knee and torn knee ligaments at the hands of another practitioner. In the past when a horse broke its, leg it was shot. The horse was useless and had to be put down. The challenge Wilder faced was simple: Was he going to quit at that point, or was he going to push on?

Having almost no money as a young man, he faced an enormous challenge to his training because of the injury, yet he refused to give up on his dream of becoming a black belt. Here is the path he chose: once home he splinted his injured knee with a wooden yardstick. A torn tee shirt and masking tape helped attach this makeshift splint to the lower and upper leg, bracing the joint.

The local pharmacist was gracious, renting Wilder a pair of crutches for the seven dollars he had in his pocket. Over the next week, he applied every form of heat he could find to the knee, gently flexing it with his hands in an attempt to gradually increase his ranges of motion. After several weeks, he was finally able to afford a proper knee brace.

For rehabilitation, he began riding a stationary bike with the seat set at its highest level. Over time, he was able to set the seat at lower and lower positions as his flexibility increased and he began to recover his strength. He began walking too. As the swelling went down, it had become clear that while there had been damage to the knee, the ligaments were stretched but not completely torn. It would eventually heal without reconstructive surgery.

During this time of self-rehabilitation, Wilder continued to attend class. At first, he simply sat and watched. Soon he was back on the *dojo* floor wearing a knee brace over his uniform pants while participating as much as he could.

Kane suffered a similar injury in a skiing accident and was likewise able to recuperate without surgery. He also continued going to the judo *dojo* while he recovered, watching the class until he was healed enough to fully participate.

Either of us could have used these injuries as excuses to quit, finding something else to do with our time. One of the most important things you can do when you are injured is continue to go to class. Even if you are just watching, you will continue to learn. Experiencing the action secondhand can keep your interest and motivation high. Furthermore, your instructor and your fellow students will support and respect you for your commitment.

> **Something to think about:**
>
> Your training does not need to stop simply because you cannot physically perform your martial art. Continue to go to class if you are injured; watch, learn, and take notes. Use your "down time" to study up on your art, practice visualization exercises, perform slow work, or train uninjured body parts. With a little creativity, your training never stops.

When you are hurt, it is very easy to skip class while thinking, "Why should I pay for this when I cannot really participate," or "I'll come back when I am healthy, it only makes sense," or "These guys are too rough." You can readily insert similar rationalizations of your own. Do not fall into this trap. It will almost certainly kill your dream of becoming a black belt.

In addition to rehabilitating your injury and regularly watching class, there are varieties of creative things you can do to continue learning while you are hurt. As Wim Demeere stated in the introduction to this chapter, you can do slow work, train opposite sides or uninjured body parts, study, and perform visualization exercises. As long as you find ways to keep martial arts a vital part of your routine odds are good that the injury will not hamper your ability to earn a black belt. It may slow things down a bit if it is serious enough, but the discipline and focus you use to overcome it will help you become a stronger person and a better practitioner in the long run. After all, anything that you learn from (that does not kill you) is a good thing.

Student Perspective (by Frank Getty)

August 8, 2004 was the day my life and martial arts training were altered forever. While helping my girlfriend move, I almost lost an eye. The bungee cord I was using to secure the load in the bed of the pickup truck broke loose and the hook struck me in the eye at full speed. I was very fortunate that my eye was not ripped from the socket, but I did suffer permanent vision loss. Being a former U.S. Marine, pain is not new to me, but this took pain to the extreme. You truly learn how dependent humans are on their eyes when you suffer visual impairment.

For the next three months, I went through multiple surgeries and medical procedures to save my eye. Thanks to some very gifted and dedicated medical professionals, I was able to not only keep my eye but also regain vision up to 20/30-1. Throughout this time, I was not only unable to train in martial arts but I could not do anything physically strenuous.

I remembered something that my Krav Maga instructor had told his class over and over again, "Mental training is every bit as important as physical training." Therefore, during my physical "downtime" I ran self-defense scenarios in my mind. I could train in my head as I sat dormant waiting until I could physically train again.

In January 2005, I had the final surgery and was cleared to engage in limited physical activity. I started weight training and running along with light bag work. All the while, I continued to "practice" Krav in my head. In the fall of 2005, I was prescribed a pair of protective sports eyewear and cleared by my eye doctor to train again.

I must admit I was a bit apprehensive about "getting in the mix" again, knowing how close I came to losing my eye. Plus I was somewhat worried that my skills had greatly diminished. I met privately with my instructor and "knocked the rust off." in January of 2006. I was pleased when my private lesson was finished and my instructor informed me that not only was I as sharp as ever but that I was in better physical shape. In March 2006, I participated in a Krav Maga Law Enforcement seminar and was quite satisfied with my performance. I know that I was able to retain my skills due to all my mental practice.

I cannot stress enough the importance of mental preparation and training. You can have the best physical skills in the world but if you are mentally untrained, they are not only useless but also potentially dangerous.

– Frank Getty [59]

Summary

Injury is a serious thing. With life expectancy higher that it has ever been, it is very important that you do not do something that causes you to spend the next fifty years or more in pain with a poorly functioning body because you were not attentive to an injury. Even simple injuries can become complicated as they can ripple throughout the body, affecting surrounding areas beyond the point of initial damage. Pay attention to pain and resist the temptation to tough things out.

Upon evaluation, if you do not have any signs of significant injury, it may be safe to take care of things by yourself at home. Nevertheless, if the pain or other symptoms become worse, you should call your doctor. A common self-treatment method involves rest, ice, compression, and elevation or RICE for short. It is a good idea to follow these four steps right after an injury and continue them for at least 24 to 48 hours afterward.

Take preventive measures to avoid injury. Warm up thoroughly before vigorous exercise, maintain good flexibility, stay in shape, use good body mechanics, and drink plenty of water. If you are injured, use your down time to work non-physical aspects of your art such as visualization and study.

Action Plan

If you are injured, your action item is simple: TREAT IT SERIOUSLY. The more attentive you are and the sooner you attend to the problem, the faster and better you are likely to heal.

• Have the injury evaluated by competent medical personnel.

_____

_____

_____

• Develop a recovery and rehabilitation plan with your doctor, seeing a specialist such as a sports medicine physician as necessary.

_____

_____

_____

• Continue to go to class even if you cannot actively participate. Watch, take notes, and continue to learn.

_____

_____

_____

• Find creative ways to continue training while you heal.

_____

_____

_____

Suggested Reading

Coseo, Marc. *The Acupressure Warm-Up for Athletic Preparation and Injury Management.* Brookline, MA: Paradigm Publications, 1992.

This unique and insightful book is written and illustrated in a clear, practical format. You will learn to identify, understand, and treat various symptoms of imbalance, working specific problem areas with tennis balls and your own bodyweight pressure to relieve aches and pains. The techniques are very well explained and really do work. Meridian stretches are also covered.

Stark, Dr. Steven D. *The Stark Reality of Stretching: An Informed Approach for All Activities and Every Sport.* Richmond, BC, Canada: The Stark Reality Publishing Group, 1997.

Guard against acute pain, strain, and permanent damage through proper warm-up and stretching. This book does an excellent job of analyzing the stretching process while illustrating the anatomy and basic biomechanics in an easy to read and understand format. The author's strategies can help keep you healthy while building strength and power, and preventing injury.

Levy, Allan M. and Mark L. Fuerst. *Sports Injury Handbook: Professional Advice for Amateur Athletes.* Hoboken, NJ: John Wiley and Sons, Inc., 1993.

A team doctor for the New York Giants football team and other professional sports franchises, the author has treated just about every kind of sports injury you can imagine from strains to sprains to muscle tears to fractured bones. Writing in everyday English, he outlines proven strategies to prevent, treat, and rehabilitate common sports injuries. Contents include special precautions for men, women, children, and older athletes, along with conditioning, nutrition, and training tips. The book also discusses what to do (and not do) in the critical seconds following an injury. Well-written and very practical.

Tsatsouline, Pavel. *Relax Into Stretch: Instant Flexibility Through Mastering Muscle Tension.* St. Paul, MN: Dragon Door Publications, Inc., 2001.

The author is a former physical training instructor for the Soviet Special Forces who works as a strength and endurance trainer for SWAT teams and elite martial artists. His book covers practical ways to increase your flexibility to help protect yourself from injury. The book covers all aspects of stretching, including which exercises are best for your situation, how much flexibility you really need, how to relax and breathe properly while stretching, and how to stretch when injured. Tsatsouline offers very practical and useful advice.

Suggested Web Sites

American College of Sports Medicine (www.acsm.org)

The American College of Sports Medicine promotes and integrates scientific research, education, and practical applications of sports medicine and exercise science to maintain and enhance physical performance, fitness, health, and quality of life. Working in a wide range of medical specialties, allied health professions, and scientific disciplines, its members are committed to the diagnosis, treatment, and prevention of sports-related injuries and the advancement of the science of exercise.

MedicineNet.com (www.medicinenet.com)

MedicineNet.com is an online, healthcare media publishing company. It provides easy-to-read, in-depth, authoritative medical information for consumers via its robust, user-friendly, interactive Web site. Topics cover the whole gambit of medical information, including dealing with sports injuries.

U.S. Department of Health and Human Services (www.pueblo.gsa.gov/cic_text/health/sports/injuries.htm)

An online resource for understanding and preventing various sports-related injuries, this Web site has excellent overview information and links to in-depth research and information.

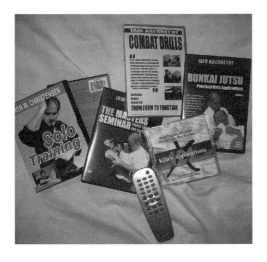

TODAY'S VIDEOS AND DVD'S ARE GREAT AIDS, BUT NOT REPLACEMENTS, TO ACTUAL ON THE FLOOR OR MAT TIME. YOU CAN USE TO SUPPLEMENT YOUR HANDS-ON TRAINING.

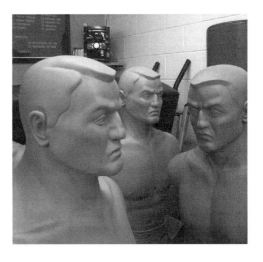

HIT THESE GUYS AS HARD AS YOU WANT. THEY NEVER SAY, "OUCH!," GET MAD, OR QUIT. BODY OPPONENT BAGS FACILITATE REALISTIC TARGETING AND HEAVY IMPACT TRAINING WITHOUT THE RISK OF INJURY.

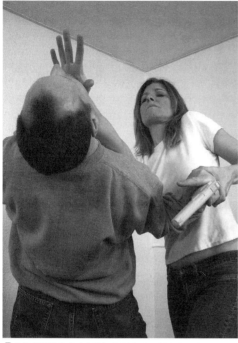

THE TRAINING GUN IS DESIGNED TO SIMULATE THE WEIGHT AND FEEL OF A REAL GUN. IT'S HEAVY ENOUGH TO STRIKE WITH YET FLEXIBLE ENOUGH TO BRUISE RATHER THAN BREAK YOUR TRAIN-ING PARTNER. ITS REALISTIC SHAPE GIVES AN EXTRA ADRENALINE CHARGE THAT FACILITATES REALISTIC PRACTICE. THIS IS AS CLOSE AS YOU'LL WANT TO GET TO THE REAL THING.

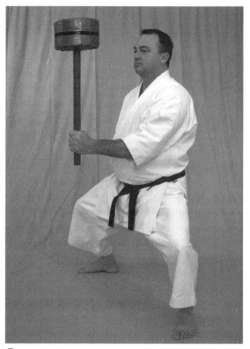

THE *CHIISHI*, A STONE-LEVERED WEIGHT, IS A TRADITIONAL TOOL THAT IS USED TO BUILD STRENGTH AND MUSCLE COORDINATION. TRADITIONAL TRAINING EQUIPMENT CAN OFTENTIMES TARGET MARTIAL ARTISTS NEEDS BETTER THAN MODERN WEIGHTLIFTING DEVICES.

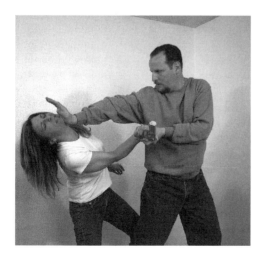

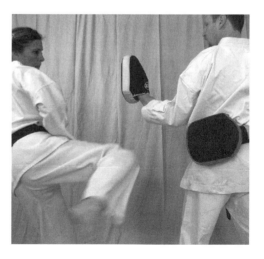

A MODERN PRACTICE GUN MADE OF YELLOW PLASTIC IS UNABLE TO CHAMBER OR FIRE A REAL BULLET. THE BRIGHT YELLOW COLOR CLEARLY IDENTIFIES IT AS A NON-FUNCTIONING TRAINING MODEL. THIS AFFORDS AN OPPORTUNITY TO PRAC-TICE HIGHLY DANGEROUS TECHNIQUES IN RELATIVE SAFETY.

MODERN STRIKING PADS MADE WITH SYNTHETIC MATERIALS PRO-VIDE EXCELLENT PROTECTION, BOTH FOR THE PERSON DELIVERING THE BLOWS AND FOR THE ONE RECEIVING THEM.

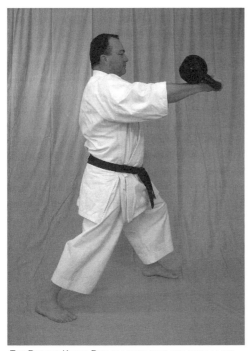

THE RUSSIAN KETTLE BELL IS A SOLID IRON BALL WITH A HANDLE. SIMPLE TECHNOLOGY AND SIMPLY HARD, IT OFFERS A GREAT WORKOUT.

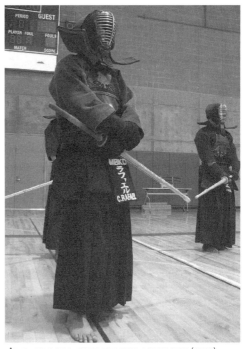

AN EXAMPLE OF A *KENDO-KA* IN FULL SAFETY GEAR (*BOGU*).

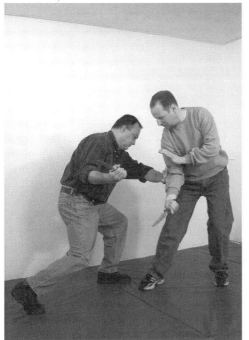

REAL KNIVES? HARDLY. THEY ARE MADE OF THE FINEST RUBBER AVAILABLE. ALMOST ANY SIZE AND SHAPE OF RUBBER KNIFE CAN BE PURCHASED TODAY FOR YOU TO TRAIN SAFELY. THERE ARE NO GOOD REASONS TO TRAIN WITH WEAPONS WHEN YOU CAN SUBSTITUTE A SAFER DEVICE WITH THE SAME WEIGHT AND BALANCE.

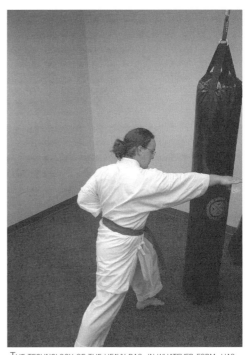

THE TECHNOLOGY OF THE HEAVY BAG, IN WHATEVER FORM, HAS BEEN TESTED OVER TIME. IT IS A RELATIVELY INEXPENSIVE PIECE OF EQUIPMENT THAT IS REALLY POWERFUL FOR SOLO TRAINING.

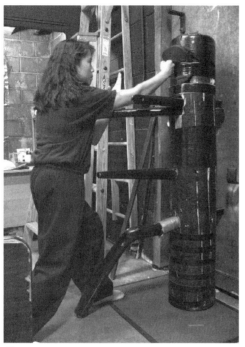

THE CLASSIC, *MUK YAN JONG,* OR WOODEN MAN, IS AN EXAMPLE OF TRADITIONAL TECHNOLOGY THAT HAS THE ADVANTAGE OF HAVING ARMS TO WORK ON AND AROUND.

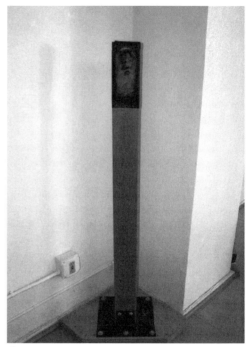

ANOTHER EXAMPLE OF TRADITIONAL TECHNOLOGY, THE *MAKI-WARA* STRIKING POST IS USED TO CONDITION THE BODY AND DEVELOP EXPLOSIVE STRIKING POWER.

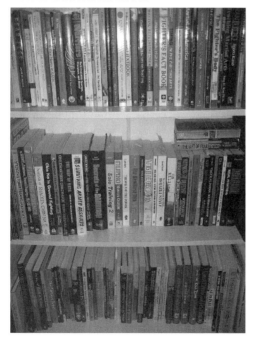

BOOKS ARE A FANTASTIC RESOURCE. GENERALLY MORE IN-DEPTH THAN A VIDEO PRODUCTION, THEY ARE EASILY TRANSPORTABLE AND ONLY REQUIRE A LITTLE AMBIENT LIGHT TO OPERATE.

CHAPTER 8

Use Technology

"No sensible decision can be made any longer without taking into account not only the world as it is, but the world as it will be..."
– Isaac Asimov [60]

Introduction (by Loren W. Christensen)

I began training in the martial arts in the summer of 1965. Months earlier, I had broken my lower back in a weightlifting contest and the doctor had told me to stop lifting weights and to try something less violent on the body. Therefore, I began karate training.

In the United States in the mid-1960s the martial arts, karate in particular, was in its infancy. Most people had not heard of it and would furrow their brow in confusion when they did. "Karate? Is that some kind of Chinese food?"

"No," I'd say with growing impatience. "Chow mein is Chinese food. Karate is a fighting art." Then I would quote the late Peter Urban, an eccentric karate master who helped bring Goju Ryu *to the East Coast in the 1960s: "Karate is the art of fightin' real good."*

Many of the fighting styles that sprang up all over the country in the 1960s were brought here by returning servicemen, military folks who had served in exotic Asian locales. They brought home this new fighting art and, along with it, the same teaching methods under which they had learned. Most often, their ways were extreme, harsh, and injurious. It was not that these martial arts pioneers were cruel, though some were; it was that they were simply employing the only teaching methods they knew.

My first few years of diligent training were done without protection for the hands, shins, feet, teeth, head, and the groin. Our white uniforms were often splattered with blood, our blood and our partner's, which we wore unwashed to show the world our red badges of warriorhood. The delicate tops of our hands and feet, our shinbones and fore-arms, and our foreheads were almost always covered with "walnuts," a name we gave those swollen lumps that littered our bony surfaces. And bruises? We had so many that our bruises had walnuts and some of our bruises had their own bruises.

One day one of us got an idea of going to a mattress warehouse and buying a large square of foam rubber. We cut off chunks and taped them to the backs of our hands and over our shins to protect especially swollen injured areas. My instructor—a product of old school training—would not let us cover anything that was not already injured.

Most of us took our broken fingers to a doctor while busted toes were just shrugged off and taped to a healthy one on either side. A hand with a broken finger would be stuffed in our belts behind our backs and we would train with the remaining arm. I remember several occasions when I had to place both arms behind my back and spar with only my feet.

Old-fashioned exercises and training methods hurt many of us, too: Exercises like squatting with a training partner on our shoulders, "duck walking" (squatting down and running laps), training-partner-assisted forced stretches, and pushing our bodies past fatigue and into the red zone of overuse.

We did not know any better, nor did our teachers. We were pioneers, forging a path littered with torn muscles and strained ligaments, broken bones and, in some cases, irreparable damage, damage that cut short martial art careers or that still haunt us old warriors years later. As I begin my fifth decade of martial arts training, I give thanks every day for over-the-counter pain killers.

Let us jump ahead to the new millennium. With today's vast array of marvelous safety equipment, you would be hard pressed to find a martial artist with mattress padding taped to his shins. For less than a hundred dollars, you can pad your critical body areas with lightweight, space-age material in a rainbow of color options. If you want to invest a thousand dollars, you can cover your entire person in the stuff, though your mobility is pretty much limited to a slow, simple shuffle.

Back in the early years, constant injuries slowed progress, sometimes stopped it. Students either stayed home until they healed, or they struggled through classes picking and choosing what they could and could not do. This rarely happens today. With ever-improving protective equipment, sprains, jams, hyperextensions, and breaks are few and far between. Sure, stuff still happens. After all, the study of martial arts is the study of fighting, not flower arranging. Nonetheless, today's injury count is nowhere near the scale of the old days. Now that students can practice in relative safety, they have greater confidence to push themselves, to try new things, to take chances.

When American service members and Asian masters first brought the fighting arts to the United States, few debated the science and wisdom (or lack of it) of what was taught. Thankfully, that was not to last. American martial artists began to ask questions, to debate, and to challenge. Martial art techniques were to be scrutinized in the scientific community: Where do they get their power? Their speed? How can martial artists get faster, stronger, better? Meditation seemed to work, but why? How can it be made more relative to the fighting arts?

Sports medicine entered the picture and along with it modern training methods. Nutritionists told us how to eat better for growth and recovery. Trainers with master's degrees and doctorates taught us the value of recuperative sleep, healthful and stamina-building nutrition supplementation, weight training for speed and explosiveness, specificity of movement exercises, aerobic and anaerobic training, and the importance of cross training. Psychologists taught us about the powerful link between mind and body.

When I began training in the mid-1960s, there were only a few books on the market. Video and DVD technology were still a few years off from their invention, as was the internet and sharing of information through Web sites, blogs, and streaming film clips. By the end of that decade, there were dozens of books on the subject and numerous magazines. Jump ahead to the present and today's modern martial artists can avail themselves to hundreds, perhaps thousands, of books, training videos, and DVDs.

Today we are in the information age and it can be happily reported that the martial arts have kept up. Today's kicking taekwondo *student can learn exotic hand techniques from kung fu by simply inserting a disc into a DVD player. A hard-punching karate stylist and his training buddy can add to their grappling techniques by garnering applications from books on standup* jujitsu *locks, Brazilian ground fighting techniques, Chinese* chin-na *moves, and gravity defying* aikido *throws. A grappler can learn powerful* muay Thai *kicks from videos taught by well-known champions.*

Can't remember how to hold your foot when you sidekick? Unlike just 15 years ago, you no longer have to lose training time by having to wait until next week to ask your instructor. Simply Google "sidekick" into your computer and you are instantly bombarded with thousands of Web sites that show experts throwing that same move.

As modern technology continues to affect the martial arts field with new and improved training equipment and teaching aids, the one aspect of martial arts training that has not changed is the one that is arguably the most important. Without it, all the fancy schmancy workout gear, books, videos, and DVDs are meaningless, worthless. I'm talking about discipline. You have got to train and then train some more. Then you must train some more after that.

When you can say no to parties, the movies, and the undeniable pleasure of sprawling on the sofa and surfing the channels to make yourself train one more time, you are on the way to being the best you can be. Making that journey just a little bit easier and virtually pain free is a vast amount of modern safety equipment and training information to take you to heights unimagined when the Asian fighting arts landed on our soil just a few decades ago.

– Loren W. Christensen [61]

Taking Advantage of Modern Technology

This chapter is about modern technology, but let us place things in context by beginning with a brief history lesson. The *samurai* of feudal Japan were easily recognized by the *daisho* (paired long- and short-swords) they wore at all times. In certain situations, other *bushi* (nobles) and *ashigaru* (infantry soldiers) could carry a single *katana* (long sword) or *wakizashi* (short sword), but matched sets were only worn by the elite *samurai*. These exquisitely crafted implements of destruction were so well-made that many centuries-old examples are still fully functional and deadly to this day, arguably the best blades ever forged by man despite the poor raw materials with which the Japanese bladesmiths had to work. These swords were more than mere weapons. They were symbols of status and power. The *samurai* who carried them were the elite of the elite, the best-trained and equipped warriors of their time.

That all changed suddenly and dramatically at the end of the 1800s. Confronted by technologically superior Western powers, Emperor Meiji came to the realization that swordsmen, no matter how well armed and trained, were really no match for gunmen, steamships, and artillery. Some of the events of that tumultuous time were more or less accurately depicted in the movie *The Last Samurai*. Emperor Meiji's reforms ultimately abolished the *samurai* class and conscripted commoners as rifle-bearing soldiers for the Japanese army. While the martial arts used by the *samurai* still exist, along with examples of their swords, Japanese culture and society were forever changed due to imported foreign technology.

While we are sometimes forced to adapt to technological innovation, oftentimes we can bend technology to suit our purposes. An excellent example of this can be found in most martial arts schools, where modern students excel at ancient arts through facilitation of modern technology. Books, articles, Web sites, videos, DVDs, podcasts, blogs, and streaming videos make ancient secrets and training methods widely available for practitioners. Japanese, Okinawan, Chinese, Korean, Thai, Filipino, and other foreign language texts are easily and inexpensively translated into English and a host of other languages. State-of-the-art protective equipment, advanced nutritional counseling, and scientifically designed strength and conditioning programs are all available to stave off injury and speed the

"Almost everybody today believes that nothing in economic history has ever moved as fast as, or had a greater impact than, the Information Revolution. But the Industrial Revolution moved at least as fast in the same time span, and had probably an equal impact if not a greater one."

– Peter Drucker [62]

development of modern martial artists. Technology lets us make the most of our training time, speeds our progress, and helps us master the martial arts in ways practitioners could not fathom even a few short years ago.

We will briefly discuss some of these items. Depending on learning style predilections (e.g., visual, auditory, or kinesthetic), you may be drawn toward some knowledge sources more than others. Pick and choose whatever appeals to you and aids your progress but be sure to take advantage of this powerful information by adding appropriate use of technology to your repertoire.

Gather Information from Articles and Books

Magazines such as *Black Belt*, *Journal of Asian Martial Arts*, *Martial Arts Professional*, *Traditional Karate*, *Taekwondo Times*, *Grappling Magazine*, and many others provide useful articles about training methods, tactics, techniques, legal aspects of martial arts, and other valuable information such as equipment reviews and *dojo* directories. Even if you do not subscribe to these periodicals, it is useful to browse through a copy on occasion or pick one up at a library.

If you would like to explore any given topic more in depth, there are a variety of books available from various publishers like Frog Limited, Kodansha International, Ohara Publications, Paladin Press, Turtle Press, Tuttle Publishing, and YMAA Publication Center. You can also search e-Bay, bookfinder.com, and used bookstores for historical tomes and rare, out-of-print editions written by the founders of many styles. There is an abundance of martial knowledge out there that you can take advantage of, including style-specific fundamentals (e.g., basic techniques and advancement requirements), *kata* performance and analysis, fitness and conditioning essentials, martial arts history and genealogy, internal energy manipulation, self-defense applications, and more.

All arts have certain elements in common. Karate, for example, includes throwing, grappling, and choking applications in addition to punches and kicks. If you are a *karateka* and want to learn more about the lesser-used aspects of your art, you can easily pick up books on *aikido*, judo, *jujitsu*, or wrestling. Likewise, Mixed Martial Arts (MMA) enthusiasts facilitate their cross training by studying techniques from a variety of styles.

There are so many books available, in fact, that it is oftentimes challenging to find quality materials for your specific area(s) of interest. Just as we point you to additional resources at the end of each chapter in this book, many instructors maintain recommended reading lists or lending libraries to facilitate your studies. That is the best place to start since your instructor should know what works best to augment his or her hands-on instruction. Book reviews found in the aforementioned magazines as well as at online sources such as Amazon.com can also help you find quality materials.

Some of our favorite authors are listed below. These folks are not "*dojo* darlings" by any stretch of the imagination. They are the real deal—experienced practitioners, street fighters, and professionals who are not only superior martial artists but also gifted writers, adept at communicating their knowledge clearly and effectively. There are dozens of other excellent authors in the field, of course, but these folks made our short list because they have penned multiple outstanding books (and DVDs in most cases) rather than one or two high-quality works, giving you a better chance of finding something of theirs that you will like.

Iain Abernethy

Iain Abernethy holds a 5th *dan* in karate with both Karate England and the British Combat Association. Iain is the author of numerous books on applied martial arts and personal development. He has also produced many popular DVDs on practical martial arts and the realistic application of traditional karate *kata*.

Dan Anderson

Since beginning his martial arts training in 1966, he has earned a 7th *dan* black belt in karate, a 6th *dan* black belt in Filipino Modern Arnis, and an 8th *dan* black belt in Modern Arnis – 80. He is a four-time National Karate Champion, having won over 70 Grand Titles! Anderson is the founder of American Freestyle Karate, a uniquely American martial art as well as the author of the best selling book, *American Freestyle Karate: A Guide To Sparring*, which has been in print for 20 years. His eight other books and four DVDs have proven popular with serious martial artists world wide.

Loren W. Christensen

Loren Christensen began his martial arts training in 1965, earning 10 black belts over the years, seven in karate, two in *jujitsu*, and one in *arnis*. He is a retired police officer with twenty-nine years of experience in military and civilian law enforcement, where he specialized in street gangs, defensive tactics, and dignitary protection. A prolific author, he has written more than thirty books and hundreds of articles on the martial arts, self-defense, law enforcement, nutrition, prostitution, gangs, and post-traumatic stress disorder. He has also produced several DVDs.

Peter Consterdine

Peter is acknowledged as one of the world's leading authorities on personal security and unarmed combat. He has written numerous books and produced many DVDs on the subject, giving seminars on security awareness and defensive tactics throughout the world. An 8th *dan* black belt in karate, he has over forty continuous years of martial arts training behind him. Along with Geoff Thompson, Peter is joint Chief Instructor of The British Combat Association, Europe's leading association for the promotion of self defense and practical combat.

Sang H. Kim

Sang H. Kim holds an M.S. degree in sports science and a Ph.D. in media studies. He is an internationally respected expert and author of several martial arts books and star of over seventy instructional DVDs. A former Korean National Champion, he was named instructor of the year in Korea in 1983. His articles are featured in over one hundred publications worldwide.

Dave Lowry

Dave Lowry has devoted his life to studying all things Japanese, immersing himself in the art and culture since 1968. He practices the martial arts of *Yagyu Shinkage Ryu* (swordsmanship), karate, *Shindo Muso Ryu* (short staff), and *aikido* as well as the peaceful arts of *go* (a board game), *shodo* (calligraphy), *kado* (flower arrangement), and *chado* (tea ceremony). He has authored numerous books on martial arts and Japanese culture. His articles have appeared in numerous magazines throughout the world. His column, *The Karate Way* (found in *Black Belt* magazine), is a must-read.

Marc "Animal" MacYoung

Growing up on gang-infested streets not only gave Marc MacYoung his street name "Animal," but also extensive firsthand experience about what does and does not work for self-defense. Over the years, he has held a number of dangerous occupations, including director of a correctional institute, bodyguard, and bouncer. He was first shot at when he was 15 years old and has since survived multiple attempts on his life, including professional contracts. He has studied a variety of martial arts since childhood, teaching experience-based self-defense to police, military, civilians, and martial artists around the world. His has written dozens of books and produced many DVDs covering all aspects of this field.

Peyton Quinn

Peyton Quinn is considered by many the "dean" of barroom brawling. He began his training in formal martial arts systems in 1964, eventually achieving black belts in karate, judo and *aikido*. While he continues to respect and explore Asian martial arts systems, his real-world experience has shown him that for most people, training in martial arts alone is not enough for real fighting. He has written numerous books and created several DVDs on the subject.

Martina Sprague

Martina Sprague has studied and taught the martial arts for twenty years, earning black belts in *Kenpo* karate, kickboxing, and street freestyle. She is a scholar of warfare and combat, having written several books on sports science, martial arts, Scandinavian history, and Norse warfare.

Dr. Yang Jwing-Ming

Dr. Yang Jwing-Ming is a prolific author as well as one of the world's foremost kung fu experts. Highly skilled in *Shaolin* White Crane (*Bai He*), *Shaolin* Long Fist (*changquan*), and *taijiquan* and other forms, he has spent more than thirty years teaching his art to others. He has published more than thirty-five books and seventy-five videos on the martial arts. Dr. Yang is currently president of Yang's Oriental Arts Association headquartered in Boston, Massachusetts.

Depending on which martial art you study, you may also wish to look for books written by the founder of your style, one of his direct disciples, or other significant figures in the art. For example, Professor Jigoro Kano, the founder of judo, outlined nearly every aspect of his art in his book *Kodokan Judo*. It is a very well written and illustrated tome. While Chojun Miyagi, the founder of *Goju Ryu* karate, did not put much of his art in writing, Seikichi Toguchi, one of his disciples, did. His books *Okinawan Goju Ryu* and *Okinawan Goju Ryu II: Advanced Techniques of Shorei-Kan Karate* are outstanding. They do not cover all of the art but do provide step-by-step instructions on much of the curricula. Supplementing this with works by preeminent practitioners like Morio Higaonna gives a reasonably complete picture of the style.

Gichin Funakoshi, the founder of *Shotokan* karate, was a prolific writer. Books such as *Karate-Do: My Way of Life* and *Karate-Do Kyohan: The Master Text* are well worth reading, even if you are not a practitioner of that style. Compilations of his work such as *The Twenty Guiding Principles of Karate: The Spiritual Legacy of the Master* are excellent and appeal to multiple styles. If you are a *Shotokan* practitioner and would like a step-by-step guide to your art you should consider *25 Shotokan Kata* by Shojiro Sugiyama. Although it does not delve into applications, it does a wonderful job describing the sequence of the forms.

> *"The man who does not read good books has no advantage over the man who cannot read them."*
>
> – Mark Twain [63]

Visit Martial Arts Web Sites

There are thousands of martial arts-related Web sites. As with everything else on the Internet, some are good and some are bad. As some of the highly publicized inaccuracies of Wikipedia.com postings have graphically illustrated, just because information is published online does not necessarily guarantee that it is accurate (or worthwhile). To the extent you can, it is important to validate any information you discover through more than one source.

Taking what you find with a grain of salt aside, the Internet is an excellent source of free (or inexpensive) research and useful data. You can easily find martial arts articles, film clips, podcasts, streaming videos, photos, book reviews, and much more.

Some authors and publishers offer sample chapters that you can download to pre-view books before you buy them. Some even offer e-books at a fraction of the cost of printed materials if you would like to go that route. You can often find audio books and podcasts as well.

Many instructors maintain their own Web sites, providing relevant information and links to sources applicable to your training. This is an excellent place to start. You can also look to the wider Web for additional data as you need it. When it comes to martial arts, there are three types of Web sites on which you may wish to focus your research:

- Style-specific sites such as www.gojuryu.net or www.judoinfo.com that can help you with basic techniques, historical information, promotion require-ments, step-by-step *kata* procedures, sparring tips, and self-defense appli-cations related to whatever art you practice. A Google or Yahoo search of your style's name will help you find relevant sites.

- General sites such as www.fightingarts.com that provide a wide range of martial arts-related topics, discussion forums, book reviews, articles, and advice. There is a growing community of martial artists on the Web, many of whom freely share their knowledge on these types of sites.

- Targeted sites exist such as www.iainabernethy.com (Iain Abernethy's site) ,which focuses on analysis of traditional karate *kata* or www.nononsense-selfdefense.com (Marc MacYoung's site), which focuses on street-worthy self-defense and personal safety topics. If there is a specific area of martial arts that interests you, odds are good that someone has a site devoted to it.

Video Record Training Sessions

Making movies in the *dojo* can be a very effective training tool. They can be used to help you record and memorize new forms, analyze your performance during *kata* practice or sparring sessions, critique the performance of your training partners, and correct bad habits. There is nothing like seeing yourself on video to truly understand how you are doing. This is particularly true during sparring sessions where you are going full speed and all your attention is focused on your training partner through-out the encounter.

Some instructors periodically set aside time for video recorded training sessions while others let you set up a camera and leave it running whenever you like. Others ban the practice altogether. Always obtain permission before recording anything and be respectful of those with whom you train. Keep anything you record within your training group unless you have express permission to share with outsiders. Just because your own instructor encourages video recording does not necessarily mean that any guest instructors he or she invites on occasion will feel the same way. Some *sensei*, particularly traditional ones, are very sensitive to having their forms recorded even by their own students, so it is always good to ask ahead of time. When you are dealing with folks who can crush you like a grape without breaking a sweat, it pays to be polite.

When analyzing your performance, it is useful to look for erroneous actions, loss of stance integrity, unbalanced (uncoordinated) movements, and improper breathing. When performing *kata*, it is relatively easy to spot mistakes such as missing, added, or incorrect techniques, but it is also important to pay attention to subtleties such as improper weight shifts, imprecise angles, poor posture, and incorrect breathing. When sparring, look for "tells," tiny gestures that telegraph what you are about to do. Common errors include dropping your shoulder, tensing your neck, over-shifting your weight, making facial gestures such as visibly flaring your nostrils, or exhaling loudly when you are about to throw a punch or launch a kick. For grappling and throwing techniques, look for improper body positioning, open space between you and your opponent that can allow him or her to counter or evade your technique.

Review DVDs Relevant to Your Art

While static pictures and descriptions in books, articles, or Web sites can provide step-by-step descriptions of *kata*, *bunkai*, or drills, some things are simply easier to understand when you can see all the motions in real time. There are a wide variety of DVDs for sale covering just about everything you need to know to earn your black belt. A recent search of martial arts DVDs carried by Amazon.com alone displayed 940 titles. You can learn *kata*, solo drills, tandem exercises, sparring techniques, and more. Clearly DVDs are no substitute for hands-on instruction, but they can be very useful to help you remember what you have learned in class.

Some organizations will also record seminars and special events, making DVDs available to attendees for a nominal fee. Taking advantage of these opportunities helps you remember what you have learned and also lets you see anything that you may have missed. Like booklists, many instructors maintain a list of recommended DVDs for their students. Most of our favorite book authors produce DVDs too, so that is another potential source of materials that you will find valuable.

Take Advantage of Podcast Learning Opportunities

Podcasting, a blend of the words "iPod" and "broadcasting," is the distribution of audio and/or video files over the internet. Podcasts can be downloaded to an iPod, laptop, or PC on demand or may be automatically delivered via a subscription service.

> **Something to think about:**
>
> In traditional schools, padding and other safety devices are generally discouraged as they limit ranges of movement and ability to perform certain techniques. Further, there are important conditioning aspects to being hit with a healthy amount of force in non-vital areas. In tandem exercises, the senior partner controls the speed and takes responsibility for safety of both practitioners, obviating the need for most protective gear.

This technology is an excellent way to receive rich content such as interviews with world-class martial arts easily and inexpensively.

A couple of free podcasts that are truly enlightening include *Martial Secrets* (www.westseattlekarate.com/podcast.shtml), hosted by *Sensei* Kris Wilder and *The Applied Karate Show* (www.karate.thepodcastnetwork.com) hosted by *Sensei* Des Paroz. These broadcasts include interviews with world-class martial artists whose experiences are easy to learn from. Many sites dedicated to martial topics include podcasts in their content. You can also search iTunes for martial arts-related broadcasts.

Utilize Appropriate Protective Equipment and Safety Gear

Martial arts are, by definition, warlike and dangerous. Mixed martial arts, tournament, and combative schools frequently utilize protective equipment to help practitioners learn hazardous techniques in a safe and controlled manner. If you plan to focus primarily on full-contact free sparring, it is important to be able to "tee off"* on each other without inadvertently sending anyone to the hospital. The use of protective gear and/or safety rules creates very different dynamics between sparring practice and actual combat, yet it is essential for assuring your ability to make it through each training session in one piece while learning as much as you can from the encounter.

In traditional schools, on the other hand, padding and other safety devices are generally discouraged as they limit range of movement and ability to perform certain techniques. Further, there are important conditioning aspects to being hit with a healthy amount of force (in non-vital areas, of course). Being able to absorb a blow is important; a black belt who is not used to contact will often be unable to present an adequate defense in a real fight. In tandem exercises, the senior partner controls the speed and takes responsibility for safety of both practitioners, obviating the need for most protective gear.

Every martial art requires a certain degree of physical contact, frequently violent physical contact. While the level of contact varies by the type of sparring that you are actually undertaking in class, *kumite* (sparring) is common in most martial styles. Use of protective equipment, where appropriate, facilitates the ability to train hard

---

* Work at full speed and power.

without seriously injuring your training partners. The basics include things like headgear, mouthpieces, groin protectors, gloves, and shin/instep/foot pads.

Common derivative forms of sparring include *kiso kumite* (prearranged sparring), *fuku shiki kumite* (freestyle sparring with *kata* emphasis), *sanbon shobu kumite* (three-point, tournament-style match), and *randori* (freestyle sparring). While none of these variations reaches the level of violence you would typically find in a street fight, the amount of contact can get close. The closer it gets, the more likely you are to need protective gear.

Kiso kumite is prearranged sparring with an emphasis on technique. It is a set of attack and counterattack sequences designed to teach self-defense skills without the dangers inherent in free sparring. Utilized frequently in traditional *dojo*, techniques are pulled from a variety of *kata* and grouped by theme (such as evasion, nerve strikes, short techniques, and so on). *Ippon kiso kumite*, a common derivative, uses only the last attack and defense from each set, followed by an additional set of freeform attacks by the original defender. Because both attacker and defender know exactly what the other partner will do and are able to absorb blows with their arms and legs, participants can execute techniques safely without the need for protective gear, while using great quickness and power. As training progresses, the patterns are burned into the practitioner's muscle memory, facilitating automatic responses in pressure situations.

Fuku shiki kumite is freestyle sparring with an emphasis on *kata*. Similar to *ippon kiso kumite,* advanced practitioners often use it to practice *bunkai oyo* (principles of *kata* application) in an unchoreographed manner. Partners may decide to use only techniques for specific *kata* or may select a more freeform manner, but either way the emphasis is on employment of *kata bunkai* (applications). *Kata*-based sparring reinforces what you learn in forms practice while building the spontaneity and timing required for executing *kata* applications in tournament and self-defense situations.

Sanbon shobu kumite is a three-point, tournament-style match. Padding and safety gear are more frequently used with this application, though certainly not in every case. Strict safety rules outlaw anything truly dangerous (e.g., eye gouges, nerve strikes, joint kicks). Even if a competitor is rendered unconscious in a match, referees and medical personnel are close at hand to safely revive him or her. Similarly, joint locks do not generally lead to hyperextension or dislocation in a tournament. Weight classes frequently match competitors of similar size/age, and mixed gender competitions are rare occurrences. While not much like street fights, tournaments are great for conditioning. They build reflex action and refine a practitioner's timing and reaction skills.

Randori is freestyle sparring, similar to a practice tournament where points are not counted or recorded. This activity is commonly used in grappling arts such as judo or *jujitsu*, includes high intensity attacks, and counterattacks drawn from anywhere within the martial system. The focus is on movement, combinations, timing, and balance. Unlike *kiso kumite*, *randori* can help practitioners enhance their ability to react instantaneously to surprise attacks. Like *sanbon shobu kumite*, however, vital areas are left alone in *randori* and blows are struck only with sufficient force to score a "victory," even when protective gear is utilized. In the grappling arts, for example, chokes are released when a practitioner taps (the ground, the mat, or a body part), often before he or she loses consciousness.

If you include full-contact sparring in your training regimen, your instructor will either provide the equipment you will need to use or give you a list of things you will have to obtain, or both. Despite safety precautions, padding, and protective gear, you will undoubtedly get bruises, abrasions, and minor cuts during practice. You may even break a bone, hyperextend a joint, suffer an inadvertent eye injury, or accidentally receive other serious damage. Be sure to use safety gear such as braces, splints, protective eyewear, or other devices when necessary to safeguard your injuries while you recover. See Chapter 7 for more information on working through injuries.

Ensure That Your Nutritional Needs Are Met

Professional athletes, martial artists, and highly active individuals have different nutritional requirements than ordinary couch potatoes. In general, you need to balance eating and exercise to stay in shape. The more active you are, the more calories you can (and need to) consume without expanding your midsection. You must ensure that all your nutritional requirements are being met with your diet too. For example, two thousand calories of fast food from your local hamburger joint is not likely to be as beneficial or healthy as the same number of calories found in a home-cooked meal.

Martial artists can burn as many as five hundred to a thousand calories per hour of activity, depending on the weight of the individual and the level of intensity of the workout. Carbohydrates are a primary source of this energy, yet adding protein and fat to your diet lowers the glycemic level of your meal so that the energy lasts longer. Protein, carbohydrates, and fat are all essential components of a healthy diet but the recommended proportions will vary depending on how active you are.

Before we go into those proportions, it is important to understand that protein is vital to maintain and build strong muscles, repairing damage done during a strenuous workout. Consuming protein shortly after exercise is quite helpful. Carbohydrates are a necessary source of quick energy to fuel your routine. Fat is effectively an energy storage system that sustains you throughout aerobic activity. Unsaturated fat is healthy in moderation, supporting your immune system and protecting vital organs as well. Saturated fat, on the other hand, is linked to LDL (bad cholesterol), an excess of which can lead to heart disease or cancer, or both.

Active martial artists frequently split their food intake in proportions of roughly 40 percent carbohydrates, 30 percent protein, and 30 percent fat. You will probably vary the exact mix based on your body type, fitness level, and training regimen at any given time. For example, if you are about to enter a tournament, take an advancement test, or attend an intense seminar, you may require proportionally more carbohydrates or even more calories than you would normally consume. If you are overweight and trying to get in better shape, you will probably lower those aspects of the mix.

To find out more about proper nutrition and tailor a diet that best supports your training regimen, you may wish to read *The Fighter's Body: An Owner's Manual: Your Guide to Diet, Nutrition, Exercise and Excellence in the Martial Arts* by Loren Christensen and Wim Demeere. The book is an outstanding resource, packed with practical advice that is easy to understand and implement.

Incorporate Strength and Conditioning Training

While practitioners with advanced martial skill can overcome larger, stronger opponents, all things equal the person in the best physical condition has the best chance to win. *Yudansha* (black belts) do not necessarily need to be Olympic-caliber athletes yet there is a certain degree of strength, endurance, and flexibility that is required to perform at black-belt level. The better shape you are in, the easier it is to get there.

Even though fitness is an important aspect of your training, while resources for getting in shape are ubiquitous, you must go to a *dojo* for specialized martial arts instruction. Consequently, some instructors include *daruma* (warm-up exercises) with every class session while many expect you to take care of that aspect on your own. Either way, you need to know how to do it safely and effectively. *Daruma* in and of itself is generally not sufficient to get you into black belt shape, so you will undoubtedly need to do some work on your own.

The first thing you will want to focus on is stretching. Flexibility is essential for quickness, balance, and injury prevention. Stretching should be completed before and after strenuous physical activity. Many practitioners stretch before their workout but forget (or are too tired) to do so afterward. You will recover better if you remember to stretch before and after training sessions.

To ensure that stretching will not cause injury to cold muscles, exercises should always begin with light aerobic activity such as jumping jacks, cross-marching (alternately raising right leg/left arm and vice versa), or jogging in place to warm up and loosen your muscles. A good analogy might be to think of the muscles as strips of bacon. When cold, they tear easily. Once warmed even a little (e.g., by cooking), they become much more elastic and are harder to break. If you are a vegetarian or have some objection to pork products, think cabbage leaves. They tear easily at room temperature yet blanched in hot water they become much more resilient.

It is best to begin by stretching your joints first and then your tendons, and finally proceeding to build your muscles, in that order. When stretching joints or moving tendons, it is best to work from the ground up so you do not miss anything. Muscles can only contract, so it is important to ensure that you always work opposing muscle groups during strength building exercises (e.g., when doing sit-ups, also do back lifts; when building biceps, also work triceps).

Body-weight exercises such as push-ups, scoop-ups (sometimes called Hindu push-ups), sit-ups, back lifts, leg lifts, trunk rotations, pull-ups, mountain-climbers, dips, and squats are performed at most martial arts schools, typically at the beginning of each class. For peak performance, it is important to complement these activities with endurance-building exercises such as distance running, hill sprinting, swimming, or jumping rope, typically done on your own outside of class. Always check with your physician before engaging in a new exercise routine, of course.

Weight-based training can be important too. *Kigu hojo undo*, or supplementary training with various tools, is part of the conditioning routine at many traditional schools. This practice can help martial artists develop tremendous physical strength and flexibility, particularly once high repetition bodyweight exercises become relatively easy to perform.

So how do you know if you are ready for weight-based exercises? If you can do the following exercise set (Martina Sprague calls this the body-weight challenge pyramid) in rapid succession without feeling like you are about to keel over from exhaustion afterward, you are probably ready to add training tools or weights of some type to your routine:

- 30 push-ups, 30 crunch sit-ups, 30 squats
- 25 push-ups, 25 crunch sit-ups, 25 squats
- 20 push-ups, 20 crunch sit-ups, 20 squats
- 15 push-ups, 15 crunch sit-ups, 15 squats
- 10 push-ups, 10 crunch sit-ups, 10 squats
- 5 push-ups, 5 crunch sit-ups, 5 squats

Okinawan training equipment traditionally includes devices such as *makiwara*, *ishisashi*, *tan*, *chiishi*, *makiage kigu*, *nigiri game*, *tetsu geta*, and *kongoken*. Many practitioners believe that these devices target the portions of the body that need the most work more effectively than modern weight training equipment, especially more than weight machines. Free weights, according to many, tend to be more effective at building functional muscle, tendon, and ligament strength than machines that target narrow muscle groups. Functional strength and endurance are necessary for most martial arts techniques.

Traditional or modern, the use of training equipment greatly increases your propensity for becoming injured. Consequently, it is vital to complete a thorough warm-up prior to the commencement of *kigu hojo undo* or modern weight training. Additionally, you should only use such specialized training equipment under the watchful eye of your instructor or personal trainer until you have developed a sufficient level of proficiency to handle the various pieces of equipment in a controlled and safe manner on your own.

Most readers should have at least a passing familiarity with modern training equipment such as heavy bags, speed bags, jump ropes, medicine balls, free weights, and so on, yet you probably do not know all that much about traditional *kigu hojo undo* devices. Here is a brief rundown:

- *Makiwara* is a striking post* with a straw, cloth, leather, or rubber covering for contact padding. It is used for practicing striking techniques as well as for conditioning the hands, elbows, knees, and feet.

- *Ishisashi* is a stone padlock resembling the shape of an old-fashioned clothes iron. It is used for strengthening arms and wrists.

- *Tan* is typically a sanded wooden log or a wooden fabrication resembling a barbell with weights on the ends. It is usually rolled over the forearms or twisted over the hips to strengthen and condition these areas.

- *Chiishi* is a concrete or stone weight at the end of a wooden handle used to strengthen the grip, as well as the joints of the elbows, wrists, and shoulders. *Chiishi* exercises condition tendons and joints and help develop the muscles used for blocking, striking, and grappling techniques. If the *chiishi* is too heavy to control appropriately, you should "choke up" on the handle† so that the weight is closer to your body.

- *Makiage kigu* is a wrist roller made from a wooden handle with a weight hung in the center on a rope. By twisting the handle to wrap and unwrap the rope, the weight is lowered and raised, strengthening the forearms, wrists, and grip. This is one of the few training tools that were found in both Europe and Asia during feudal times.

---

* The Korean for this device is *dallyon joo*, which translates as "forging post." There is no traditional Chinese equivalent, though the *muk yang jong* (wooden dummy) plays much the same role in some types of kung fu training.
† Sliding your hands toward the heavy end to increase your mechanical leverage as you might do with a baseball bat.

- *Nigiri game* are gripping jars, usually made of clay with a rim around the top to grip with the fingers. Water, sand, or small stones are often added to increase the weight. Exercises with these jars are designed to strengthen the fingers for gripping and tearing applications.

- *Tetsu geta* are iron clogs used to strengthen kicking techniques. Much like ankle weight wraps used by modern athletes, *tetsu geta* add a few extra pounds to the end of your leg as you perform your kicking routines, facilitating faster, more powerful strikes once they are removed. Some argue that they are less prone to damaging the joints than modern ankle weights.

- *Kongoken* is a heavy rectangular hoop. Used alone or with a partner, *kongoken* techniques strengthen and condition your body for physical contact.

These items are traditional implements used by karate practitioners for supplemental weight training exercises. Morio Higaonna's book *Traditional Karatedo – Okinawa Goju Ryu Vol. 1: Fundamental Techniques* demonstrates in detail how to use all the *kigu hojo undo* devices described herein. If you are interested in more modern methods, Martina Sprague's book *Strength and Power Training for Martial Arts* is an outstanding resource, which not only describes the proper use of body-weight and machine exercises but also provides tailored workout routines for common martial styles.

Keep a Training Journal

For centuries, oral tradition was used throughout the Orient to pass martial traditions from master to student. Very little was written down, partly because literacy was quite rare outside the nobility and certain privileged merchant classes and partly to keep confidential practices from becoming public knowledge. Neither of these inhibiting factors continue to be relevant today. Modern martial arts students are not only capable of researching all aspects of their art, but also of recording their findings, tracking their own progress, and documenting their discoveries in a way that can help them advance their own training more rapidly.

Many martial forms require advanced students to complete a thesis or research project concurrent with testing for black belt rank. This is an excellent opportunity for these individuals to advance the knowledge base of their organization while clarifying and adding depth to their own understanding of their chosen martial arts. As students progress through the lower ranks, it is very useful for them to document what they have learned in journals or notebooks. The mere process of writing things down facilitates internalization and understanding of the knowledge that is written.

A training journal is not only a good way to document what you have learned, but also a good way of working through plateaus in your development. As you chart

Advice for New Students

by Loren W. Christensen [64]

There are four complex elements critical to achieving the coveted black belt: right mind-set, proper physical training, dynamic fuel, and movement-specific weight training.

There is no argument that you need unparalleled discipline, vision, sensible goal setting, an intelligent training program, proper instruction, and an absolute burning desire to be the best that you can be. When these elements are in place and held constant, your journey will be enjoyable, productive, and rewarding.

On the physical level, know that overtraining hurts more students, especially new and hard-charging ones, than just about any other cause. Doing too much too often leads to injury, illness, and a lack of desire to train. You must seek a proper balance between hard training and sufficient rest so that your body grows progressively stronger, faster, and aerobically fit each week, each month, and each year.

It is mandatory that you take in proper nutrition to refuel. Just as you should never put cheap gasoline in a Cadillac, you should never, or rarely, put fast food burgers, soda pop, and fries into your body. Reduced to their crude basics, these "foods" are nothing more than sugar, grease, fat, sodium, and other chemicals that only hinder the recuperation of your fatigued muscles and the repair of your injuries.

Lastly, it is absolutely mandatory to supplement weight training in your workout regimen. When all other aspects of training are the same, students who lift weights and employ other forms of resistance exercises are superior to those who do not. In my mind, there is no debate about this. Correct weight training will not make you muscle bound or in any way inhibit your movements. It will, however, increase your power, explosiveness, raw speed, stamina, and resistance to blows. The science of weight training for martial arts has come a long ways in the last few years, ways that will dynamically help you reach your optimum skill level and that all-important black belt.

your progress, you will frequently realize that it is greater than you might have guessed, even when you feel stuck in a rut with little perception of progress. Furthermore, if your record includes video clips, your improvement over time will be even more readily apparent.

"People who keep journals have life twice."

– Mary Jessamyn West [65]

Student Perspective (by T. K. Nelson)

I have been using videotape as a training aid for at least 12 years. I currently have approximately 37 hours of footage of myself, training partners, and students performing various applications.

I normally do not waste my time just taping random training. If during the training, we come across a combination we want to remember, discover new bunkai, *or have an epiphany of some sort, I grab the camera I keep close by, that always has a martial arts miscellaneous tape in it ready to go, and put it down on film real quick. I may view it right away, or I may wait until the tape is full, but either way it is there to run across another day.*

By the time the tape is full, you have a whole lot of short, to-the-point, relevant footage at your disposal. There is no having to watch hours of a bunch of boring workout footage to find a glimmer of something good or progressive. Just keep your camera ready and then tape what you want.

How many times have you had a great idea in the dojo, *and by the time you are in the* dojo *again all you can remember is that at one point you had a great idea? No clue what it is now, but you remember it was great.*

You would be surprised how little you need to view your footage to remember it. It really helps add to your knowledge base, as well as retaining that knowledge. I will find myself looking for something in particular on a tape, and come across three or four really cool ideas I had maybe gotten away from, and it helps me get back to them.

In addition, I will come home right after a seminar and fire up my camera trying to catch whatever I have left over floating in my brain and on my notepad, from the instructor's lesson that day. If you attend any regular seminars from one specific person, it really helps you track your progress as well as understand his teaching progression better.

I once had an instructor who was very good, but would always bombard you with so many technique combinations in one class, and give you so little time to work them, that you always walked away feeling like he was this bottomless well of knowledge, and you could not remember anything. He never gave you enough time to work on one thing.

So I started to keep a notepad in my car and as soon as I could get out there after class, I would write down every technique I thought I could remember from that day's class. I would then go directly over to a friend's house, a guy who lived three blocks away from the dojo, *and he would record me trying to remember as many of the techniques off the list I could, performing them on him, of course.*

Within a year, I began to see that my instructor was not the bottomless well I thought, but instead he was using the principles of about 10 to 15 different techniques and just applying them various ways. Once I understood this, my comprehension level skyrocketed and I quickly advanced in the classes.

When my relationship with this instructor ended, I had the content of almost every class for the last three years on videotape, and I am still able to train in those techniques because of this video journal, despite the fact that I am no longer his student. It has also helped me with noticing and drawing comparisons between the various systems I study. Sometimes the principles of one style can help aid in the effectiveness of a technique in another style.

Videotaping has been a GREAT tool for me and my students.

– T. K. Nelson [66]

Summary

Modern technology can make your life much easier as a martial arts student. Books, articles, Web sites, videos, DVDs, streaming videos, and podcasts make ancient secrets and training methods available and affordable for just about anyone. Japanese, Okinawan, Chinese, Korean, Thai, Filipino, and other foreign language texts are easily and inexpensively translated into English (and other languages as well). State-of-the-art protective equipment, advanced nutritional counseling, and scientifically designed strength and conditioning programs are all available to stave off injury and speed the development of modern martial artists.

Technology lets us make the most of our training time, speeds our development, and helps us master the martial arts in ways practitioners could not fathom even a few short years ago. Take advantage of it in your quest to become a black belt.

Action Plan

• Create a reading list of books, articles, and Web sites relevant to your art and learning objectives. Spend a little time each week expanding your martial knowledge even as you develop your physical skills.

_____

_____

_____

• Develop a fitness and nutritional regimen to achieve optimal physical conditioning and fuel your body in a manner that facilitates your ability to endure the rigors of martial arts training.

_____

_____

_____

• Document what you will need to know for your next rank promotion. Simply writing down the requirements will help you set goals, but if your instructor is willing it is even better to video record him/her performing the *kata* that you will need to learn and *bunkai* you will need to know for each advancement test.

_____

_____

_____

• Record portions of a training session, *kata* performance, or sparring matches on video and spend some time diagnosing your performance. You probably will not want to wade through hours of tape so plan in advance what you are interested in and record only the important stuff. Look for strengths to build on as well as areas for improvement. Discuss what you find with others in your class.

_____

_____

_____

- Create a training journal to collect your notes and chart your progress. Take a little time each month to review what you have learned.

_____

_____

_____

Suggested Reading

Christensen, Loren and Wim Demeere. *The Fighter's Body: An Owner's Manual: Your Guide to Diet, Nutrition, Exercise and Excellence in the Martial Arts.* Wethersfield, CT: Turtle Press, 2003.

Ever wish you came with an owner's manual like your car does? Wouldn't it be nice if you knew what, when, and how to keep yourself running at peak performance? Well guess what, the answers to all these questions are in this outstanding book. Christensen and Demeere cut through the fads and hype to provide solid, practical, and most importantly factual advice for martial artists and athletes of all kinds. Those of us who train regularly find customized, easy to read and understand support to keep us at the top of our game.

Christensen, Loren. *Speed Training: How to Develop Your Maximum Speed for Martial Arts.* Boulder, CO: Paladin Enterprises, Inc., 1996.

The adage "speed kills" has never been truer than in a street fight. Speed is one of the most important assets a martial artist can have. Unfortunately, few of us are born with lightning reflexes and natural speed, yet anyone can improve their innate quickness if they know how to do so. This outstanding book helps you develop instantaneous reflexes and explosive speed for punching, kicking, grappling, and defensive tactics. The book includes hundreds of useful tips to improve your perception, polish your timing, and significantly increase your fighting speed. Chapters not only cover how to develop and refine your own techniques, but also how to defend against faster opponents.

Christensen, Loren. *Fighting Power: How to Develop Explosive Punches, Kicks, Blocks, and Grappling.* Boulder, CO: Paladin Enterprises, Inc., 1996.

Miyamoto Musashi, arguably the greatest swordsman who ever lived, advocated quickness and power as superior to strength and speed. Exceptional martial artists in every style demonstrate both quickness and power in all their applications, overwhelming opponents with seemingly little effort. Mr. Christensen's best-selling book *Speed Training* covered the quickness aspect. This outstanding book covers power. It is well written, easy to follow, and easily incorporated into your martial training. Subjects covered include *ki* power, ancient (traditional) exercises, modern weight resistance training, plyometrics (elastic strength/explosiveness), isometrics (resistance training), dynamic tension, developing a powerful neck, push-ups, abdominals, kicking power, punching power, bag work, timing, and defending against power. You will learn how to use proper body mechanics and hip rotation to increase your power markedly. Even Bruce Lee's famous "1-inch" punch is explained with sufficient clarity that most martial artists will be able to perform it themselves.

Higaonna, Morio. *Traditional Karatedo – Okinawa Goju Ryu Vol. 1: Fundamental Techniques.* Tokyo, Japan: Minato Research and Publishing Co., Ltd., 1985.

This outstanding tome covers *kihon*, the fundamental basics, in a fashion that is applicable to almost all striking arts, particularly karate. More importantly, it is the most comprehensive and holistic resource available for practitioners who wish to understand how to properly utilize traditional *kigu hojo undo* equipment for strength and conditioning. A bit hard to find since it is no longer in print, yet we have found it a very worthwhile volume nevertheless. You may wish to search e-Bay, bookfinder.com, or used bookstores to obtain a copy.

Sprague, Martina. *Fighting Science: The Laws of Physics for Martial Artists.* Wethersfield, CT: Turtle Press, 2002.

Practitioners have known for years that sheer size and brute strength mean very little to accomplished martial artists, yet many never truly understood why. Read this excellent book and you will know. Sprague's book helps us reach our full potential in the fighting arts, martial sports, and even in every day conditioning by successfully explaining in straightforward terms how the laws of physics can be applied to generating maximum power from martial technique. She describes how things like balance, momentum, rotational speed, friction, direction, impulse, and conservation of energy can work for or against us in executing striking, kicking, throwing, grappling, and joint manipulating techniques. That pretty much covers all the bases. There are tons of great illustrations, summaries, and even quizzes to supplement the materials. This is an easy to read, easy to implement text that can only help you become a better martial artist.

Sprague, Martina. *Strength & Power Training for Martial Arts.* Wethersfield, CT: Turtle Press, 2005.

Strength and power training is important. If you want to perform in the ring, on the street, or in just about any martial endeavor, functional strength is an essential component of success. As the author so eloquently states, martial arts skill, background and experiences are not substitutes for strength; they are complementary qualities. If you are overweight, under-conditioned, or lazy, you must condition yourself above the basic requirements of your art, regardless of what kinds of hurdles stand in your way. So how do you build muscular strength, endurance, and power? By reading this outstanding book, of course... Well, that and making a concerted effort to regularly perform the exercise routines contained therein. The author's scientific approach to martial arts is a breath of fresh air in a field often filled with hype and hyperbole. Her writing is insightful, easy to understand, and, most importantly, her ideas really do work. The photos are clear and do a good job of reinforcing the text. It is a great resource for the novice and expert alike. Well laid out, easy to read, and straightforward to implement.

Recommended Web Sites

Aiki Productions (www.aikiproductions.com)

Aiki Productions was started by world-class martial artists Tony Gamell and Alain Burrese. They produce instructional DVDs as well as provide free articles, podcasts, and video clips. Topics include self-defense, martial arts training, physical conditioning, martial styles, countries and cultures, martial arts history, and more.

Blauer Tactical Systems (www.tonyblauer.com)

Blauer Tactical Systems is a world-leader in the design of force-on-force training equipment, as well as program management for police defensive tactics, military combative training, close quarter combatives, and personal defense training. Their products HIGH GEAR, Ballistic Micro-fights, and S.P.E.A.R. SYSTEM are used by many defensive tactics and self-defense instructors to augment their self-defense skills.

Book Finder (www.bookfinder.com)

BookFinder.com is an engine that searches over 100 million books for sale—new, used, rare, out-of-print, and textbooks. They save you time and money by searching every major catalog available online and letting you know which booksellers are offering what you want, with the best prices and selection. When you find the book you were searching for, you can buy it directly from the original seller without any markup or search fee. Their Web site is produced by a team of high-tech librarians and programmers based in Berkeley, California, and Düsseldorf, Germany. It was originally launched as a personal Web site in 1997 by then-19-year-old University of California at Berkeley undergraduate Anirvan Chatterjee.

Peter Consterdine (www.peterconsterdine.com)

Peter Consterdine is an 8th *dan* black belt. A former British Full Contact Champion, bouncer, and bodyguard, he works around the world on close protection operations. He co-founded the British Combat Association, Europe's leading association for the promotion of self-defense and practical combat. This Web site accesses not only Peter Consterdine's home page, but also the British Combat Association and Protection Publications home pages as well. It is a great source of books, DVDs, and articles about martial arts and self-defense.

Gavin DeBecker and Associates (www.gavindebecker.com)

Gavin DeBecker is acknowledged by many as the world's greatest expert on the prediction and prevention of violence and the management of fear. He wrote an international bestselling book, *The Gift of Fear*. His consulting firm advises media figures, public figures, police departments, transnational corporations, government agencies, universities, and at-risk individuals on the assessment and management of situations that might escalate to violence.

Fighting Arts (www.fightingarts.com)

Fightingarts.com is an online community and network of traditional martial artists, historians, and writers dedicated to the promotion and understanding of their arts. The site is not associated with any specific school, style or organization, nor limited to Asian martial arts. Their goal is to provide timely and historical information, reporting, video presentations and interviews that are reliable, objective, and presented by knowledgeable experts. This site was founded by Christopher Caile.

The All Goju Ryu Network (www.gojuryu.net)

The All *Goju Ryu* Network is an online educational community and international reference portal for *Goju Ryu* Karate and Okinawa Martial Arts. This portal caters to *Goju Ryu* practitioners world wide, including association members of Okinawa *Goju Kai*, *Jundokan*, JKF *Gojukai*, *Doshinkan*, *Kenbukan*, *Okinawa Goju Ryu Karatedo Kyokai*, *Eibukan*, *Seiwakai*, *Meibukan*, JKGA & IKGA, *Seigokan*, *Eidokan*, *Shudokan*, *Jitsueikai*, *Yuishinkan*, *Seishikan*, *Shiseikan*, *Ryushinkan*, *Kuyukai*, *Butokukai*, *Uchiagekai*, IOGKF and many more. They offer a variety of books, articles, *dojo* directories, and online forums for *karateka*.

The Grinding Shop (www.grindingshop.com)

Wim Demeere is a martial artist, personal trainer, fitness expert, and massage therapist. His Web site offers a variety of excellent books, videos, and articles as well as an interesting blog. Information provided is both useful and entertaining.

International Society of Close Quarter Combatants (www.survive-the-street.com)

The ISCQC is an international organization dedicated to providing the skills necessary to survive a street attack. It provides access to weekly live and recorded self-defense video training sessions from knowledgeable self-defense experts. Subjects covered include reality-based martial arts, combat martial arts, military special operations units, law enforcement, Special Weapons And Tactics (SWAT), counterterrorism, and "no holds barred" fighting.

Judo Information Site (www.judoinfo.com)

The Judo Information Site is a virtual *dojo* with comprehensive information about the sport and art of judo. They offer a variety of books, articles, *dojo* directories, and products (e.g., uniforms) for *judoka*. There is even a humor section.

Rocky Mountain Combat Applications Training (www.rmcat.com)

Created by famed author and martial artist Peyton Quinn, this site offers books, videos, and applications for hands-on courses covering adrenal stress training. It offers very solid, proven content for real world self defense against open hand brawls, guns, knives, and other weapons.

West Seattle Karate Academy (www.westseattlekarate.com)

This is Kris Wilder's Web site. It contains useful articles and podcasts that can help expand your martial knowledge. There are sample chapters of various books available for free download as well as links to recommended readings.

YMAA (www.ymaa.com)

Dr. Yang Jwing-Ming founded YMAA Publication Center in 1984 with the goal of producing the highest quality books and instructional videos on traditional martial arts and health. Ymaa.com is not only the official Web site of this publisher, but also an excellent resource for training information and interactive content. It is segmented by Publishing (e.g., Books, DVDs, etc.), Training (e.g., school information, classes, instructors, community forum), Seminars (e.g., opportunities to learn from Master Yang or other teachers), and Articles (e.g., free newsletters, videos, and training tips).

Conclusion

"Karate as a means of self-defense has the oldest history, going back hundreds of years. It is only in recent years that the techniques which have been handed down were scientifically studied and the principles evolved for making the most effective use of the various moves of the body. Training based on these principles and knowledge of the working of the muscles and joints and the vital relation between movement and balance enable the modern student of karate to be prepared, both physically and psychologically, to defend himself successfully against any would-be assailant."
– Motoo Yamakura [67]

You have set a very high goal for yourself. Earning a black belt truly is a challenging endeavor, one that an awful lot of folks fail to accomplish. It is also something that millions of people have proven themselves worthy of worldwide. You can do it, too. Unlike most tests in the traditional education system, however, you simply cannot cram for your black belt exam. You can expedite the process, but you cannot master the prerequisites overnight. A black belt is earned through steady, consistent training over a very long period of time.

The amount of time it takes can vary with the system you study, how naturally talented you are, the quality of instruction you receive, and how effectively you practice. You cannot do a whole lot about the aptitudes you were (or were not) born with, of course, but you certainly can use what you have learned here to choose a quality instructor and take responsibility for your own training. Know how you learn and utilize this insight to optimize your time and attention both in the *dojo* and during your solo practice.

Diligence and hard work are paramount, but if forced to select only one, we choose diligence as most important. There is simply no substitute for conscientious practice to build the knowledge, skill, and abilities that you will need to earn your black belt. Finding creative ways to learn at least a little new information each day will really help. Martial artists today have access to an unprecedented level of information from books, DVDs, Web sites, podcasts, and a host of other sources that can help expedite the process.

Martial arts training is a long process, so stand back from time to time to assess what you have done and make sure that you are still on track. Document your objectives, set stretch goals, keep a training log, and monitor your performance against specific, measurable, achievable, realistic, and time-bound goals throughout your training. Both authors are big believers in notebooks as an aid in training and tracking. Keeping notebooks not only keeps you from going astray, but also helps you bridge plateaus in your training. Visualize success, and take proactive steps to eliminate the inevitable obstacles that will pop up along the way.

Of all the obstacles you may face on the road to your black belt, injuries can be the most challenging to overcome. It is easy to take the inevitable bumps and bruises in stride, yet serious damage can derail your progress or even stop it altogether. Take preventive measures to safeguard yourself. Warm up thoroughly, maintain good flexibility, stay in shape, eat right, utilize good body mechanics, and drink plenty of water. If you do become injured, be sure to use your downtime to work the non-physical aspects of your art such as visualization and study.

"We are what we repeatedly do."

– Aristotle [68]

Earning a black belt can be one of the toughest things you will ever do. It will also be one of the most rewarding. Your perspective of martial arts will likely be very different once your black belt has been tied around your waist than it was when you first got started. You will be stronger, faster, better educated, and more skillful, yet it is important to remain humble and never stop training. Your journey has just begun.

APPENDIX A

Common Terminology

All the foreign language terms used in this book can be found in the glossary. We primarily used Japanese, but your art might utilize a different language. The following is a list of some common martial arts words that you might encounter during your training. It is by no means a complete or all encompassing list. Because there are several dialects of Chinese to choose from, we decided to use Cantonese. It is also important to note that there may be several names for any given technique. For example, a "knife hand" can also be referred to as a "sword hand." Although the essence of the technique is the same, the term when translated may be different.

English	Japanese	Korean	Cantonese
Stance	*Dachi*	*Sogi*	*Ma*
Back Stance	*Kokutsu Dachi*	*Fugul Sogi*	*Hau Ma*
Cat Stance	*Neko Ashi Dachi*	*Beom Sogi*	*Dui Ma*
Crane Stance	*Sagi Ashi Dachi*	*Haktari Sogi*	*Daan Goek Ma*
Cross Leg Stance	*Bensoku Dachi*	*Koa Sogi*	*Quai Ma*
Front Stance	*Zenkutsu Dachi*	*Chongul Sogi*	*Ji Ng Ma*
Horse Stance	*Kiba Dachi*	*Kima Sogi*	*Tu Ma*
Hourglass Stance	*Sanchin Dachi*	*Not Applicable*	*Not Applicable*
Sumo Stance	*Shiko Dachi*	*Annun Sogi*	*Sei Ping Ma*
Kicking	*Geri*	*Chagi*	*Tek*
Back Kick	*Ushiro Geri*	*Dwit Chagi*	*Hau Tek*
Front Kick	*Mae Geri*	*Ap Chagi*	*Chin Tek*
Jump Kick	*Tobi Geri*	*Twimyo Chagi*	*Tiu Tek*
Roundhouse Kick	*Mawashe Geri*	*Tolyo Chagi*	*Lun Wan Tek*
Side Kick	*Yoko Geri*	*Yop Chagi*	*Zak Tek*
Punching/Striking	*Tsuki* (or *Zuki*)		
Hook Punch	*Kagi Tsuki*	*Bandal Taeragi*	*Gau Kyun*
Lunge Punch	*Oi Tsuki*	*Bandae Jirugi*	*Chop Choy*
Reverse Punch	*Gyaku Tsuki*	*Baro Jirugi*	*Hau Kyun*
Backfist Strike	*Uraken Uchi*	*Joomuk Taerigi*	*Hau Sau Kyun*
Elbow Strike	*Hiji Ate*	*Palkup Taerigi*	*Sau Janng*

| Finger Strike | *Nukite* | *Sonkut Tulgi* | *Caap Zi* |
| Knife-Hand Strike | *Shuto Uchi* | *Sonkal Taerigi* | *Sau Dou* |

Blocking/Receiving — *Uke* — *Makgi* — *Dong*

Blocking/Receiving	*Uke*	*Makgi*	*Dong*
Downward Block	*Gedan Uke*	*Najunde Makgi*	*Haa Dong*
Middle Block	*Chudan Uke*	*Kaunde Makgi*	*Zung Dong*
Sword Hand Block	*Shuto Uke*	*Han Sonal Makgi*	*Sau Dong*
Upper Block	*Jodan Uke*	*Nopunde Makgi*	*Soeng Dong*

General Terms

Bow	*Rei*	*Kyungyet*	*Guk Gung*
Instructor	*Sensei*	*Sabumnim*	*Sifu*
Lower Belt Practitioner	*Kohai*	*Kup*	*Si Di*
Rank of Black Belt (1st – 10th)	*Dan*	*Dan*	*Dyun*
Refers to the Rank of Lower Belts	*Kyu*	*Kup*	*Kap*
Senior, Higher Rank Practitioner	*Sempai*	*Sunbaenim*	*Si Hing*
Spirit Shout (loud, focused yell—from the diaphragm for power)	*Kiai*	*Kiyup*	*Daai Giu*
Student	*Deshi*	*Panjanim*	*Hok Daang*
To be (or make) Ready	*Yoi*	*Pyeonhi Sogi*	*Jyu Bei*
Training Hall	*Dojo*	*Dojang*	*Kwoon*

Counting

One	*Ichi*	*Hana*	*Yat*
Two	*Ni*	*Dul*	*Yi*
Three	*San*	*Set*	*Sam*
Four	*Shi (Yon)*	*Net*	*Sei*
Five	*Go*	*Daseot*	*Mm*
Six	*Roku*	*Yeoseot*	*Look*
Seven	*Shichi (Nana)*	*Ilgop*	*Chat*
Eight	*Hachi*	*Yeodeol*	*Baat*
Nine	*Kyu*	*Ahop*	*Gau*
Ten	*Ju*	*Yeol*	*Sap*

A Brief Overview of Martial Styles

Here is a brief overview of some of the various martial arts you may find in your local area. This is not intended to be an all-encompassing list. If a form does not appear here, this in no way invalidates the system or style. Because the focus of this book is on earning a black belt rather than on comparing martial styles, it makes no sense to go into too much depth or attempt to list everything.

Common Martial Arts
Aikido
Aikido is a Japanese martial art created by Morihei Ueshiba beginning in the 1920s. It has its roots in *jujitsu*, Japanese combative wrestling, and *kenjutsu*, the way of the sword. It is known for throwing, arm locks, and spiritual development. Many forms of *aikido* exist today but they all trace their lineage directly to Ueshiba, who is often referred to as *O-Sensei*, or "greatest *sensei*" in English.

Arnis
One of the characteristics of Filipino martial arts is the use of weapons from the very beginning of training. Arnis incorporates striking, locking, and throwing techniques performed with short rattan staves, knives, short swords, and empty hand. "Modern *Arnis*," a widely popular style, was founded by Remy Presas.

Baguazhang
Baguazhang (*Pau Kua Chang*) is a form of kung fu. Referred to as the "Eight Palm Changes," *baguazhang* is considered an internal Chinese martial art because it uses deceptive circular footwork and flowing hands to gain position on opponents. Throws and multiple forms of striking with the hands are also used.

Brazilian Jiu-Jitsu
Brazilian *jiu-jitsu* is a version of Japanese *jujitsu* that has changed significantly enough to become its own system. Brazilian *jiu-jitsu* places great importance on ground fighting, called *ne waza*, in Japanese judo and *jujitsu* schools. Popularized by the Gracie family from Brazil, its practitioners have won many "No holds barred" fights worldwide.

Capoeira
Capoeira was developed around the 1600s by African slaves in Brazil. It uses music to aid in training and it emphasizes kicking, take downs, and slipping of oncoming attacks. It does not seem to be as popular as other forms of martial arts in the United States and Europe, possibly due to its unique methodologies of combining music and dance as part of the training process.

Catch Wrestling

Catch Wrestling (also called shoot wrestling/fighting) is a form of barnstorming wresting popular in America at the turn of the twentieth century. Popular wrestlers of the time included Martin "Farmer" Burns and Frank Gotch. Modern professional wrestling grew out of the sport, becoming popular in the 1950s in America. Catch Wrestlers where classified as "hookers," who had very strong skills and took on all comers as they traveled, and "shooters," who were wrestlers with a background in real fighting.

Escrima

Escrima is a Filipino martial art that uses rattan sticks and knives to deliver attacks from multiple angles. A combination of weapons is also used (e.g., one stick and a free hand). Aggressive and offensive in nature *escrima* masters were well known for fighting with one another to prove their point of superiority. These matches were discouraged by the Filipino government and are not common today.

Hapkido

Hapkido is a Korean martial art that uses punches, kicks, and throws with joint locks. *Hapkido* is also known for it aerial displays of throwing, leaping, and rolling. It is similar to *aikido* in some ways such as the use of throwing applications. *Hapkido* uses a traditional karate-type uniform and belt ranking system.

Hung Gar

Hung Gar is a southern Chinese style made famous in Hong Kong films. *Hung Gar* is also known as the "Tiger Crane" form, noted for its powerful stances and rooting to the earth.

Hwa Rang Do

Hwa Rang Do (The Flower-Man Way) is Korean and was developed by the Lee Brothers. Similar to *taekwondo*, *Hwa Rang Do* emphasizes pursuits of self-betterment through other classical pursuits to form a well-rounded person, not just a martial artist.

Jeet Kune Do

Jeet Kune Do (The Way of the Intercepting Fist) was created by Bruce Lee. It was developed out of *Wing Chun* kung fu and grew to be an assembly of ideas and concepts based on adapting what is useful to the practitioner and discarding what is deemed as useless. No real forms or classical patterns (i.e., *kata*) are used.

Judo

Judo (The Gentle Way), a Japanese martial art and now an international and Olympic sport that consists of throwing, grappling, choking, and arm locks. Founded by Jigoro Kano, who began his martial arts studies in *jujitsu*, judo evolved into a distinct form of fighting. It emphasizes throwing while removing some of the most dangerous techniques of *jujutsu* to ensure safety and the longevity of the sport.

Jujutsu

Jujutsu is a general term used to describe unarmed combat using throwing, grappling, choking, and joint locks. It was developed for the Japanese *samurai* to use on the battlefield should they lose their weapon(s). The classic grips and attacks reflect the opponent wearing battlefield armor. Classic *jujutsu* was not introduced into the general public until the Meiji restoration when the *samurai* began to teach it as a means of earning a living.

Kajukenbo

Kajukenbo is derived from karate, *jujutsu*, *kenpo*, and Chinese boxing takes its name from the arts that comprise its techniques: *Ka* = karate, *Ju*= jujitsu, *Ken*=kenpo, *Bo*=boxing. *Kajukenbo* was developed in Hawaii in the late 1940s. It can alternatively be translated as *ka* (long life), *ju* (happiness), *ken* (fist), *bo* (style), or "through this fist style, one gains long life and happiness."

Karate

Karate, meaning "empty hand," was originally called "*Te*" or hand. Karate takes on many forms today and is very popular worldwide. Karate is a striking art dominated by hand and foot techniques, yet it also includes joint locks, chokes, and throws. Examples of the many styles include *Shito-Ryu*, *Goju-Ryu*, *Uechi-Ryu*, *Shotokan*, *Shorin-Ryu*, *Isshin-Ryu*, and *Wado-Ryu*.

Kenpo

Kenpo is a martial art that resembles karate. Developed by Edmund K. Parker, *Kenpo* is based on Chinese and Japanese styles of martial arts he studied in his youth in Hawaii. *Kenpo* is a striking art and uses a large amount of pins and traps, but like all arts, contains throws and joint manipulations as well. After Parker's death, the IKKA, International Kenpo Karate Association, split into several organizations.

Kendo

Kendo is the Japanese sport of sword fighting. *Kendo* uses a *shinai* (bamboo sword) and armor that protects the practitioner. A national sport in Japan, it is taught in schools where both males and females participate.

Krav Maga

Krav Maga is a form of self defense and hand-to-hand combat created in Israel. Israeli security forces and Special Forces use *Krav Maga* because it is fast to learn, effective and swift. *Krav Maga* might not be considered a "martial art" in the classical sense, but more of a self-defense structure. Since its inception, it has been modified for civilians, becoming popular throughout the world.

Kuk Sool Won

Kuk Sool Won is a Korean art founded in the early 1960's by In Hyuk Suh. The name translates to "National Martial Art." *Kuk Sool Won* uses traditional fighting methods and is progressive in its adoption of modern techniques and weapons.

Kung Fu

Kung fu or *gung-fu* is a general term that refers to many various forms of martial arts that are Chinese in origin. Some, but not nearly all, of the styles of *gung fu* include: *Wing Chun, taijiquan, Choy Lay Fut*, and *Hung Gar*. The word *gung-fu*, which translates as "hard work," can be used to explain a person's skill in any activity, not just the martial arts.

Kyudo

The Japanese art of archery, *kyudo* translates as "the way of the bow." More than mere marksmanship, *kyudo* is often seen as a path to spiritual enlightenment. The *yumi* (bow) used by *kyudo* practitioners often reach nearly eight feet in length. They are traditionally made of bamboo, wood, and leather using techniques that have not changed for centuries. *Ya* (arrow) shafts were traditionally made of bamboo, with either eagle or hawk feathers for fletching.

Mixed Martial Arts (MMA)

Mixed Martial Arts is a sport that uses many martial arts disciplines to create a freestyle form of fighting that adheres to the few rules that govern the sport. Popular in Japan, Brazil, and the United States, some forms of events are called PRIDE Fighting Championships and UFC (Ultimate Fighting Championship).

Muay Thai

Muay Thai is a Thai art that can be classified as kickboxing. *Muay Thai* boxers are able to use knees, elbows, shins, and feet while fighting. Boxing-type gloves are also used. *Muay Thai* is an extraordinarily physical art requiring a high level of physical conditioning. It is similar to western boxing in that is has stables of fighters, rings for competition, and trainers.

Ninjutsu

Ninjutsu is a Japanese style of martial arts in the sense of combat, but *ninjutsu* also incorporates the tools of an advance scout or spy. Practitioners, called a *ninja*, learn the skills of survival, concealment, and espionage. *Ninja* are popular in the movies and are often portrayed as villains because their ways were cloaked in secrecy.

Sambo

Sambo, an abbreviation of the Russian words *Samozashchita Bez Oruzhiya*, means "self defense without a weapon." *Sambo* was heavily influenced by judo as well as indigenous Russian wrestling. Developed for the Russian military, the jacket and uniform used in competition reflects a military uniform in design, including belt loops on the fighting jacket.

Shaolin Kung Fu

Shaolin kung fu is a form of kung fu that is based in animal systems. Fighting forms come from mimicking animals such as tigers, snakes, or cranes, as well as others.

The history of the *Shaolin* temple is intertwined with lore and fact. *Shaolin* kung fu uses weapons such as spears, sticks, and swords, in addition to open-hand applications.

Shorinji Kempo

Shorinji Kempo is Japanese and incorporates Buddhism into the art, adding a distinctly spiritual emphasis. *Shorinji Kempo* contains the strikes, joint locks, throws, and other aspects of what would be considered a traditional martial art from an Eastern perspective.

Silat

Silat or *Pencak Silat* is an art from Indonesia and the adjacent regions. A varied and creative art, it allows for and encourages personal adaptation of technique. Virtually all parts of the body are used to attack and defend. Mapped lines of attack and defense are often placed on the training floor to serve as training aids regarding movement.

Southern Praying Mantis

Southern Praying Mantis is a form of kung fu that mimics the insect called a praying mantis. Designed for fighting close the arms are used to trap, pin, and strike. This form also uses both hard and soft movements.

Sumo

Sumo is an ancient Japanese sport surrounded by ceremony and Shinto ritual. Professional Sumo can trace its roots back to the Edo Period in Japan as a form of sporting entertainment. The original *sumo* wrestlers were probably *samurai*, often *ronin*, who needed to find an alternate source of income. The rules of *sumo* are fairly simple: the first wrestler to step out of the ring or to touch the ground with any part of his body other than the soles of his feet loses.

Systema

Systema is a Russian martial art that has no *kata* and no ranking system (e.g., badges or belts). *Systema* uses movement joined with breathing to create a means of fighting and controlling one's body during conflict. With no weapons per se, *Systema* uses anything available to create an impromptu weapon.

Taijiquan

Taijiquan (*Tai Chi Chuan*) is a system of martial arts that is often practiced for health but can also be a powerful form of self-defense in the hands of a skilled practitioner. Characterized by slow movements this serves to integrate the patterns of movement into the person doing the art. Popular forms of *taijiquan* are *Wu*, *Chen*, and *Yang*, but the art is not limited to these three.

Taekwondo

Taekwondo is Korean in origin. It translates as, "The way of the foot and the hand." Since becoming an Olympic sport it has grown into one of the most popular martial arts in the world. Emphasizing kicking over hand striking, *taekwondo* is known for creative kick combinations and powerful kicks.

Tang Soo Do

Tang Soo Do is Korean in origin. It translates as, "The Way of the Chinese Hand." Standardized by Grandmaster Hwang Kee, it used what would be considered traditional forms to transfer fighting techniques. Chuck Norris, *Tang So Do*'s most well-known practitioner, learned the art while in Korea.

Wing Chun

Wing Chun is sometimes spelled *Ving Tsun* or *Wing Tsun*. It is a Chinese martial art that, as legend has it, was created by a woman monk. Characterized by hand and fist techniques with low kicks, its most famous practitioner was Bruce Lee, who went on to found his own art, *Jeet Kune Do*.

Xingyiquan

Xingyiquan (*Hsing I Chuan*) is a Chinese form of western boxing. It is popular and sometimes considered one of the three sisters of Chinese martial arts composed of *xingyiquan*, *taijiquan*, and *baguazhang*. *Xingyiquan* uses aggressive and direct footwork as well as explosive striking.

Martial Arts Movies We Like

Let's face it; we all enjoy a good martial arts flick now and again. While wider audiences might thrill at the lighting-fast kung-fu fighting action, even experienced martial artists who know how unrealistically Hollywood typically portrays this stuff can still enjoy the choreography. Certain movies might even teach us a little something about the history or traditions of the martial arts, using period costumes, brilliant dialog, and high drama to enrapture us with the intricate story line and complex plot. Or they might simply be a lot of fun.

Without further ado, here is a short list of some of our favorite movies:

Kris Wilder's List

The Challenge (1982)

Starring Scott Glenn as an American boxer on the down side of his career and Toshiro Mifune as an adherent of the traditional ways of the *samurai*, the story revolves around an old Japanese *katana* sword. The American finds himself caught in the middle of a battle between two Japanese brothers, one a defender of the old ways and the other a modern businessman. Their violent fight over the valuable heirloom has some great drama and lots of fun.

Seven Samurai (1954)

Akira Kurosawa directed this classic film about seven *samurai* that have no master and are now classified as *ronin* or "wave men." These *ronin* join forces and set out to protect a village from marauders. Truly a classic, it runs three and a half hours. Shot in black and white and with subtitles, it has wonderful character development and a great story. Considered the best of its kind, *Seven Samurai* was imitated in the West and made into a western gunfighter film called *The Magnificent Seven*. If you love *samurai* movies, this is a must see.

The Last Samurai (2003)

Starring Tom Cruise and Ken Watanabe, *The Last Samurai* is the story of a Western warrior that loses his integrity, and ultimately himself, after violently putting down multiple Indian rebellions in the Old West. He is then remade and redeemed via a *samurai* and his band of rebels who fight against the Emperor's attempts to modernize feudal Japan. While the story is not entirely true, the movie affords a very realistic and incredibly well acted portrayal of how Emperor Meiji's reforms ultimately abolished the *samurai* class and westernized Japan.

Police Story (1985)

A ton of light-hearted fun! Jackie Chan directed, choreographed, and starred in this wild ride. He runs from the law in an attempt to clear his name. In the meantime he bounces off everything around him while fighting a wonderful assortment of bad guys in interesting ways. It is a real treat to see Chan perform all his own stunts.

Return of the Dragon (1972)

Okay, everybody is always talking about *Enter the Dragon* sure, but *Return of the Dragon* is the one I keep going back to. Tang, played by Bruce Lee, travels to Rome to keep organized thugs from taking his relative's property. The culmination of the movie is the fight between Bruce Lee and Chuck Norris in the Roman Coliseum. Lee wrote, directed, choreographed, and starred in this martial arts thriller. Outstanding fight scenes make it worth watching again and again.

Above the Law (1988)

Above the Law was Steven Seagal's movie debut. He plays a Vietnam veteran, trained in covert operations, who has become a cop. He gets wind of illegal operations that the Feds are watching and goes his own way. This one has got attitude to spare and lots of cool fights. Though the production is average and the story line shallow, it makes up for its deficits through tons of fun action.

The Heroic Trio (1992)

Starring Michelle Yeoh, *The Heroic Trio* goes way over the top. The women superheroes set out to save kidnapped babies while wearing outfits that are half lingerie and half superhero costume. The suspension of the laws of physics and human abilities in this movie is just goofy fun. Look for the horizontal airborne spinning motorcycle inside a warehouse; oh, and the ability to fight from said motorcycle too. Kung fu on wires at its best!

Street Fighter (1974)

Very violent and classic, starring Sonny Chiba as an anti-hero willing to fight first and ask questions later. Terry, Chiba's character, is a mercenary who takes on a contract and then switches sides when the plot does not suit his needs, incurring the wrath of the *Yakuza*, the Chinese mob, and Western thugs to boot. As good as any Italian "spaghetti western" movie from the '70s, Chiba uses fists and kicks instead of a gun.

Lawrence Kane's List

Mortal Kombat (1995)

Based on a video game of the same name, but so much fun that you will hardly notice that there is virtually no plot. Lightning God Rayden (Christopher Lambert) guides warrior Liu Kang (Robin Shou), police detective Sonja Blade (Bridgette Wilson), and action movie star Johnny Cage (Linden Ashby) to a remote island in a parallel universe to compete in the ultimate martial arts tournament, Mortal Kombat. If the evil forces of Outworld led by Shang Tsung (Cary-Hiroyuki Tagawa) win ten times in a row, they can invade the Realm of Earth. Because they have been victorious nine times in a row, our heroes cannot afford to fail… Cool music, great sets, fun costumes, exceptional pacing, and stunning fight choreography make this one a whole lot of fun. A riotous, rockin' good time!

James Clavell's Shogun (1980)

Starring Richard Chamberlain, Toshiro Mifune, Yoko Shimada, and a host of other fine actors, this is one of the most amazing recreations of early seventeenth century Japan ever produced on film. It closely follows Clavell's outstanding book of the same title. English Pilot Major John Blackthorne (Chamberlain) is shipwrecked during a storm. A hated foreigner, he eventually earns the trust of Lord Toranaga (Mifune). A feudal warlord, Toranaga struggles to become *Shogun*, military ruler of all Japan, outwitting the malevolent Lord Ishido. The price of failure is death…, by ritual suicide. Stunning cinematography, brilliant dialog, intricate plot, magnificent acting, enjoyable music, and some of the best *samurai* battle sequences ever filmed, this movie is not only wonderful to watch, but it also gives terrific historical insight into feudal Japanese culture. You will not only be entertained but you will pick up a bit of the Japanese language too. It is nearly ten hours long, yet I have seen it at least a dozen times…, 'nuff said.

Enter the Dragon (1973)

Bruce Lee's most famous film, the incredible success of this movie blazed the trail for hundreds of similar works and inspired a whole generation of practitioners to study the martial arts. Recruited by an intelligence agency, kung fu artist Lee enters a deadly karate tournament to infiltrate a drug operation and take down the reclusive crime lord Han (Shih Kien). Sizzling action and fantastic choreography by Lee himself more than make up for spotty dialog and bad acting in this king of the chop socky flicks!

Highlander (1986)

"He fought his first battle on the Scottish Highlands in 1536. He will fight his greatest battle on the streets of New York City in 1986. His name is Connor MacLeod. He is immortal." That's one outstanding tagline, is it not? Starring Christopher Lambert, Clancy Brown, and Sean Connery, and featuring a stellar soundtrack by the rock group Queen, this fantasy adventure is packed with action, yet has a solid plot and excellent acting. If you enjoy classic good versus evil battles, and well-choreographed swordsmanship, this one is for you. This movie spawned a bunch of wretched sequels and a couple of pretty good television shows, yet it is by far the best of the series. Highly recommended!

Romeo Must Die (2000)

A modern day *Romeo and Juliet* kung fu style, this movie features well-choreographed fight sequences, wry humor, witty dialog, and solid pacing with just enough plot to keep your attention. Martial artist Jet Li stars alongside hip-hop singer Aaliyah, who also produced the soundtrack. An avenging cop, Han (Li), seeks out his brother's killer only to fall in love with the daughter of a mob boss who did him in (Aaliyah). Not only is there everyday martial arts action, but some unusual pressure point sequences as well. Great fun!

Ong-Bak – The Thai Warrior (2003)

There are no computer images or hidden wires in this one, only well-choreographed martial arts action. Somewhat unique to the action movie genre, Tony Jaa utilizes impressive *Muay Thai* applications in the superb fight sequences. When the head of the villager's sacred statue, *Ong-Bak*, is stolen a young warrior (Jaa) must go to Bangkok to retrieve it. Discovering that the thief is connected to an illicit underground fight club, he is unwillingly drawn into the competition where he takes on the criminal underworld with his elbows, knees, fists, and feet. Solid rock 'em sock 'em action!

Under Siege (1992)

A former Navy Seal working as a cook is the only person who can stop a gang of terrorists from seizing control of a battleship and stealing its nuclear arsenal. Starring Steven Seagal and Tommy Lee Jones, this movie is a true action classic. Former Playboy Playmate Erika Eleniak not only pops out of a cake, but also hurls grenades at the bad guys when Seagal needs a little help. You gotta love that!

Lone Wolf McQuade (1983)

Starring Chuck Norris as a butt-kicking Texas Ranger, David Carradine as a drug kingpin, and Barbara Carrera as their mutual love interest, this movie is packed with martial arts action. From the opening scene where Norris single-handedly wipes out an entire gang of horse thieves to the climactic face-off at the end, the action never stops. It just does not get any better than this. Do not mess with Chuck's armadillo!

Glossary

Romaji (Romanization) note—We have primarily used the *Hebon-Shiki* (Hepburn) method of translating Japanese writing into the English alphabet and determining how best to spell the words (though accent marks have been excluded), as it is generally considered the most useful insofar as pronunciation is concerned. We have italicized foreign terms such that they can be readily differentiated from their English counterparts (e.g., *dan* meaning black belt rank versus Dan, the male familiar name for Daniel). As the Japanese and Chinese languages do not use capitalization, we have only capitalized those words that would be used as proper nouns in English.

Japanese is a challenging language for many English speakers to pronounce correctly. A few hints—for the most part, short vowels sound just like their English counterparts (e.g., a as in father, e as in pen). Long vowels are essentially double-length (e.g., o as in oil, in the word *oyo*). The u is nearly silent, except where it is an initial syllable (e.g., *uke*). Vowel combination e + i sounds like day (e.g., *bugeisha*), a + i sounds like alive (e.g., *bunkai*), o + u sounds like float (e.g., *tou*), and a + e sounds like lie (*kamae*). The consonant r is pronounced with the tip of the tongue, midway between l and r (e.g., *daruma*). Consonant combination ts is pronounced like cats, almost a z (e.g., *tsuki*).

Although there are a few words here from other languages such as Chinese, Korean, or Latin, the vast majority of words listed in this glossary come from Japanese. Where another language is used it is noted.

Foreign Terminology	**English Definition**
ap chagi	front kick, Korean
ap hurya chagi	hook kick, Korean
ashigaru	infantry soldiers in feudal Japan
ashi uke	leg block
ashi waza	foot techniques (e.g., kick)
budo	martial ways (martial arts)
bunkai	martial applications found in *kata* (forms)
bunkai oyo	principles of *kata* application, as demonstrated in tandem exercises
bushi	Japanese nobility during feudal times
carpe diem	"seize the day," Latin
caveat emptor	"let the buyer beware," Latin
century	Roman military unit of approximately 80 men, Latin

chiishi	weighted stick
chiki chagi	crescent kick, Korean
chudan uke	chest block
cohort	Roman military unit of approximately 480 men, Latin
corvus	gang plank, Latin
curriculum vitae	a longer, more comprehensive version of a résumé listing the credentials, background, and qualifications of an instructor
dachi	stance
daisho	paired long- and short-swords worn by the *samurai* in feudal Japan
dallyon joo	"forging" post, identical to the Japanese *makiwara*
dan	black belt rank
daruma	warm-up exercises
do	the "way"
dojang	training hall, Korean
dojo	training hall, literally "the place to learn the way"
dojo kun	precepts or virtues of a school
dollyo chagi	roundhouse or turning kick, Korean
dwet chagi	spinning kick, Korean
fuku shiki kumite	freestyle sparring with *kata* emphasis
furi uchi	swing strike
gedan uke	down block
geri	kick
gladius	Roman short sword, Latin
go	a Japanese board game
Goju Ryu	an Okinawan form of karate founded by Chojun Miyagi
Go Rin No Sho	*The Book of Five Rings*, a book of strategy by famous Japanese swordsman Miyamoto Musashi
haiku	a traditional epigrammatic Japanese poem based on 17 syllables which are arranged 5 – 7 – 5
hakama	divided skirt worn by the *samurai* in feudal Japan
haori	coat worn by the *samurai* in feudal Japan
happo no kuzushi	eight directions of imbalance
harai uke	sweeping block
hiji ate	elbow strike
hiji uke	elbow block
hiki uke	pulling/grasping block
hiza geri	knee strike

hiza uke	knee block
hodoki	"unleashing of the hands," a probationary period prior to training
ippon kiso kumite	"one move" pre-arranged sparring
ishisashi	stone padlock
jari bako	sand bowl
jodan uke	head block
judan	tenth-degree black belt, the highest possible rank in most martial arts
judoka	judo practitioner
jutsu	technique
kado	Japanese art of flower arranging
kakai uke	hooking block
kappo	resuscitation techniques
karateka	karate practitioner
kasai no genri	the theory of deciphering fighting applications from *kata*
kata	"formal exercises," a logical series of offensive and defensive techniques performed in a particular order
katana	Japanese long sword
keppan	blood oath
ki	internal energy
kiba dachi	horse stance
kigu undo	supplementary exercises performed with traditional equipment
kihon	basics or fundamentals of a martial art
kimono	jacket worn by the *samurai* in feudal Japan
kiso kumite	pre-arranged sparring
koken tsuki	wrist strike
koken uke	wrist block
kongoken	heavy rectangular loop
kuchi waza	disruptive chatter; literally "mouth" technique
kukinage	air throw or "wind" technique
kumite	sparring
kuroi-obi	black belt
kuzushi	imbalance
kwoon	training hall, Chinese
kyu	colored belt rank
legion	Roman military unit of approximately 5,240 men, Latin
mae geri	front kick

makiage kigu	wrist roller
makiwara	striking post
mawashe geri	wheel kick
mawashe uke	circular or wheel block
mikazuki geri	hook kick
monjin	"person at the gate," one who has proven worthy of martial arts training
mudansha	those not yet having earned a *dan* (black belt) rank
muk yang jong	wooden training dummy, Chinese
mushin	empty mind, a meditative state
naeryo chagi	axe kick, Korean
Nage no Kata	A formal tandem exercise developed in 1884 at the *Kodokan*. This *kata* consists of 5 sets of three throws, each performed on both the left and right sides. It includes a progression of attack styles demonstrating how practitioners must adjust to differing actions by an opponent.
ne waza	grappling or groundwork techniques
neko ashi dachi	"cat leg" stance
nigiri game	gripping jars
obi	belt
okuden	hidden teachings or secrets of a martial art
omote	surface training
osae uke	pressing block
pila	Roman javelin, Latin
randori	free sparring
ryu	a martial school or system
sanbon shobu kumite	three-point, tournament-style sparring match
sanchin dachi	"hourglass" stance
sashi ishi	stone weight
scutum	Roman shield, Latin
seiken tsuki	fore fist punch
seiza	kneeling position
sensei	teacher, literally "one who has come before"
shiai	competition; literally "to try each other"
shiko dachi	"*sumo*" or straddle stance
shinai	bamboo practice sword used primarily in *kendo*
shodan	first-degree black belt, literally "least" of the *dan* ranks
shodo	Japanese art of calligraphy

shogo	teaching titles; these include honorifics such as: *Hanshi* (model teacher), *Kyoshi* (master teacher), *Renshi* (senior expert), and *Shihan* (expert teacher)
shotei uchi	palm heel strike
shugyo	hardship or austere training, typically a week long intensive period
shuto uchi	sword hand strike
signifer	Roman standard bearer, Latin
sukui uke	scooping block
tachi waza	throwing techniques
tamashiwara	breaking techniques (e.g., board breaking with your fist or target cutting with a sword)
tan	wooden log
tatami	traditional training mats
tate tsuki	standing fist punch
tetsuarei	dumbbells
tetsui uchi	hammerfist
te waza	hand techniques (e.g., punch)
tetsu geta	iron clogs
tonfa	*kobudo* weapon, looks much like a side-handled police baton
tou	bundle of sticks
twimyo chagi	jumping kick, Korean
uchi uke	inside forearm block
ude uke	"wing" block
uke	"to receive," a defensive or blocking application
ura waza	"inner ways," an understanding of why techniques work
uraken tsuki	backfist
ushiro geri	back kick
wa uke	"valley" block
wakizashi	Japanese short sword
waza	technique
yama uke	"mountain" block
yoko geri	side kick
yop chagi	side kick, Korean
yudansha	those having earned a *dan* (black belt) rank
zenkutsu dachi	"front" (forward) stance

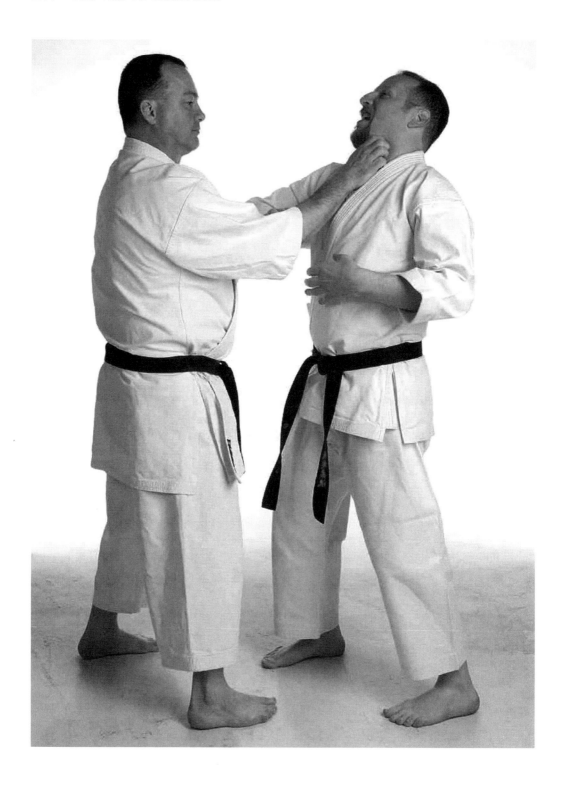

Endnotes

1 Morio Higaonna is the Chief Instructor of the International Okinawan *Goju Ryu* Karate-Do Federation (IOGKF). A direct disciple of Chojun Miyagi, who founded the system, Higaonna is one of *Goju Ryu*'s most famous practitioners. He has published numerous books and videos about his art.

2 Antoine de Saint-Exupéry (1900 – 1944), French aviator and writer. He was the author of eight books including *Le Petit Prince* (The Little Prince), his most famous work. He became one of the pioneers of international postal flight in the days when aircraft had few instruments and pilots flew by instinct, complaining later that those who flew the more advanced aircraft were more like accountants than pilots. He was shot down by the Germans during WWII.

3 *Haiku* is a traditional epigrammatic poem based on 17 syllables which are arranged 5 – 7 – 5. The original Japanese reads *toshu kuken hatsukaminari wo toriosou*. Translation was done by Patrick McCarthy. This episode retold in the book *Tales of Okinawa's Great Masters* by Shoshin Nagamine (translated by Patrick McCarthy), North Clarendon, VT: Tuttle Publishing, 2000.

4 Sir Arthur Charles Clarke (1917 –), British author, futurist, and inventor. While he has written over fifty books, his most famous novel is probably *2001: A Space Odyssey*, which was later converted into a movie. In the 1940s, he forecast that man would reach the moon by the year 2000, an idea "experts" totally dismissed at the time. When Neil Armstrong landed on the moon in 1969, NASA administrators reportedly stated that Clarke had "provided the essential intellectual drive that led us to the moon." The Clarke Belt, or geosynchronous orbit that satellites are placed into, was named in his honor along with an asteroid. Similarly, the Mars Odyssey orbiter was named after his work.

5 Iain Abernethy holds a 5th *dan* in karate with both Karate England and the British Combat Association. Iain is the author of a number of books on applied martial arts and personal development. He has also produced many popular DVDs on practical martial arts and the realistic application of traditional *kata*. His Web site is www.iainabernethy.com.

6 Arnold Joseph Toynbee (1889 – 1975), British historian. His most famous work was a twelve-volume analysis of the rise and fall of civilizations entitled *A Study of History*.

7 Martina Sprague has studied and taught the martial arts for twenty years, and has black belts in *Kenpo* karate, kickboxing, and street freestyle. She is a scholar of warfare and combat. She has written several books on sports science and the martial arts as well as two books on Scandinavian history and Norse warfare. She is pursuing a Master of Arts in Military History at Norwich University. You can reach Martina through her Web site, www.modernfighter.com.

8 George Washington Carver (1864 – 1943), African American botanist. He reputedly discovered three hundred uses for peanuts and hundreds more uses for soybeans, pecans and sweet potatoes. Among the listed items that he suggested to southern farmers to help them economically were his recipes and improvements to/for: adhesives, axle grease, bleach, buttermilk, chili sauce, fuel briquettes, ink, instant coffee, linoleum, mayonnaise, meat tenderizer, metal polish, paper, plastic, pavement, shaving cream, shoe polish, synthetic rubber, talcum powder, and wood stain.

9 Johann Wolfgang von Goethe (1749 – 1832), German poet, novelist, playwright, and natural philosopher. He served as Chief Minister of State for the Duchy of Weimar for ten years. His most famous works were *The Sorrows of Young Werther*, *Theory of Colors*, and *Faust*.

10 Graham Wendes lives in Chelmsford, Essex U.K. where he is a Senior Site Manager for the Metronet Alliance working on the London Underground refurbishment contract. He earned his *shodan* (1st degree black belt) in Okinawan *Goju Ryu* karate in 2004, 28 years after receiving his 1st *kyu* brown belt.

11 Publilius Syrus (~46 BC), Latin poet and philosopher. A native of Syria, he was brought to Italy as a slave yet won his freedom (and education) by impressing his master with his talent and wit.

12 Graham Wendes (see note 10).

13 Albert Einstein (1879 –1955) a German-born physicist regarded as the greatest scientist of the twentieth century. He authored the general theory of relativity and made other contributions to the quantum mechanics and cosmology. He was awarded the 1921 Nobel Prize for Physics for his explanation of the photoelectric effect.

14 Martin Westerman, is a Lecturer at the University of Washington Business School in Seattle, Washington USA.

15 Carl Jung (1875 - 1961), Swiss psychiatrist. Jung developed the field of analytical psychology, exploring the human psyche through dreams, art, mythology, religion, and philosophy. Some of the concepts he championed included the archetype, collective unconscious, and synchronicity.

16 Dr. William Arthur Ward earned Ph.D., D. Litt., and D.D. degrees. He preached for sixty years, ministering in every state in the United States, in 84 countries, and in nearly every major city of the world. A dedicated scholar, he is the author of numerous books, was the editor for many years of a popular Christian magazine, and served as pastor and teacher.

17 Jeff Stevens started his *Goju-Ryu* training in 1989. In his earlier years he competed and placed in events locally and in Europe. He has taught *Goju-Ryu* karate for several years at various local Parks and Recreation Departments. He is currently a contributing instructor at the West Seattle Karate *Dojo*. He is employed as a supervisor in flight operations for an air transport company.

18 Marc "Animal" MacYoung teaches experience-based self-defense to police, military, civilians, and martial artists around the world. A former bouncer and street fighter, and all around dangerous guy, his advice is available at www.nononsenseselfdefense.com.

19 Mason Campbell began practicing karate while attending college in the early eighties. He has used his martial arts skills in real life to capture a criminal, physically subduing the perpetrator until police arrived. He lives with his son in Washington State, USA.

20 Aristotle (384 – 322 BC), Greek philosopher. Aristotle was a major contributor in determining the orientation and content of Western intellectual history. He was the author of a philosophical and scientific system that served as a foundation for scholastic thought until the end of the seventeenth century.

21 Aaron Fields is a professional firefighter in a major metropolitan area. He operates and is the head instructor for the Seattle *Ju-jutsu* Club, *Hatake Dojo*. His combative background is in *Meiji* period *ju-jutsu*, judo, and Russian *Sambo*. He lived and trained in the former Eastern Bloc for a period of time. Prior to his career in the fire service, Aaron was a schoolteacher of all grade levels and a variety of subjects. Today, he continues his teaching experience in both *budo* and the academic arena. Also, as a fire service instructor, he teaches firefighting skills at a number of departments. He has continued to lecture and write in his academic field of Mongolian History.

22 Peter Drucker (1909 – 2005), business guru. Drucker promulgated the idea that companies have three responsibilities: 1) make a profit, 2) satisfy employees, and 3) be socially responsible. He was an editorial columnist for *The Wall Street Journal* and a frequent contributor to the *Harvard Business Review* who wrote 31 books, including *Concept of the Corporation*, *The New Society*, *The Practice of Management*, *The Temptation to Do Good*, *The Frontiers of Management*, *The Theory of Business*, *Managing Oneself*, and *The Effective Executive in Action*. His works are very popular worldwide and have been translated into more than twenty languages.

23 Eugene S. Wilson (1906 – 1981), Dean of Admissions, Amherst College. Once described as a "Jeep with a sixteen-cylinder Cadillac engine," Eugene "Bill" Wilson was known for his sense of humor and his genuine interest in the welfare of each student. In addition to his duties in the Admission Office, at various times Dean Wilson also served Amherst as Alumni Secretary, teacher of English, Secretary to the Board of Trustees, and was an avid sports fan. He wrote several books, including *After College What?* and *The College Student's Handbook*.

24 General Colin Luther Powell (1937 –), United States Army (Ret.). During his military service Powell served as National Security Advisor (1987 – 1989) and Chairman of the Joint Chiefs of Staff (1989 – 1993). As a civilian, he served as United States Secretary of State (2001 – 2005).

25 Benjamin S. Bloom (1913 – 1999), American educational psychologist. Bloom was very influential in the field of educational psychology, contributing theories of learning mastery and talent development. His most famous works were *Taxonomy of Educational Objectives* and *All Our Children Learning*.

26 Elizabeth J. Simpson, educational psychologist. Simpson developed her theories primarily from Bloom's work, most impressively by fleshing out the psychomotor domain. Her most famous works were *The Classification of Educational Objectives in the Psychomotor Domain*, *Educating for the Future in Family Life*, and *The Home as a Learning Center for Vocational Development*.

27 Martina Sprague (see note 7).

28 John McNally recently passed his test and was promoted to the rank of *shodan* (1st degree black belt) in *Goju Ryu* karate. An engineer by training, with financial management experience, he supports sales for an internet commerce software company. John wrestled in high school and college, but has otherwise been a casual athlete through tennis, racquetball, windsurfing, and now karate.

29 Benjamin Franklin (1706 – 1790) was a U.S. author, inventor, politician, diplomat, and printer. He is considered a "Founding Father" of the United States of America.

30 *Sifu* Phillip Starr is the author of *The Making of a Butterfly*. He began martial arts training in 1956, studying traditional *Xingyiquan*, *Baguazhang*, and Northern *Shaolin* boxing under Master W. C. Chen. In 1976, he became a U.S. National Champion of the U.S.K.A., the only kung fu stylist to be awarded that title. In 1982, he founded *Yiliquan*, an amalgamation of traditional *Xingyiquan*, *Baguazhang*, *Taijiquan*, and northern *Shaolin*. In 1991, he was elected as National Chairman of the AAU Chinese Martial Arts Division and developed that organization into the largest kung fu organization in America at that time. In 1991 and 1992, he won the title of AAU U.S. National Champion in the *Xingyiquan* Division and was named to the AAU's All-American Team. In 1992, he was named to the Kung Fu Hall of Fame by *Inside Kung Fu* magazine. In 1995 he left the AAU and now resides in Omaha, Nebraska, where he teaches *Yiliquan*, serving as Chairman of the *Yiliquan* Martial Arts Association, and writes about martial arts.

31 Bruce Lee (1940 – 1973), founder of *Jeet Kune Do*. He is widely regarded as one of the most influential and famous martial artists of all time. His films helped mainstream martial arts movies for Western audiences, paving the way for other notables such as Chuck Norris, Jackie Chan, and Jet Li.

32 Carl Philipp Gottfried von Clausewitz (1780 –1831), Prussian general and military theorist. Writing at the time of Napoleon's campaigns, Clausewitz developed his landmark treatise on the art and philosophy of warfare entitled *Vom Kriege* (*On War*). Distinguishing between war and politics, he describes not only when war is appropriate but how to assure victory as well.

33 Miyamoto Musashi (1584 – 1645), arguably the greatest swordsman who ever lived. Considered *Kensei*, the sword saint of Japan. Musashi killed more than sixty trained *samurai* warriors in fights or duals during the feudal period where even a minor battle injury could lead to infection and death. Two years before he died, Musashi retired to a life of seclusion in a cave where he codified his winning strategy in the famous *Go Rin No Sho* (*Book of Five Rings*).

34 Sun Tzu (544–496 BC) was the author of *The Art of War* a Chinese book on military strategy.

35 Martina Sprague (see note 7).

36 Dan Keith is an instructor at the Okanogan Valley Martial Arts and Cariker's Academy of Self Defense in Tonasket, Washington. He began training in 1972 in kung fu. He has also trained in *Kempo* karate and is a 4th *dan* black belt in *taekwondo*.

37 Lao Tzu (~604 BC – 531 BC), Chinese philosopher and founder of Taoism, his famous work is the *Tao Te Ching* (*The Way of All Life*). Lao Tzu was purportedly not his real name, but rather an honorific title, meaning "Old Master."

38 Iain Abernethy (see note 5).

39 Miyamoto Musashi (see note 33).

40 Christopher Morley (1890 – 1957), American journalist, novelist, and poet. Author of more than fifty books, he is best known for his work *Kitty Foyle*, which was made into an Academy Award-winning movie. Other famous books include *Thunder on the Left*, *The Haunted Bookshop*, and *Parnassus on Wheels*.

41 Confucius (551 BC – 479 BC), Chinese philosopher. His teachings emphasized personal and governmental morality, social relationships, justice and sincerity. These values gained preeminence in China during the *Han* Dynasty, hundreds of years after his death and are still respected today.

42 Gichin Funakoshi (1868 – 1957), founder of *Shotokan* karate. Funakoshi *Sensei* learned both *Shuri Te* and *Naha Te* in Okinawa, combining these styles to form his *Shotokan* School. He traveled to Japan to demonstrate his art to no lesser dignitaries than the emperor himself, remaining there to teach and promote karate.

43 Shoshin Nagamine (1907 – 1997) was the founder of *Matsubayashi-Ryu Karate-Do*. He wrote *The Essence of Okinawan Karate-Do* and *Tales of Okinawa's Great Masters*. Practicing his art for more than 70 years, he achieved the rank of *Hanshi* (10th *dan* black belt) in karate and also earned black belts in judo, *kendo*, and *sumo*. He was president of the Okinawan Police Station, and served as police chief of Naha City, and as an instructor of police judo teams in Okinawa, Japan.

44 Wim Demeere began training at the age of 14, studying the grappling arts of *judo* and *jujitsu* for several years before turning to the kick/punch arts of traditional kung fu and full-contact fighting. Over the years he has studied *sanshou, muay Thai, kali, pentjak silat,* and *shootfighting.* Since the late 1990s, he has been studying *tajiquan* and its martial applications. Wim's competitive years saw him win four national titles and a bronze medal at the 1995 World *Wushu* Championships. In 2001, he became the national coach of the Belgian *Wushu* fighting team. A full-time personal trainer, Wim instructs both business executives and athletes in nutrition, strength and endurance, and a variety of martial arts styles. He co-authored two books with Loren W. Christensen: *The Fighter's Body* and *Timing in the Fighting Arts.* He can be reached at www.wimdemeere.com or www.grindingshop.com.

45 Sir Winston Churchill (1874 – 1965), British Prime Minister. Churchill became the voice of Britain during WWII, his emotional speeches inspiring his nation to endure hardship and sacrifice necessary to win the war. He also won a Nobel Prize for Literature in 1953 for his six-volume history of World War II.

46 Irene Doane currently holds the rank of *i-kyu* (brown belt) in *Shotokan* karate and expects to test for her *shodan* (black belt) this coming summer. She currently works event security and teaches karate classes for children.

47 Miyamoto Musashi (see note 33).

48 Sgt. Rory Miller has studied martial arts since 1981. He has received college varsities in *judo* and fencing and holds *Mokuroku* (teaching certificate) in *Sosuishitsu-ryu jujutsu.* He is a tactical team leader and teaches and designs courses in defensive tactics, close quarters combat and the Use of Force policy and application for Law Enforcement and Corrections Officers. He lectures on realism and training for martial artists and writers.

49 Confucius (551 BC – 479 BC), Chinese sage. As he traveled widely throughout China, his ideas for social reform made him the idol of the people but made him many powerful enemies as well. His moral teaching stressed the importance of the traditional relations of filial piety and brotherly respect.

50 Marc MacYoung (see note 18).

51 Michael Thue is a twenty-year student of the Asian martial arts, primarily as experienced in the form of karate and *kobudo.* Mr. Thue holds a third-*dan* black belt in *Kobayashi Shorin-Ryu* under *Sensei* Tadashi Yamashita. He trains regularly under *Sensei* Brian Lentz of Grand Rapids, Michigan at Professional Karate, LLC. Mr. Thue can be reached via email at lmac29@tm.net.

52 Mark "Blackwood" Swarthout is an attorney working in contract management. A student of *Shido Kan Shorin Ryu* karate under his *Sensei* Robert Menders and *Hanshi* Seikichi Iha, Mark earned his *shodan* (first degree black belt) at age 47. He instructs youth classes with his daughter. Swarthout in Dutch means "Blackwood" hence, Blackwood *Dojo.* He maintains his instructors' Web site at www.mendersdojo.com.

53 Miyamoto Musashi, (see note 33).

54 Hippocrates of Cos (~ 460 BC – 377 BC) was a Greek physician. He is often deemed the "the father of Western medicine." Hippocrates is regarded as one of the most important figures in the history of medicine. He wrote the *Corpus Hippocraticum,* the Hippocratic writings. These writings laid the foundation for medicine to move into the sciences, away from the influence of magic and superstition. A saying often attributed to Hippocrates is, "There are in fact, two things: science, and opinion; the former begets knowledge, the latter ignorance."

55 Wim Demeere (see note 44).

56 Christopher Reeve (1952 – 2004), American actor and director. He is best known for his motion picture role as Superman. Since becoming paralyzed by a fall from a horse at an equestrian competition in 1995, Reeve not only put a human face on spinal cord injury but he motivated neuroscientists around the world to conquer the most complex diseases of the brain and central nervous system. His books *Still Me* and *Nothing is Impossible* have proven inspirational for those suffering from physical and/or emotional injuries.

57 Dr. Allan M. Levy is team physician for the New York Giants, and formerly the New Jersey Nets and New York Islanders. He runs a successful New Jersey-based sports medicine practice for high school and recreational athletes.

58 Jeffery Cooper, M.D., is a fellow of the American Academy of Emergency Medicine and a clinical instructor of emergency medicine. He has been involved in the martial arts for some twenty-five years, achieving the rank of *yodan* (4th degree black belt) in *Goju Ryu* karate. As tactical medical director of Toledo (Ohio) SWAT, he has received advanced training in hostage extraction, hand-to-hand combat, firearms, and knife fighting. Dr. Cooper is also a commander in the U.S. Naval Reserve Medical Corps.

59 Frank Getty is currently a green belt in *Krav Maga*. A former Marine MP, he currently works in corporate security for an aerospace company. He is featured on the cover and in many of the pictures in Lawrence Kane's book, *Surviving Armed Assaults*.

60 Isaac Asimov (1920 – 1992), Russian-born American author and biochemist. He is best known as an award-winning science fiction novelist, and scholar. His most famous works include *Foundation*, *Foundation and Empire*, *Second Foundation*, *The Gods Themselves*, and *I, Robot*. The Oxford English Dictionary credits his science fiction for introducing the words *positronic*, *psychohistory*, and *robotics* into the English language.

61 Loren Christensen began his martial arts training in 1965, earning ten black belts over the years, seven in karate, two in *jujitsu*, and one in *arnis*. He is a retired police officer with twenty-nine years of experience in military and civilian law enforcement, where he specialized in street gangs, defensive tactics, and dignitary protection. He is the author of more than thirty books on the martial arts, self-defense, law enforcement, nutrition, prostitution, gangs, and post-traumatic stress disorder. His book *On Combat*, which he co-authored with Lt .Col. Dave Grossman, is mandatory reading at the United States War College in Washington, DC. Loren's Web site is www.lwcbooks.com.

62 Peter Drucker (1909 – 2005), business guru. Drucker promulgated the idea that companies have three responsibilities: 1) make a profit, 2) satisfy employees, and 3) be socially responsible. He was an editorial columnist for *The Wall Street Journal* and a frequent contributor to the Harvard Business Review who wrote 31 books, including *Concept of the Corporation*, *The New Society*, *The Practice of Management*, *The Temptation to Do Good*, *The Frontiers of Management*, *The Theory of Business*, *Managing Oneself*, and *The Effective Executive in Action*. His works are very popular throughout the world and have been translated into more than twenty languages.

63 Mark Twain (1835 – 1910) was the pen name for Samuel Langhorne Clemens. He was an American humorist, novelist, writer, and lecturer. His most famous works include *The Adventures of Tom Sawyer*, *The Adventures of Huckleberry Finn*, and *A Connecticut Yankee in King Arthur's Court*.

64 Loren Christensen. (see note 61)

65 Mary Jessamyn West (1902 – 1984), American novelist. Her most famous works include *The Friendly Persuasion* (which was made into a movie starring Gary Cooper in 1956), and *Except for Me and Thee*.

66 T. Kent (T.K.) Nelson teaches martial arts in Lansing, Michigan, running a school called the *Kai Shin Kan Dojo* (roughly translates to "House of an Open Mind"). He has over 22 years of experience with a variety of Okinawan, Filipino, Chinese, Indonesian, and Korean martial arts. His Web site is www.tkentnelson.com.

67 From the book, *Goju Ryu Karate-Do: Volume 1 Fundamentals for Traditional Practitioners* by Motoo Yamakura, Monroe, Michigan: G.K.K. Productions, 1989.

68 Aristotle (see note 20).

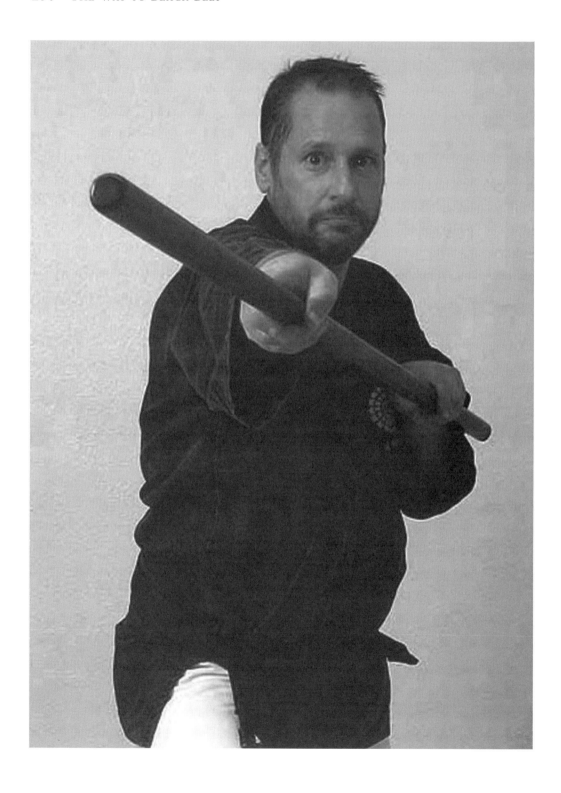

Bibliography

Books

Abernethy, Iain. *Mental Strength: Condition your Mind, Achieve your Goals.* Cockermouth, UK: NETH Publishing, 2005.

Armstrong, Lance. *It's Not About the Bike: My Journey Back to Life.* New York, NY: Penquin Putnum, Inc., 2000.

Baum, Kenneth and Richard Trubo. *The Mental Edge: Maximize Your Sports Potential with the Mind-Body Connection.* New York, NY: Berkley Publishing Group, 1999.

Christensen, Loren and Wim Demeere. *The Fighter's Body: An Owner's Manual: Your Guide to Diet, Nutrition, Exercise and Excellence in the Martial Arts.* Wethersfield, CT: Turtle Press, 2003.

Christensen, Loren. *Fighter's Fact Book: Over 400 Concepts, Principles, and Drills to Make You a Better Fighter.* Wethersfield, CT: Turtle Press, 2000.

Christensen, Loren. *Fighter's Fact Book 2: Street Fighting Essentials.* Wethersfield, CT: Turtle Press, 2007.

Christensen, Loren. *Fighting Power: How to Develop Explosive Punches, Kicks, Blocks, and Grappling.* Boulder, CO: Paladin Enterprises, Inc., 1996.

Christensen, Loren. *Solo Training 2: The Martial Artist's Guide to Building the Core for Stronger, Faster and More Effective Grappling, Kicking and Punching.* Wethersfield, CT: Turtle Press, 2005.

Christensen, Loren. *Solo Training: The Martial Artist's Guide to Training Alone.* Wethersfield, CT: Turtle Press, 2001.

Christensen, Loren. *Speed Training: How to Develop Your Maximum Speed for Martial Arts.* Boulder, CO: Paladin Enterprises, Inc., 1996.

Clausewitz, Carl von and J. J. Graham (translator). *On War.* New York, NY: Penguin Books, Ltd., 1968.

Coseo, Marc. *The Acupressure Warm-Up for Athletic Preparation and Injury Management.* Brookline, MA: Paradigm Publications, 1992.

Gendlin, Eugene T., Ph.D. *Focusing.* New York, NY: Bantam Books, 1978.

Funakoshi, Gichin. *Karate-Do: My Way of Life.* New York, NY: Kodansha International, 1975.

Funakoshi, Gichin. *Karate-Do Kyohan: The Master Text.* New York, NY: Kodansha International, 1973

Funakoshi, Gichin and Jotaro Takagi and John Teramoto (Translator). *The Twenty Guiding Principles of Karate: The Spiritual Legacy of the Master.* New York, NY: Kodansha International, 2003.

Heckler, Richard Strozzi. *Aikido and the New Warrior,* Berkeley CA, North Atlantic Books 1985.

Higaonna, Morio. *Traditional Karatedo – Okinawa Goju Ryu Vol. 1: Fundamental Techniques.* Tokyo, Japan: Minato Research and Publishing Co., Ltd., 1985.

Kane, Lawrence A. *Martial Arts Instruction: Applying Educational Theory and Communication Techniques in the Dojo.* Boston, MA: YMAA, 2004.

Kane, Lawrence A. *Surviving Armed Assaults: A Martial Artists Guide to Weapons, Street Violence, and Countervailing Force.* Boston, MA: YMAA, 2006.

Kane, Lawrence and Kris Wilder. *The Way of Kata: A Comprehensive Guide to Deciphering Martial Applications.* Boston, MA: YMAA Publication Center, 2005.

Kano, Jigoro. *Kodokan Judo.* New York, NY: Kodansha International, 1986.

Kaufman, Stephen F. *The Art of War: The Definitive Interpretation of Sun Tzu's Classic Book of Strategy.* North Clarendon, VT: Tuttle Publishing, 1996.

Lawrence, Gordon D. *Looking at Type and Learning Styles.* Gainesville, FL: CAPT, 2004.

Loehr, James E., Ed.D. *The New Toughness Training for Sports, Mental Emotional and Physical Conditioning from One of the World's Premier Sports Psychologists.* Plume/Penguin, New York, NY. USA, 1995.

Lovret, Fredrick, J. *The Way and the Power: Secrets of Japanese Strategy.* Boulder CO: Paladin Enterprises, Inc., 1987.

Levy, Allan M. and Mark L. Fuerst. *Sports Injury Handbook: Professional Advice for Amateur Athletes*. Hoboken, NJ: John Wiley and Sons, Inc., 1993.

Lowry, Dave. *In the Dojo: A Guide to the Rituals and Etiquette of the Japanese Martial Arts*. Boston, MA: Shambhala Publications, 2006.

Maynard, Kyle. *No Excuses: The True Story of a Congenital Amputee Who Became a Champion in Wrestling and in Life*. Washington, DC: Regnery Publishing, 2005.

Morgan, Forrest. *Living The Martial Way*. Fort Lee, NJ: Barricade Books, Inc., 1992.

Nagamine, Shoshin and Patrick McCarthy (translator). *Tales of Okinawa's Great Masters*. North Clarendon, VT: Tuttle Publishing, 2000.

Pearl, Bill and Gary T. Moran, PhD. *Getting Stronger, Sports Training – General Conditioning – Body Building*. Shelter Publications Inc., Bolinas, CA, USA 1986.

Powell, Goran. *Waking Dragons: A Martial Artist Faces His Ultimate Test*. Chichester, U.K.: Summersdale Publishers, 2006.

Rosenbaum, Michael. *Kata and the Transmission of Knowledge: In Traditional Martial Arts*. Boston, MA: YMAA Publication Center, 2004.

Siddle, Bruce. *Sharpening the Warrior's Edge: The Psychology and Science of Training*. Millstadt, IL: PPCT Research Publications, 1995.

Sprague, Martina. *Fighting Science: The Laws of Physics for Martial Artists*. Wethersfield, CT: Turtle Press, 2002.

Sprague, Martina. *Strength & Power Training for Martial Arts*. Wethersfield, CT: Turtle Press, 2005.

Stark, Dr. Steven D. *The Stark Reality of Stretching: An informed Approach for All Activities and Every Sport*. Richmond, BC, Canada: The Stark Reality Publishing Group, 1997.

Sugiyama, Shojiro. *25 Shotokan Kata*. Chicago, IL: J. Toguri Mercantile Company, 1984.

Thompson, Geoff. *Dead or Alive, The Choice is Yours: the Definitive Self-Protection*. Boulder, CO: Paladin Enterprises, Inc., 1997.

Toguchi, Seikichi. *Okinawan Goju Ryu*. Santa Clara, CA: Black Belt Communications, 1979.

Toguchi, Seikichi. *Okinawan Goju Ryu II*. Santa Clara, CA: Ohara Publications, 2001.

Tsatsouline, Pavel. *Relax Into Stretch: Instant Flexibility Through Mastering Muscle Tension*. St. Paul, MN: Dragon Door Publications, Inc, 2001.

Twigger, Robert. *Angry White Pajamas: A Scrawny Oxford Poet Takes Lessons From the Tokyo Riot Police*. New York, NY: HarperCollins, 1997.

Vactor, Karen Levitz and Susan Lynn Peterson, Ph.D. *Starting and Running Your Martial Arts School*. Boston, MA: Tuttle Publishing 2002.

Wiley, Carol A. *Martial Arts Teachers on Teaching*. Berkeley, CA: Frog, Ltd., 1995.

Wiley, Mark V. *Filipino Martial Culture*. North Clarendon, VT: Tuttle Publishing, 1997.

Wilson, Scott William. *The Lone Samurai: The Life of Miyamoto Musashi*. New York, NY: Kodansha International, Ltd, 2004.

Yamakura, Motoo. *Goju-Ryu Karate-Do Vol. 1: Fundamentals for Traditional Practitioners*. Monroe, MI: G.K.K. Publications, 1989.

Web Sites

Aiki Productions (www.aikiproductions.com)

American College of Sports Medicine (www.acsm.org)

Blauer Tactical Systems (www.tonyblauer.com)

Center for Applications of Psychological Type (www.capt.org)

Dan Anderson's Web site (www.danandersonkarate.com)

Fighting Arts (www.fightingarts.com)

Gavin DeBecker and Associates (www.gavindebecker.com)

Grapple Arts (http://grapplearts.com/)

Iain Abernethy's Web site (www.iainabernethy.com)

International Society of Close Quarter Combatants (www.survive-the-street.com)

Judo Information Site (www.judoinfo.com)

Loren Christensen's Web site (www.lwcbooks.com)

MedicineNet.com (www.medicinenet.com)

Minnesota State University – Mankato: What Makes a Good Teacher Article (http://www.mnsu.edu/cetl/teach-ingresources/articles/goodteacher.html)

Peter Consterdine (www.peterconsterdine.com)

Rocky Mountain Combat Applications Training (www.rmcat.com)

Steve Pavlina: Personal Development for Smart People (http://www.stevepavlina.com/index.htm)

Study Guides and Strategies (http://www.studygs.net/)

System for Adult Basic Education Support: What Makes A Good Teacher Article (http://www.sabes.org/resources/adventures/vol12/12hassett.htm)

The All *Goju Ryu* Network (www.gojuryu.net)

The American Success Institute (www.success.org)

The Art of War (www.chinapage.com/sunzi-e.html)

The Book of Five Rings (http://www.samurai.com/5rings)

The Clausewitz Homepage (www.clausewitz.com)

The Grinding Shop (www.grindingshop.com)

UNICEF Teachers Talking (http://www.unicef.org/teachers/teacher/teacher.htm)

U.S. Department of Health and Human Services (www.pueblo.gsa.gov/cic_text/health/sports/injuries.htm)

West Seattle Karate Academy (www.westseattlekarate.com)

YMAA (www.ymaa.com)

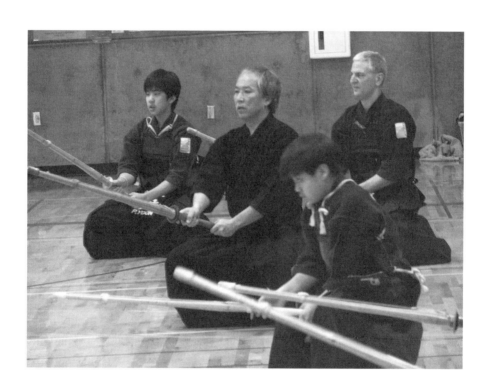

Index

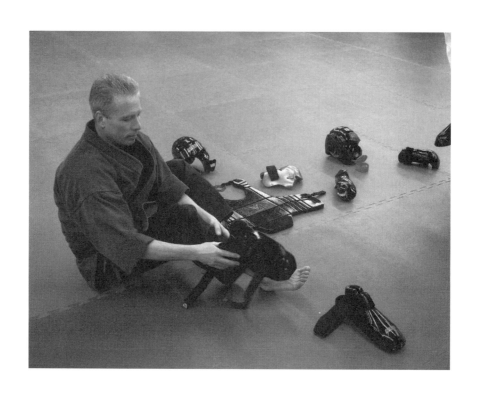

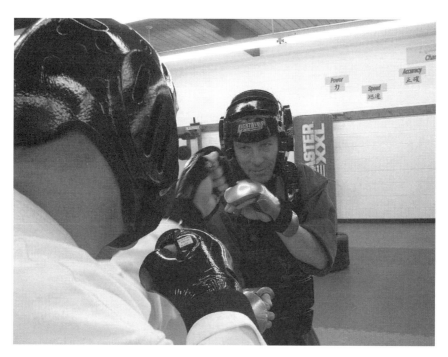

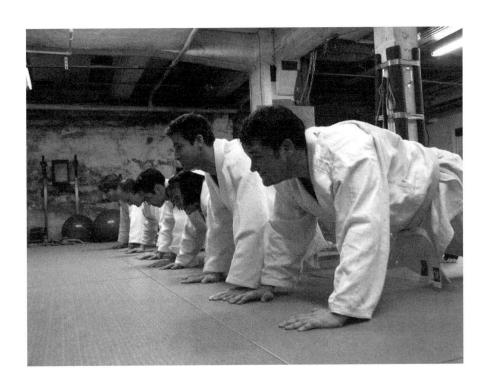

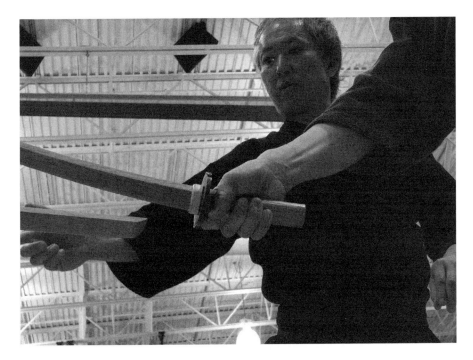

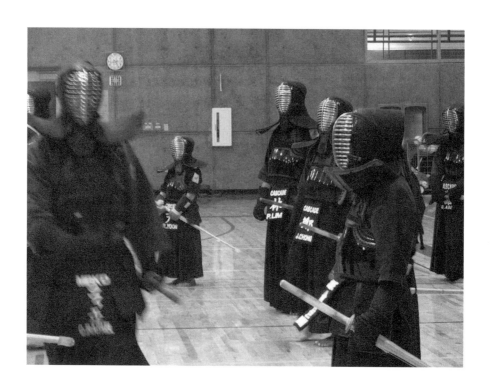

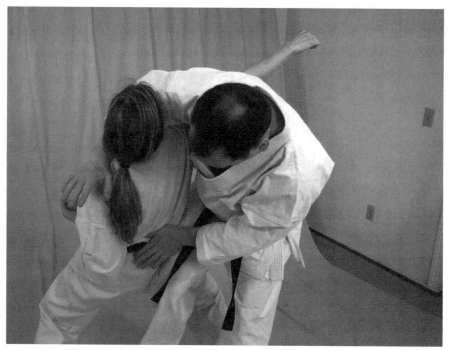

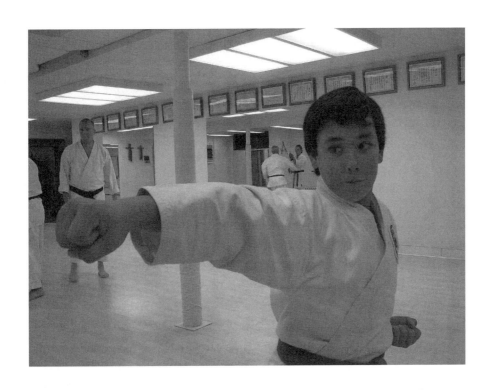

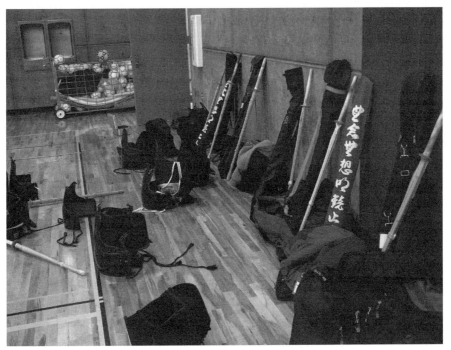

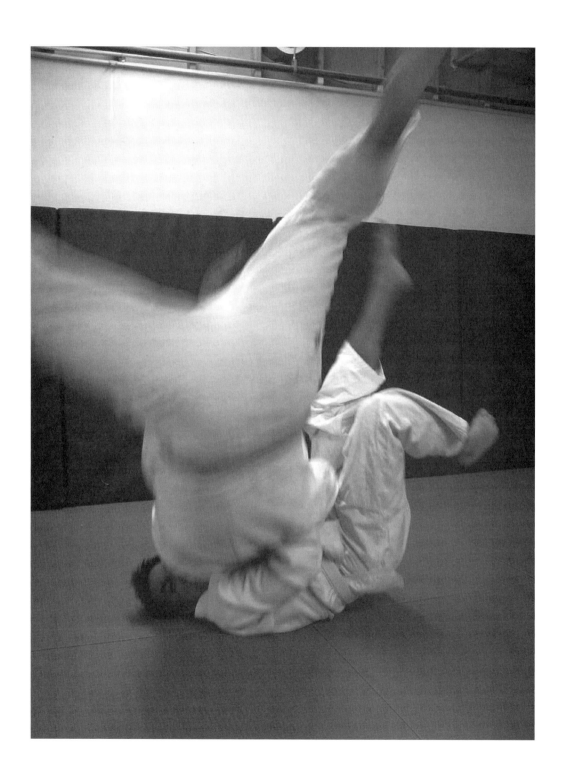

About the Authors

Kris Wilder

Beginning his martial arts training in 1976 in the art of *taekwondo*, Kris Wilder has earned black belt-level ranks in three arts: *taekwondo* (2nd Degree), *Kodokan* Judo (1st Degree) and *Goju Ryu* Karate (4th Degree), which he teaches at the West Seattle Karate Academy. He has trained under Kenji Yamada, who as a Judoka won back-to-back United States grand championships (1954 – 1955); Shihan John Roseberry, founder of *Shorei-Shobukan* Karate and a direct student of Seikichi Toguchi; and Hiroo Ito, a student of *Shihan* Kori Hisataka (Kudaka in the Okinawan dialect), the founder of *Shorinji-Ryu Kenkokan* Karate.

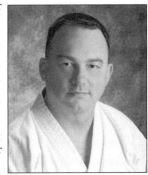

Though now retired from Judo competition, while active in the sport Kris competed on the national and international levels. He has traveled to Japan and Okinawa to train in karate and has authored several books on the martial arts, including co-authoring *The Way of Kata*. He has written guest chapters for other martial arts authors and has had articles published in *Traditional Karate*, a magazine out of the U.K. with international readership. Kris also hosts the annual Martial University, a seminar composed of multidisciplinary martial artists. He also regularly instructs at seminars.

Kris lives in Seattle, Washington, with his son Jackson. He can be contacted via e-mail at kwilder@quidnunc.net or through the West Seattle Karate Academy Web site at www.westseattlekarate.com.

Lawrence Kane

Lawrence Kane is the author of *Martial Arts Instruction* (YMAA, 2004) and *Surviving Armed Assaults* (YMAA, 2006), as well as co-author (with Kris Wilder) of the critically acclaimed book, *The Way of Kata* (YMAA, 2005). He has also published numerous articles about teaching, martial arts, self-defense, and related topics, contributed to other author's books, and acts as a forum moderator at www.iainabernethy.com, a Web site devoted to traditional martial arts and self-protection.

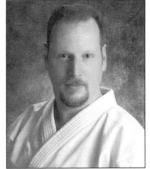

Since 1970, he has participated in a broad range of martial arts, from traditional Asian sports such as judo, *arnis*, *kobudo*, and karate to recreating medieval European combat with real armor and rattan (wood) weapons.

He has taught medieval weapons forms since 1994 and Goju Ryu karate since 2002. He has also completed seminars in modern gun safety, marksmanship, handgun retention, and knife combat techniques, and he has participated in slow-fire pistol and pin shooting competitions.

Since 1985, Lawrence has supervised employees who provide security and oversee fan safety during college and professional football games at a Pac-10 stadium. This part-time job has given him a unique opportunity to appreciate violence in a myriad of forms. Along with his crew, he has witnessed, interceded in, and stopped or prevented hundreds of fights, experiencing all manner of aggressive behaviors as well as the escalation process that invariably precedes them. He has also worked closely with the campus police and state patrol officers who are assigned to the stadium and has had ample opportunities to examine their crowd control tactics and procedures.

To pay the bills, he does IT sourcing strategy and benchmarking work for an aerospace company in Seattle where he gets to play with billions of dollars of other people's money and make really important decisions. Lawrence lives in Seattle, Washington, with his wife Julie and his son Joey. He can be contacted via e-mail at lakane@ix.netcom.com.

BOOKS FROM YMAA

more products available from...

YMAA Publication Center, Inc. 楊氏東方文化出版中心

4354 Washington Street Roslindale, MA 02131

1-800-669-8892 • ymaa@aol.com • www.ymaa.com

VIDEOS FROM YMAA

ADVANCED PRACTICAL CHIN NA — 1, 2	T0061, T007X
ARTHRITIS RELIEF — CHINESE QIGONG FOR HEALING & PREVENTION	T558
BACK PAIN RELIEF — CHINESE QIGONG FOR HEALING & PREVENTION	T566
CHINESE QIGONG MASSAGE — SELF	T327
CHINESE QIGONG MASSAGE — PARTNER	T335
COMP. APPLICATIONS OF SHAOLIN CHIN NA 1, 2	T386, T394
EMEI BAGUAZHANG 1, 2, 3	T280, T299, T302
EIGHT SIMPLE QIGONG EXERCISES FOR HEALTH 2ND ED.	T54X
ESSENCE OF TAIJI QIGONG	T238
NORTHERN SHAOLIN SWORD — SAN CAI JIAN & ITS APPLICATIONS	T051
NORTHERN SHAOLIN SWORD — KUN WU JIAN & ITS APPLICATIONS	T06X
NORTHERN SHAOLIN SWORD — QI MEN JIAN & ITS APPLICATIONS	T078
QIGONG: 15 MINUTES TO HEALTH	T140
SHAOLIN KUNG FU BASIC TRAINING — 1, 2	T0045, T0053
SHAOLIN LONG FIST KUNG FU — TWELVE TAN TUI	T159
SHAOLIN LONG FIST KUNG FU — LIEN BU CHUAN	T19X
SHAOLIN LONG FIST KUNG FU — GUNG LI CHUAN	T203
SHAOLIN LONG FIST KUNG FU — YI LU MEI FU & ER LU MAI FU	T256
SHAOLIN LONG FIST KUNG FU — SHI ZI TANG	T264
SHAOLIN LONG FIST KUNG FU — XIAO HU YAN	T604
SHAOLIN WHITE CRANE GONG FU — BASIC TRAINING 1, 2, 3	T440, T459, T0185
SIMPLIFIED TAI CHI CHUAN — 24 & 48	T329
SUN STYLE TAIJIQUAN	T469
TAI CHI CHUAN & APPLICATIONS — 24 & 48	T485
TAI CHI FIGHTING SET	T0363
TAIJI BALL QIGONG — 1, 2, 3, 4	T475, T483, T0096, T010X
TAIJI CHIN NA IN DEPTH — 1, 2, 3, 4	T0282, T0290, T0304, T031
TAIJI PUSHING HANDS — 1, 2, 3, 4	T505, T513, T0134, T0142
TAIJI SABER	T491
TAIJI & SHAOLIN STAFF — FUNDAMENTAL TRAINING — 1, 2	T0088, T0347
TAIJI SWORD, CLASSICAL YANG STYLE	T817
TAIJI WRESTLING — 1, 2	T037, T038X
TAIJI YIN & YANG SYMBOL STICKING HANDS–YANG TAIJI TRAINING	T580
TAIJI YIN & YANG SYMBOL STICKING HANDS–YIN TAIJI TRAINING	T0177
TAIJIQUAN, CLASSICAL YANG STYLE	T752
WHITE CRANE HARD QIGONG	T612
WHITE CRANE SOFT QIGONG	T620
WILD GOOSE QIGONG	T949
WU STYLE TAIJIQUAN	T477
XINGYIQUAN — 12 ANIMAL FORM	T310

DVDS FROM YMAA

ANALYSIS OF SHAOLIN CHIN NA	D0231
BAGUAZHANG 1, 2, 3 — EMEI BAGUAZHANG	D0649
CHEN TAIJIQUAN	D0819
CHIN NA IN DEPTH COURSES 1 — 4	D602
CHIN NA IN DEPTH COURSES 5 — 8	D610
CHIN NA IN DEPTH COURSES 9 — 12	D629
EIGHT SIMPLE QIGONG EXERCISES FOR HEALTH	D0037
THE ESSENCE OF TAIJI QIGONG	D0215
QIGONG MASSAGE—FUNDAMENTAL TECHNIQUES FOR HEALTH AND RELAXATION	D0592
SHAOLIN KUNG FU FUNDAMENTAL TRAINING 1&2	D0436
SHAOLIN LONG FIST KUNG FU — BASIC SEQUENCES	D661
SHAOLIN WHITE CRANE GONG FU BASIC TRAINING 1&2	D599
SIMPLIFIED TAI CHI CHUAN	D0630
SUNRISE TAI CHI	D0274
TAI CHI CONNECTIONS	D0444
TAI CHI ENERGY PATTERNS	D0525
TAI CHI FIGHTING SET—TWO PERSON MATCHING SET	D0509
TAIJI BALL QIGONG COURSES 1&2—16 CIRCLING AND 16 ROTATING PATTERNS	D0517
TAIJI PUSHING HANDS 1&2—YANG STYLE SINGLE AND DOUBLE PUSHING HANDS	D0495
TAIJI PUSHING HANDS 3&4—YANG STYLE SINGLE AND DOUBLE PUSHING HANDS	D0681
TAIJIQUAN CLASSICAL YANG STYLE	D645
TAIJI SWORD, CLASSICAL YANG STYLE	D0452
UNDERSTANDING QIGONG 1	D069X
UNDERSTANDING QIGONG 2	D0418
UNDERSTANDING QIGONG 3—EMBRYONIC BREATHING	D0555
UNDERSTANDING QIGONG 4—FOUR SEASONS QIGONG	D0562
WHITE CRANE HARD & SOFT QIGONG	D637

more products available from...
YMAA Publication Center, Inc. 楊氏東方文化出版中心
4354 Washington Street Roslindale, MA 02131
1-800-669-8892 • ymaa@aol.com • www.ymaa.com